Tradition and Reality

Everything that's happened, everything that's gone on, is all traditional, but now we're face to face with a modern society, which is reality. I mean, we're in a different world altogether…Now we find professional people going out on strike, and starting to do all the things we wouldn't have a bar of.

Marjorie Connor to Isabell Collins and BMcC, 1990

Tradition and Reality

Nursing and Politics in Australia

Brigid McCoppin RN RM BSW MA
Senior Lecturer, School of Behavioural Health Sciences,
La Trobe University, Melbourne

Heather Gardner MA
Senior Lecturer, School of Behavioural Health Sciences,
La Trobe University, Melbourne

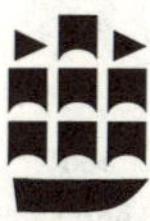

CHURCHILL LIVINGSTONE
MELBOURNE EDINBURGH LONDON MADRID NEW YORK TOKYO 1994

CHURCHILL LIVINGSTONE
Medical Division of Longman Group UK Limited

Distributed in Australia by Longman Cheshire Pty Limited,
Longman House, Kings Gardens, 95 Coventry Street,
South Melbourne 3205, and by associated companies,
branches and representatives throughout the world.

First edition 1994

ISBN 0 443 04217 9

National Library of Australia Cataloguing in Publication Data

McCoppin, Brigid,
Tradition and reality

Bibliography,
Includes index.
ISBN 0 443 04217 9.

1. Nursing - Australia. 2. Nursing - Political aspects - Australia. 3. Nurses - Australia. 1. Gardner, Heather. ii. Title.

362.1730994

Produced by Churchill Livingstone in Melbourne
through Longman Malaysia, VVP

For Churchill Livingstone in Melbourne
Publisher: Judy Waters
Co-ordinating Editor: Maja Ingrassia, John Macdonald
Copy Editor: Maja Ingrassia, John Macdonald
Desktop Preparation: Sandra Tolra
Typesetting: Designpoint
Indexer: Master Indexing
Production Control: Peter Hylands
Design: Churchill Livingstone

The publisher's policy is to use **paper manufactured from sustainable forests**

Contents

Preface

This book is the product of four years of reading and thinking about Australian nursing and above all of listening to Australian nurses, and others, who gave their time and energies in talking to us about their work, past and present, their hopes and ideas. We acknowledge here with gratitude their generosity and candour.

The book is about Australian nursing in its relation to the political system, and it is an account of nurses' efforts to become a recognised part of that system, an accepted voice in policy making, so that they can enlarge their control over their occupation and its future. We have concentrated on general registered nursing, and much work remains to be done on the political and industrial activity of psychiatric nurses, midwives and enrolled nurses. Future accounts may challenge and contradict what is written here—we hope so, since contradictory findings and differing ideas will lead to debate and added interest.

Australian nursing is more complex than would appear from interpretations depicting it as advancing steadily towards the beacon of professionalism, or as the victim of medical oppression; and it goes beyond nursing itself, for Australian nursing is part of the history of women, of work and of medicine. These dimensions are for the most part only suggested here. Australian nursing must also be assessed in relation to nursing elsewhere, not only because we can learn from other nurses while not necessarily accepting their practices without question, but also because they may learn from us.

We have tried to balance our admiration and appreciation of the achievements of Australian nurses with a wish to give them the respect which is their due in the form of a critical and partly detached (never wholly objective) assessment. As Carolyn Emden writes (1991), inquiry can become a collaborative process between researcher and research *participants* (not 'subjects'). The voices of nurses themselves are introduced throughout the text to comment and explain from their own points of view—they are true participants in the research endeavour and their story is at the centre of the book.

Melbourne 1993

BMcC
HG

Emden C 1991 Becoming a reflective practitioner. In: Gray G, Pratt R (eds) Towards a discipline of nursing. Churchill Livingstone, Melbourne

Acknowledgements

We owe special thanks to the many nurses who have talked to us over the last four years. We hope they enjoy the result even if they do not always agree with it. Diane Mackay assisted in collecting the large volume of research material necessary for this study. Dr Arthur O'Neill of the Department of Health Administration and Health Education, Lincoln School of Health Sciences, La Trobe University, read drafts and made many valuable comments and suggestions. The staff of the Library, Department of Nursing, La Trobe University, have given their usual expert and friendly help on many occasions, and thanks are due also to Josie Mauro who typed part of the final manuscript. We sincerely thank Judy Waters of Churchill Livingstone for her help and frequent encouragement, and above all for her patience. The Royal College of Nursing, Australia generously provided a research grant, which contributed to our travelling and research expenses, and is gratefully acknowledged.

BMcC
HG

Abbreviations

ACSPA	Australian Council of Salaried and Professional Associations
ACT	Australian Capital Territory
ACTU	Australian Council of Trade Unions
ALP	Australian Labor Party
AMA	Australian Medical Association
ANA	American Nurses Association
ANF/RANF	Australian Nursing Federation/Royal Australian Nursing Federation
ANFES	Australian Nursing Federation Employees Section
ANJ	Australian Nurses' Journal
ATNA	Australasian Trained Nurses Association
AUNA	Australian United Nurses Association
BMA	British Medical Association (in Australia)
CAE	College of Advanced Education
C of N,A	College of Nursing, Australia (see RCNA)
CPD	Commonwealth Parliamentary Debates
CTEC	Commonwealth Tertiary Education Commission
HEA/HEF	Hospital Employees Association/Hospital Employees Federation
HREA	Health and Research Employees Association
ICN	International Council of Nurses
ILO	International Labour Organisation
LPN	Licensed practical nurse (USA)
NEB	Nurses Education Board (NSW)
NFNC	National Florence Nightingale Committee
NNED	National Nursing Education Division (RANF)
NORC	Nursing Organisations Representative Committee
NSC	National Steering Committee (of the 'Goals in Nursing Education')
NSWNA	New South Wales Nurses Association
NSWPD	New South Wales Parliamentary Debates
PTS	Preliminary Training School
QNA	Queensland Nurses Association
QNU	Queensland Nurses Union
QPD	Queensland Parliamentary Debates
RBNA	Royal British Nurses Association
RCN	Royal College of Nursing (London)
RCNA	Royal College of Nursing, Australia
RN	Registered nurse
RVCN	Royal Victorian College of Nursing
RVTNA	Royal Victorian Trained Nurses Association (see VTNA)
SA	South Australia
SAPD	South Australian Parliamentary Debates
SEN	State enrolled nurse
TAFE	Technical and Further Education
TLC	Trades and Labour Council

TNG	Trained Nurses Guild
TPD	Tasmanian Parliamentary Debates
VPD	Victorian Parliamentary Debates
VTHC	Victorian Trades Hall Council
VTNA/RVTNA	Victorian Trained Nurses Association/Royal Victorian Trained Nurses Association
WA	Western Australia
WAIT	Western Australian Institute of Technology
WANA	Western Australian Nurses Association
WAPD	Western Australian Parliamentary Debates
WHO	World Health Organization

1. Building a tradition: Australian nursing to 1960

European settlement in Australia began as an extension of 18th century English society, but as a penal colony it reflected the 'worst aspects of the mother country' (Kiddle 1951). The men in charge of the convicts brought with them contemporary English attitudes to the sick and the poor which at home produced the 19th century workhouses, institutions in which the nurses were 'able-bodied paupers' who might be paid in gin for performing unpleasant tasks such as laying out the dead (Abel-Smith 1960:10-16). The first European attendants on the sick in Australia were convict men.

Over the next 200 years Australian nursing developed from this unpromising start. At first it kept close to English traditions, especially under the Nightingale influence, but gradually it established its own character. What follows here is a brief impression only of how it did so. Australian nursing has been continually buffeted by forces of division: the separation of the original colonies and of their successors, the states in the federal Commonwealth; the long debated question of whether nurses were professionals, as opposed to trade unionists; and the hierarchical arrangement of the workplace which subordinated all nurses to doctors and most nurses to their seniors. Perhaps the only forces to draw them together were their belief in their work as nurses, and more recently their position as women in what has always been very much a 'man's country'.

Convict and colonial nursing

There were few opportunities for women in the early settlement, but some did assume positions which had a connection with nursing. In the hospitals of the female convict 'factories' at Parramatta and Cascade much of the space was given over to 'lying-in' women, and a number of convict women probably assisted from necessity as 'accidental' midwives (Thornton 1972, Willis 1983:99).

Despite the European invasion, much Aboriginal culture survived, including that of the traditional 'medicine men'. These men had high standing and were trained for local conditions, but there was little they could do for people whose material means of existence were taken from them, and who often caught imported diseases from which they had no natural protection.

Many Aboriginal women were experts in preparing and using herbal remedies, and some assisted European women in childbirth in the early settlement—a rare example of interracial co-operation (Rowley 1972:10-11, 22-3; Willis 1983:99-100).

Governor Macquarie founded Sydney Hospital in 1811 as a convict hospital, where the nurses were selected convicts who received no pay but were maintained at public expense. Female convict nurses as well as male were mentioned first in 1816, but were described as 'usually a dissolute class' who often came drunk on duty (Brodsky 1968:18). This description may reflect the enduring 'damned whores' image of the convict women, but as in England there were probably many conscientious if untrained nurses before the 19th century reforms.

Care of the mentally ill was purely custodial, and before the establishment of lunatic asylums they were often housed in part of a gaol, as at Port Phillip (Melbourne), with no treatment and no nursing care. The more violent lunatics had to be transferred to the new Tarban Creek Asylum in Sydney until the Yarra Bend Hospital opened in 1848, with a lay superintendent whose wife became matron at £50 a year, half her husband's pay (Brothers nd:11-15), a disparity which would have seemed routine at the time. The women who were styled 'matrons' of the early hospitals worked more as housekeepers than as nurses—nursing management may have developed before the job of giving bedside care. Much nursing in fact consisted of domestic cleaning tasks, though qualities such as compassion and diligence were seen as desirable in those caring for the sick (Schultz 1991:69).

Trained nursing starts as convict society ends

The first trained nurses to arrive in Australia were two of the five Irish Sisters of Charity who landed in Sydney in late 1838, shortly before the official ending of the convict system. Australia was a nascent colonial society by the 1840s rather than a penal settlement. It had the beginnings of self-government and so was able to end the transportation of convicts, except in Western Australia where it was practised up to 1868. The colonies were inevitably influenced by the changes which had taken place in Europe since the French Revolution, with the growth of industrial society, the rise of liberal bourgeois democracy and the first stirrings of socialism. The expansion of the pastoral industry and the influx of people during the gold rushes made the proportion of convicts in the population quite small. There were now settlements in Queensland, Victoria, Tasmania and South Australia (the last always without convicts) and by 1850 the inhabitants had set up hospitals in each colony. After the convict period, general hospitals were based on the English principle of public-spirited citizens subscribing charitable funds to institutions which at the time were little more than refuges for the destitute sick. The more affluent were nursed privately in the superior safety of their own homes. Most Australian hospitals departed from the English system in expecting some state financial support, but were still seen as voluntary and therefore not under direct government control. This system had future implications for nursing by giving successive governments an excuse for not interfering in hospital affairs.

The nurses who worked in these hospitals were not on the whole the dissolute harridans depicted in some accounts. The typical nurse was 'a moderately efficient maidservant. Until Florence Nightingale's principles were accepted, she was not expected to be anything else' (Inglis 1958:95). An accompanying development in the 1850s in which nurses took no part but which ultimately affected them was the start of the trade union movement. The gold rushes attracted many British workers whose unions had been crushed at home. These men and women found in Australia a more propitious climate for a labour movement. By the 1880s Australia began to acquire the reputation of a 'workingman's paradise': unions were flourishing, hours and conditions of work were far superior to those 'at home', and a voluntary system for the conciliation and arbitration of industrial disputes had emerged (Hagan 1981:6-7).

'Nightingales' migrate south

The arrival of Lucy Osburn and her four Nightingale nurses at Sydney Hospital in 1868, at the invitation of Sir Henry Parkes, is usually seen as the start of modern secular nursing in Australia. Osburn had trained at St Thomas's Hospital and was described there as 'a lady of superior birth'. The method of what became known as Nightingale nursing was inspired by German programs of training which had begun in the late 18th century, and by the work of the Quaker reformer Elizabeth Fry, developed from the 1840s by sisters of Anglican nursing orders in the London voluntary hospitals. These orders promoted the practical skills of 'applying dressings, leeching and administering enemas', combined with personal traits of 'sexual purity, punctuality, cleanliness and obedience to matron's orders' (Shyrock 1968, Smith 1982:155).

The mid 19th century spread of humanitarian ideas and patriotic feeling during the Crimean War helped promote the Nightingale principles. A concurrent influence which affected medicine and thus hospital conditions was the movement for sanitary reform. In the later 19th century, medicine adopted a more biological approach to disease as germ theory enabled it to develop antiseptic, and later aseptic, techniques. These scientific advances led directly to the need for more training for nurses, while rising standards in medical education as a response to the new science may have had an even greater though indirect effect (Shyrock 1968). The hospital itself changed from a repository for the sick poor to a place where at least some of the sick could look forward to recovery. The emergence of the modern hospital was itself the most important reason for the rise of nursing as an occupation, and was part of a general reorganisation of production in which formerly domestic activities were moved into central workplaces (Melosh 1982:8, Coburn 1988).

Nightingale recognised the need for a more expert nurse and proposed a system of training. The formidable Mrs Wardroper, Matron of St Thomas's and an early example of a working mother, actually developed the new program, while the heroine of the Crimea supplied money from a public fund collected in her name and prescribed the rules for the probationers (trainees), rules which emphasised obedience and discipline even more than learning (Smith 1982:158). This was essential, since any suspicion of sexual laxity would have deterred respectable families from allowing their daughters to train. The specifications for the new nurse therefore combined nursing as an activity, the appropriate training, and the personal qualities of the 'good nurse' (Abel-Smith 1960:20-2, Davies 1977).

The Nightingale reform was not an instant revolution. The system changed only slowly, as the chief reformer herself thought advisable—even she had to compromise with the entrenched power of the hospitals and their medical staff. The new training system departed immediately from her precepts: where she wanted the trainees to have time off for study, the hospitals quickly discovered the advantage of deploying them as part of the workforce (Baly 1985).

The founder at home

Florence Nightingale was a highly intellectual and self-willed woman. If she did not invent modern nursing (and nursing was not her chief interest) she gave it a valuable asset: she identified it in the public mind with 'sanctified duty', raising its prestige in Victorian Britain and beyond. Further, she opened up a respectable occupation which could provide 'an outlet for the social conscience and frustrated energies of the Victorian spinster', that is, for the many British women of the time who like herself remained single, though without her means (Smith 1982:155). Changing conditions required a more educated and disciplined nurse, and Nightingale successfully promoted nursing as a calling acceptable to the social groups from which she sought to recruit suitable trainees. Although of elevated social standing herself, she expected many of those trained under her system to be women of the lower middle class and even from the more respectable reaches of the working class.

It was the 'lady-pupils' however who spread the reforms, many of them as hospital matrons. Nightingale herself engineered appointments for her protégées and pursued them with copious advice, urging them to acquire her own imperious style when they met opposition. The new nurses had in effect to stake out their territory, thus coming into conflict with the lay administrators, with the doctors, and with the 'old' nurses. The foundations of her system rested especially on the position of the matrons, who as 'ladies' fitted easily into management. Nightingale had found a managerial gap in the co-ordination of hospital services, a gap which the new matrons were able to fill (Abel-Smith 1960:22-6, Davies 1977). The characteristics of the 'nursing role' also appeared early. It drew together the disparate elements that Nightingale had discerned: executing delegated medical tasks, caring for the patient's needs, and managing the staff and the ward since doctors showed no inclination to do so and lay administrators were at one remove from patient care (Carpenter 1977).

'Nightingales' at Sydney Cove

The Nightingale nurses who came to Sydney Hospital had the benefit of the founder's backing and of her continuing advice, and they had to deal with predictable opposition from those in established positions as well as dismal physical conditions in the hospital itself. Appearing before a commission of inquiry into the management of the colony's public charities in 1873, Lucy Osburn declared that as Lady Superintendent she should have sole control of the nursing staff, a basic Nightingale dictum. Instead, she said, she had endured constant interference from the manager. The commission vindicated Osburn, judging that her authority had not been clearly defined, that she had been denied sole control of the nursing staff, and that she had been discouraged in her efforts to train nurses (Brodsky 1968:57, 71; Schultz 1991:85).

In the later years of the 19th century, colonial governments carried out a number of commissions of inquiry like that in Sydney into their charitable institutions. Recommendations often included advice about the need to have trained nurses for the major hospitals, and female nurses rather than male wardsmen. The Sydney experience led the way to a general change, especially after Osburn started a training school in 1869. Trained nurses, many of them British, now spread the gospel of the new nursing to the other Australian colonies (Schultz 1991:101, 115, 228). The Melbourne Hospital proved recalcitrant until the secretary and one of the surgeons finally persuaded the committee of management that the current system was 'atrociously and scandalously bad', opening the way in 1890 for the appointment of the Scottish Isabella Rathie as Matron. Sydney-trained nurses also took charge of many country hospitals, and even of insane asylums—in the absence of a specialised training there was no barrier to moving from a general hospital to a different establishment. Midwifery training had already begun in Melbourne in 1862, but under medical control so that those trained lacked the independence of traditional midwives (Inglis 1958:98-9, Hobbs 1980:6, Willis 1983:103, Durdin 1991:23, 28).

Like Osburn, many of these women came into conflict with both lay and medical staff, and like her saw the authorities as continually frustrating their efforts to improve conditions for both patients and nurses. However sincere these feelings, as leaders of a social movement the early nurses inevitably saw opposition as obstruction, their own cause as unquestionably just. In the United States, the hospital became the scene of a struggle for authority between nurses, doctors and administrators (Reverby 1987) and the same struggle seems to have occurred in Australia. A dispute at the Adelaide Hospital in the 1890s was significant in that it demonstrated some assertiveness on the part of nurses below matron rank. The granting of the vote to women in South Australia in 1894, which nurses had supported, may have encouraged this. One of the leading figures in the dispute was Margaret Graham, later Matron of the Adelaide Hospital and a prominent figure in nursing associations. She and a colleague submitted their names in 1895 for nomination as Labor Party candidates, among the first women to do so, but owing to a misunderstanding did not actually stand in the subsequent state election. An Englishwoman of dominating character, Graham 'never deviated from her intense devotion to the British tradition' (Hughes 1967:112, Jones 1986, Durdin 1991:29, 42).

Such devotion carried to the colonies by forceful women like Graham delayed the development of a distinctively Australian nursing, though one Australian nurse thought colonial nursing was always more egalitarian than British, since 'Florence Nightingale's idea that "ladies" and educated women should care for the sick rather than ignorant servants, was extremely acceptable in a country where servant status was associated with convictism and a despised social system' (Slater 1963).

Colonial women's work and worth

The various colonial commissions of inquiry also uncovered much about nurses' work and working conditions. Long hours of heavy manual labour, were usual, with 10, 12 or even 14-hour days common. 'Time off' could be as little as half a day a week, and annual leave might be two weeks. Many of the tasks would be familiar to nurses today, such as making beds, washing patients, giving enemas, taking temperatures and distributing drugs. But these were only part of the nurse's work in the 1890s. She also spent time cleaning and polishing the floors, dusting and tidying the ward before the doctors' rounds, carrying baskets of supplies, and removing and sorting dirty linen—in spite of Nightingale's poetic admonition that 'Nurses should not scour; it is a waste of power'. The justification for many of these tasks was the sanitary idea, the notion that disease lurked in and emanated from dirt. With sanitary reform a major ideal of the 19th century, for the nurse 'even the scrubbing of floors was partly lit by the glow of medical science' (Carpenter 1977).

For this work the nurse was maintained at the hospital's expense—Nightingale had decreed 'living in' to avoid the distraction of family obligations. It also ensured constant supervision of the student nurse's conduct (Dickenson & Law 1974). In most hospitals the accommodation was at best spartan, the pay more so—first year probationers often received nothing, some even paid a premium (Keneley 1988). Hospital administrators had discovered early on that trainees cost much less to employ than domestic staff—even qualified nurses might earn less than the hospital cook (Templeton 1969:113). Matrons who attempted to get better pay and conditions for their nurses (and not all did) usually found that if the hours were reduced this required a larger staff and therefore additional accommodation which hospital boards were unwilling to fund. In the severe recession of the 1890s some hospitals even reduced nurses' pay (Schultz 1991:254, 267). Nurses suffered this in common with many other workers, including women in the 'sweated' clothing trade. Defeated in the strikes of the 1890s, trade unions began to support compulsory arbitration so that employers would be forced to negotiate with them, and they set up state and federal Labor parties for the representation of workers' interests (Hagan 1981:8-10).

Since hospitals were in theory voluntary and therefore semi-autonomous, there was no uniformity in nurses' wages and conditions even within one colony. In the 1890s hospital boards were able to ignore parliamentary debates over the eight hour day in New South Wales and Victoria. In any case, New South Wales nurses reportedly felt that public discussion of the possibility of a shorter working week was an intrusion into their affairs. At a time when both doctors and patients had begun to realise that skilled nursing was a vital adjunct to medical care, nurses' working conditions remained inferior to those of most other comparable female occupations (Mitchell 1977:109, Keneley 1988, Schultz 1991:253-9). Why then did nursing become—and remain—a popular occupation?

Florence as founder...

The image of Florence Nightingale, the popular conception of her career and good works, made nursing a respectable occupation for the daughters of the 'educated classes', assisted by the new appreciation of the benefits of skilled nursing care, and by doctors' growing interest in diagnosis so that they were prepared to delegate (while keeping control over) some treatment functions (Shyrock 1968, Carpenter 1977). The demand for trained nurses combined therefore with a readiness on the part of recruits to meet that demand in spite of the rigours of the work. The shortage of alternative work of comparable standing and the attractions of an occupation which did not deprive a girl of the chance of marriage may also have been influential (Kingston 1977:83). In the late Victorian era a woman's primary role was seen as one of duty to husband and family rather than to any sort of career, even though in England and in the US demographic factors led to a surplus of single women by the end of the century—the word 'surplus' itself implies their status as a burden. Australia did not have this surplus (in fact there was a surfeit of men) but it offered few opportunities for women with professional aspirations (Buxton 1974).

Some feminist historians (influenced by Marxism) argue that 19th century conditions created a belief that the family was the basic social unit and that a family structure in which women had a subordinate position was essential for maintaining social order. The prevailing moral code dictated the domestic sphere as proper for middle class women. Women outside this moral code (working class, immigrant and black women) could join the workforce but the code still affected them, and it brought advantages for employers by encouraging women workers to think that because their proper place was in the home, work outside it was a transient experience. They were less likely therefore to join unions to agitate for better wages and conditions, and employers could treat women's earnings as merely supplementing those of men (Kessler-Harris 1976). Women were thus seen as belonging to a secondary labour market, as in Australia's highly sex segregated workforce. Women's work was less visible than men's because it was often thought to be inessential. It was thus open to exploitation (Beaton 1982). New occupations emerge as a consequence of technical and social changes which alter the social division of labour. Most are 'sex typed' at the start, as was nursing, and without radical change in labour market or technical conditions are likely to remain so (Murgatroyd 1982).

For middle class women, or for those aspiring to their standards and values, nursing seemed desirable because it enabled them to take up a socially acceptable occupation which offered them independence but did not necessitate their relinquishing cherished aspects of their 'proper' role, that of dutiful wife and mother. They therefore carried into their work the family based ideals and values of the Victorian era which encouraged women to derive self-esteem from serving the needs of men. The job of matron as supervisor of the hospital 'household' was congenial to the expectations of middle class women: the analogy between the family and the doctor-nurse-patient triad has often been noted, though the living-in provisions made younger nurses more akin to daughters living under matron-mother's moral guidance. A further effect was that hospitals got a workforce that was docile as well as cheap. The vocational ideology of the occupation ensured that however menial the task, its performance was sanctified by being part of the work of a worthy calling, so that any expression of discontent was silenced, industrial action unthinkable (Carpenter 1977, Kingston 1977:82, Williams 1978, Trembath & Hellier 1987:27-31).

Ideology here refers to the interpretative and explanatory statements offered by the leaders of an occupation to its members concerning their activities as members, both individual and collective (Davies 1983). In nursing, the ideology of vocation was combined with a naturalistic orientation—nursing was 'naturally' a woman's occupation (Coburn 1988).

...and Florence as feminist

Nursing as an occupation was therefore compatible with 19th century ideals of womanhood. Its standing was further promoted by the image, eventually the legend, of Florence Nightingale, or by those aspects of her life and character which appealed to contemporary values. The revised version of Nightingale known today is of a woman who wanted to exercise power over men and over affairs and who chose in secluded invalidism a peculiarly Victorian way of doing so, since as a woman she was denied more orthodox methods. She was ruthless, self-assured and opinionated to a degree—like her younger rival Ethel Bedford Fenwick. Her stated impatience with the feminists of her time hid an inner turmoil that forced her to reject the conventional suffocation of family life. She was not alone in this nor in channelling her passion into religion—the revival of Anglican religious sisterhoods in mid-century has been described as one of the first signs of incipient feminism among middle-class women. Her feminism was powerful, but it was individualistic. She believed in women's emancipation, but she could not bring herself to believe in their rights (Showalter 1981).

The image which made Nightingale a celebrity in 19th century England, the authorised version, 'a saintly woman who merely wants to serve', stood for a culturally desirable femininity, desirable because it embodied 19th century romantic and humanitarian values. Attaching as it did to an upper class woman, it gave nursing respectability and had the further effect of enabling the nurse to feel that she was making a 'safe sacrifice' for a worthy cause, untainted by the baser motive of monetary reward (Whittaker & Olesen 1978). Such ideas masked the potentially demeaning nature of the work, and they encouraged a feminine meekness at odds with the founder's real character.

Training for work

Nightingale herself stressed that the skill required for nursing was not intuitive in women and must be learned. Even if the system that actually developed gave only cursory attention to learning, at least hospitals had to acknowledge the need for some training. By 1900 most larger Australian hospitals had three year courses for probationer or student nurses, again following British developments. At the Melbourne Hospital, for example, students in the 1890s followed three courses of study: anatomy, surgery, and physiology and medicine, with lectures given by an honorary surgeon and practical instruction by Isabella Rathie herself (Inglis 1958:99-100). Dr Campbell at the Adelaide Children's Hospital taught nurses 'the Art of Bandaging', the 'Administration of Medicines', and how to apply poultices, cupping and leeching (Durdin 1991:25). Textbooks gave instruction in treatments and nursing care while avoiding anatomical details that might shock the innocent (Hobbs 1980:51). Practical skills included invalid cookery, housekeeping and principles of hygiene. Yet the long hours of work made off duty learning difficult. At the Alfred Hospital in Melbourne in the 1890s lecture times were at the convenience of the honorary medical staff and nurses were often too tired to concentrate (Mitchell 1977:110). A sympathetic doctor commented in 1899 on the life of a Sydney Children's Hospital trainee: 'Most of the first year is spent in actual drudgery work more fitting for a scullery maid than an embryo nurse. There is so much routine work that has to be got through that there is not much time for training' (Hamilton 1979:49).

The pattern of nursing work and education was thus laid down by the turn of the century. The shape of nursing organisation had also emerged by this time, with its clearly differentiated hierarchy from the matron down, through the ranks of senior sisters, sisters, staff nurses, and third, second and first year probationers, the last also the lowliest (Hobbs 1980:21).

A hierarchy of class...

This hierarchy was part of a larger set of differentiated relations in which nursing was subordinate to medicine. When medicine in England inaugurated its successful control over the occupation in the mid 19th century, the actual expertise of doctors by today's standards was limited, their effectiveness more so, since their seizure of control pre-dated scientific medicine. But if medicine could not demonstrate that its practitioners cured disease, it could at least show that they were men of education and social standing. The high value put on impersonal expertise (rather than personal qualities) which underpins modern professions, was probably a development of the later 19th century (Davies 1983).

A profession commonly makes a 'contract' with society: in exchange for state protection, its governing body affirms that it will ensure safe (and even ethical) practitioners. It thus at once publicly claims to safeguard its clients from dangerous imposters and less publicly protects its members by outlawing competition. The cumulative effect of these measures is to raise the status of the occupation by ensuring that its members are educated to practise safely, and to guarantee them a high degree of autonomy in their work and commensurate material reward.

Through 'ladies' like Nightingale and Fenwick, British nursing became an accepted occupation for women, and the 'ladies' dominated its senior ranks. In US nursing there was a limited attempt to counteract this, but early organisations also were élitist. Nursing leaders were conservative women whose political agenda was limited to their own educational development. It did not include social change (Ashley 1975, Davies 1983). They did not think of raising the status of all nurses by uniting with them to oppose male/medical domination. Rather, they prescribed strict obedience and loyalty to doctors (Coburn 1988). Medicine achieved a degree of collective upward mobility (Willis 1983:11), but nursing remained a stratified occupation. From the 19th century idea of nursing as a vocation, then still held by many nurses, the leaders turned increasingly in the 20th century to the idea of a career: for them, 'medical professionalisation offered a model for the control over work and the public legitimacy they sought for nurses', and they rejected the 'angel of mercy' image held dear by their more traditionally minded sisters (Melosh 1982:10-11, 26-9). Seeing themselves as socially equal to their medical colleagues, nursing leaders adopted a professionalising strategy—that is, an ideologically directed program of action through which they hoped to achieve professional status for their occupation (Davies 1983). They wanted nursing to be seen as a profession in the male mould, but the female hierarchy and the increasingly outmoded ideology of 'duty' restricted nurses' collective power (Reverby 1987:200).

...and a hierarchy of sex

Medical practice depends on a combination of diagnosis-prescription and treatment-observation. In an apparently rational division of labour, medicine delegated much of the treatment-observation function to nursing which accepted also the Nightingale hygiene functions of maintaining clean and comfortable surroundings for the patient. But this 'rational' division of tasks was based not just on the different training doctors and nurses received at the time, but on the reflection within health care of the power relations of the Victorian middle class family. This determined nursing tasks to be those considered at the time most appropriate for women in the domestic sphere, though the shift of these tasks to the sphere of paid labour did not mean discarding the idea of women's obligation to serve. The ensuing inequality was justified not by an objectively assessed lesser value of nurses' work, but by that work seeming 'natural' for their sex:

> Nursing was set up and defined as women's work, and a good nurse was seen as primarily a good woman. This 'deprofessionalised' the relations between nursing and medicine, and situated the nurse-doctor relation, characterised by the subordination of nursing to medicine, within a patriarchal structure. The occupational ideology of nursing thus genderised the division of labour: it associated science and authority with doctors, and caring—putting science into practice—with women. In this way health care based itself on allegedly sex-specific personal qualities (Gamarnikow 1978:114).

This occupational ideology, based as it was on 19th century ideas of women as having duties rather than rights, 'gave trained nursing purpose but limited its power to control or define its occupational or professional existence'. The shared experience of women's work could not become the basis of unity since hierarchy, not equal sisterhood characterised the occupation. Nurses were 'a group of women so divided by class that their common oppression based on gender could not unite them', says Reverby (1987:2, 6, 201), but as an occupational group they did not in fact reflect the social class structure of the workforce. Nurses were to some degree an élite among working women (Melosh 1982:10), so although there were class differences between the 'ladies' and the other ranks further down the hierarchy, the divisions between them probably owed less to class antagonism than to the opposing interests of superiors and subordinates created by the hierarchical organisation of the workplace.

Nightingale believed in each nurse's allegiance to herself as charismatic founder and saw no need for nursing associations or for registration (Davies 1983) but leading nurses, influenced by the example of medicine, started to organise. For the first half of this century nursing associations in Australia were fragmented and ambivalent about their industrial role, but slowly they became the foundation for later political action.

Women, and nurses, mobilise

Ethel Bedford Fenwick, former matron of St Bartholomew's Hospital, had joined with other prominent nurses and doctors (including her husband) in 1887 to form the British Nurses' Association—'Royal' from 1893 (RBNA). Dr Fenwick himself described the association in 1904 as a 'union of nurses with professional objects', unwittingly encapsulating what eventually emerged as the two central, if sometimes opposing, purposes of such associations. The RBNA was originally dominated by matrons and by senior medical practitioners. It set up a register for nurses and in 1889 stipulated that three years' training in a recognised hospital (that is, with over 40 beds) was essential for admission. The register was ineffective, but it was seen as a provisional measure only since the RBNA aimed at official registration such as doctors already had (Abel-Smith 1960:69-76).

Nine years later similar associations were set up in the United States and Canada, though in the former nurses dominated from the start (Davies 1983). Ethel Fenwick also helped found in 1899 the International Council of Nurses (ICN)—significantly, as part of an International Council of Women Congress held that year. Her bold pronouncement that 'the nurse question is the woman question' immediately connected nursing with feminism: 'The emergence of determined nursing organisations was inextricably linked with feminist revolt and was, initially, as little respectable or popular' (Minchin 1977:12).

The congress set up a nursing section whose members exhorted those attending its meetings to return to their various countries and organise national associations to push for higher standards of nursing and for registration, to enforce a proper education system with examinations. Susan McGahey, Matron of the Royal Prince Alfred Hospital in Sydney, was at the congress and on her return joined with others, including a number of doctors, to establish the New South Wales Trained Nurses' Association. Within months the association had changed its name to the Australasian Trained Nurses' Association (ATNA), its intention 'to embrace the whole of Australia and beyond' (Anon. 1968, Schultz 1974). With federation of the Australian colonies about to occur, this was a timely change. The ATNA invited the other states to set up branches, which most did, though these branches were largely autonomous and, despite the coming of the Commonwealth, nursing organisations remained state oriented (Dickenson 1971).

Margaret Graham set up a branch of the RBNA in South Australia which became almost exclusive to nurses from her own Adelaide Hospital, though after some tension between it and the local ATNA branch the two associations co-existed for some years, Graham finally joining the ATNA in 1909 (Durdin 1991:42-50). In 1907 branches in Tasmania and Western Australia were inaugurated, like those of the other states under medical patronage. Victorian nurses supported the setting up in 1901 of the Victorian Trained Nurses' Association (VTNA), deciding 'at the outset', that it should 'stand independently of the ATNA' especially as regards the proposed system of training and registration (Armstrong 1951, Kelly 1977:139, Hobbs 1980:26, Trembath & Hellier 1987:64). This was the first of a number of decisions by Victorian nurses to stand separately from their older and larger neighbour. This had long term consequences, as one of today's nursing leaders observes:

> ...when the Australasian Trained Nurses' Association had actually set itself up in 1901, they perceived that the Royal Victorian Trained Nurses' Association, set up in Victoria in direct opposition, had prevented Australia from getting a national organisation, right from the days of federation. [MP/91]

The tensions between the two major states form a constant theme in Australian nursing, perhaps its first clear departure from the British parent, though at the time an absence of national unity was usual in similar Australian associations.

Following the ICN line, the major aim of each of the new bodies was to establish systems of registration so that doctors, hospitals and the public could distinguish trained nurses from the unqualified. Fenwick was clear in her interpretation of at least some of these requirements in 1890 when she stipulated that 'the only way of organising a profession is...by having a controlling body outside [the hospitals]' (quoted Trembath & Hellier 1987:44). As well as registration to exclude the untrained, Fenwick's professionalising strategy included specified entry requirements to raise nursing's status. She thus differed from Nightingale (though not in her deference to medicine) and aroused the founder's antagonism as well as that of hospital managements, the latter because registration would limit the numbers in the nursing workforce and bring demands for higher pay (Davies 1977, 1983; Coburn 1988).

The Australian associations also aimed to raise nursing's status through registration, and they had in common with the RBNA a strong representation of matrons and doctors in their governing councils. By 1907 five states had set up examining boards which supervised three year courses and advised that those entering such courses should be examined as to their 'educational fitness' (Anon. 1968). Like other such associations, the ATNA established a journal in 1903, the *Australasian Nurses' Journal* (ANJ). The VTNA also set up a regulatory body and established uniform standards of training, but it defied the ATNA by publishing its own journal, "*UNA*", simultaneously with the first ANJ. It even went one better by acquiring the title 'Royal' in 1904, partly to pay back the ATNA for allegedly stealing the idea of a journal (Armstrong 1951; Trembath & Hellier 1987:53, 60).

In setting up organisations for regulating nursing and establishing standards for training that were modest but appropriate, Australian nurses were in line with their colleagues in Britain, the United States and Canada, and they were following the example of many other women in Australia in creating a web of organisations in the first decade after federation. The councils of these state associations were unrepresentative, but they apparently shared the aims of working nurses which were not primarily directed to improving pay and conditions. The militant feminist Vida Goldstein failed to convince Victorian nurses that they could raise economic questions without betraying their professional ideals (Encel et al 1974:6, 238, 243), though Susan McGahey had said the first aim of the ATNA was to 'promote the interests of Trained Nurses—male and female—in all matters affecting their work as a class' (Dickenson & Law 1974). Although they saw the advantages of organising, nurses were far from seeing their associations as instruments of power and certainly not as trade unions. Further, their training encouraged loyalty to the 'home hospital' rather than a broader occupational allegiance (Reverby 1987:122).

Change was also under way at this time in asylum nursing. By 1900 various acts had made it mandatory to separate the mentally retarded from the mentally ill, and both groups from the 'inebriates', and to send the mentally ill to an asylum rather than to gaol. Although care was still largely custodial, the mostly male 'mental attendants' began to receive lectures from the medical staff, and there were suggestions for employing trained female nurses (Keane 1987:4).

The nursing workforce was changing at this time in two directions: from 1900 to 1914 the proportion of trainees to trained staff in hospitals rose steadily, at least in Victoria and South Australia; and of the trained nurses, the majority worked in private practice looking after patients in their own homes. Private nursing was also common in comparable countries such as England, Canada and the US, though most attention has gone to hospital nursing. In Victoria the pay and conditions of work for private duty nurses, unlike those of hospital nurses, were prominent in RVTNA discussions, showing that it is an exaggeration to claim that nurses were not concerned with what would now be called industrial matters. They were, but not as part of the official trade union movement. The private duty nurses in fact considered themselves independent professionals since like doctors they accepted a fee for their services (Trembath & Hellier 1987:73-4, 104; Durdin 1991:46, 78). An 'extensive debate' actually took place in the pages of the ANJ in 1912 over the ethics of raising fees for private nurses, who argued that it was difficult to meet their modest needs out of two guineas (£2 2s. or $4.20) a week. Queensland nurses finally voted in 1914 for a one guinea (£1 1s. or $2.20) fee rise (Law 1980). The Australian system of wage determination rested on the 1907 Harvester judgement in the federal Arbitration Court, which specified the 'normal needs' of a family man, with women's pay usually 54% of the male rate.

Professionalism triumphs...

During the Great War of 1914-1918 over 2000 trained nurses served overseas. At home the gaps were filled by members of the Voluntary Aid Detachments (VADs) similar to the British variety. The ATNA and RVTNA saw to it that only the fully trained had the privilege of serving in military hospitals. Nurses who had served overseas were given certain military privileges, such as the right to march on Anzac Day. They became part of the Anzac legend and were the only women to do so, but this had no radical implications since they had performed what the public then saw as women's work (Trembath & Hellier 1987:106-8; Goodman 1988:102, 112).

Nursing after the war was not substantially different from nursing in 1900. The training was 'rigorous, physically demanding, and involved much repetitive work, but it lacked intellectual stimulation'. The public thought highly of them, but rank and file nurses were still mostly obedient to their superiors with little control over their own affairs (Durdin 1991:88). Like their British sisters, they led restricted lives dominated by fear, especially fear of authority (Abel-Smith 1960:141).

The war years were however crucial in the fight for state registration. In this, as in so many other matters, the ICN influenced Australian nursing (Dickenson 1971). An ATNA conference in Sydney in 1909 had discussed the subject, but before 1914 only Queensland had official registration, and there it had been sponsored by the Medical Board (Anon. 1968). In England Bills for registration had been refused a parliamentary hearing every year from 1904 to 1914, with Ethel Fenwick a familiar figure in the House of Commons lobby. The influx of briefly trained VADs made regular nurses anxious to maintain their distinction. The major push for registration came from Fenwick and her supporters in the RBNA, the 'lady' nurses. Nightingale had opposed and subverted registration from behind the scenes on the grounds that it would introduce examinations and thus test knowledge rather than personal qualities, but she had died in 1910. Most in nurses' favour was their status as women who were about to get the right to vote from a grateful government after their services during the war, and in 1919 British nursing finally achieved registration. In one scholar's view the fight for registration was 'a battle for status against a background of rampant snobbery and militant feminism' on the part of those who wished to make nursing more exclusive, against those (including some nurses) who saw that this would reduce the supply and who disliked the 'superior airs' of the lady nurses (Abel-Smith 1960:66-7; 89-97). In another view, just as the suffrage movement aimed to free women from patriarchal control at home, so registration, the leaders thought, could free nursing from medical control at work. For the 'worker nurses', registration with its stress on education was at once a threat to their status and irrelevant to their vocational ideals (Reverby 1987:126, 142).

Australia's federal constitution ensured that registration would proceed differently in the various states, though appreciation of nurses' war service was probably an advantage everywhere. Female suffrage was not an issue since women had gained the vote in all states between 1894 and 1908, partly as a result of federation and with significant agitation by women only in the two larger states (Encel et al 1974:221-35).

In South Australia, with 'no evidence of a nursing lobby', the hospitals association sponsored a registration Bill which passed in 1920, hoping that it would enable smaller hospitals to become training schools and thus acquire cheap labour (Durdin 1991:90). Western Australia was next: the Sisters' branch of the Returned Soldiers Association encouraged the 1922 Act, and though some MPs demonstrated 'ignorance and bigotry' about registration, it was supported by Edith Cowan, the first woman MP in Australia (Hobbs 1980:67, 73). The New South Wales ATNA had begun to campaign for registration in 1903, but the Act was not passed until 1924. Tasmania's was even later in 1927. The RVTNA, trying since 1914 for legislation, still failed in its aim in 1919, partly because Labor MPs tried to use the Bill to prescribe pay and a 48 hour week for trainees. The Bill finally passed in 1924, setting up a board on which the RVTNA was well represented, thus consolidating its position as the voice of nursing in Victoria (Kelly 1977:117; Castle 1987; Trembath & Hellier 1987:149).

In the case of midwifery, registration enactments in Victoria between 1915 and 1920 ensured that this once independent occupation came under medical control. Further legislation in 1928 and 1929, which both doctors and nurses supported, completed this process: midwifery became part of nursing and like it formally subordinate to medicine (Willis 1983:111-16). In New South Wales a Bill to register trained midwives was introduced in 1895 but was not passed until 1924. Again, practice was less independent than in Britain or Europe. Midwives had been held responsible for a high rate of infant mortality, but the persistence of a high rate even after doctors took over most obstetrics suggests that their level of skill was higher than some doctors (perhaps fearing competition) were willing to acknowledge (Williamson 1982).

...but the spectre of unionism haunts Australian nursing

After the war conditions at home began to change. In Victoria staff shortages had stimulated groups of nurses to protest against conditions, including the lengthening of the three year training to four years. The public and some left wing politicians were becoming more sympathetic to nurses' claims for better conditions, prompted by the activities of the war nurses, but the RVTNA was slow to respond to new demands, maintaining its policy of not interfering in hospital affairs. A major barrier to raising pay, then as now, lay in the reluctance of both government and hospitals to spend more money. The RVTNA's hesitation left the way open for a breakaway group led by Gretta Lyons, a former president and ardent feminist, who tried to persuade nurses that they would improve their working conditions through belonging to the industrial arbitration system. This was the Trained Nurses' Guild (TNG). Its revolt lasted less than two years, but it forced the RVTNA to adopt some economic goals. The TNG lived on by achieving registration as an industrial organisation in the Commonwealth Arbitration Court, despite opposition from the RVTNA. 'Brusque in manner almost to rudeness' but dedicated to improving the lives of working women, Lyons so antagonised the RVTNA that her obituary in the journal did not mention the TNG (*The Herald* 5 November 1923; *UNA Nursing Journal* December 1923:208; Trembath & Hellier 1987:109-19; 144-8).

In the north, Brisbane student nurses in 1921 formed the Queensland Nurses' Association (QNA) which demanded higher pay, a 48 hour week and penalty rates to give nurses conditions comparable with those of other workers. This forced the Queensland ATNA to take the 'revolutionary step' of registering as a union under the 1916 Arbitration Act. The branch opposed the QNA claim but the industrial court granted nurses an award, thus accepting them as workers whose conditions could be legally regulated, though the Queensland ATNA doubted that nurses could adhere to award conditions.

Representatives of the Western Australian ATNA went to a conference in Sydney in 1921 to discuss the union question, and the WA branch considered altering its constitution so that trainees could belong—presumably to prevent their joining other unions. The ATNA, the WA nurses found, was ineligible for registration because many of its members were either employers or private duty nurses (Anon. 1968; Dickenson 1975; Hobbs 1980:72). These events suggest that some nurses were less convinced than their leaders that nurses could not be classified as 'workers'.

This upsurge of industrial interest, mild though it was, took place at the time of origin of most Australian white collar unions. Nurses were experiencing the same dilemma which faced their British colleagues: was nursing a trade or a profession? In Britain, the Royal College of Nursing (RCN) had disapproved strongly when mental nurses went on strike in 1918—the first ever nursing strike. It was further perturbed during the 1920s by signs of incipient unionism among nurses at local authority hospitals (the former Poor Law workhouses). In the higher status voluntary hospitals they were less likely to join a union for reasons which were both ideological (the idea of nursing as a vocation) and class based—many nurses were ladies and 'many others had become nurses in the hope that they would be regarded as such'. They could hardly identify themselves therefore with a working class movement such as trade unionism, especially one with Labour Party connections (Abel-Smith 1960:132-3).

A national association—just

In 1922 the RVTNA Secretary, Louise Crocker, wrote to the ATNA secretary suggesting a meeting 'with a view to forming a Federated Nurses' Association'. The first meeting of the Australian Nursing Federation (ANF), attended by representatives from the six states, took place in 1924, the same year that the Canadian Nurses Association was formed. Nursing's debt to medicine was maintained: the first meeting of the ANF took place in the Sydney BMA building, its first constitution was based on that of the BMA (later AMA), and the first president was a doctor. Affiliation with the ICN proved impossible for some years, and the RVTNA refused to co-operate with the further aim of issuing a national journal. The constitution followed the principles of the Australian Senate: each state branch had two votes, a provision which the small WA branch understandably applauded (Armstrong 1951; Schultz 1974; Hobbs 1980:74; Trembath & Hellier 1987:150).

Nurses and the depression

The depression of the 1930s brought many Australians up against the misery of mass unemployment when 'a few bleak years of economic catastrophe' demolished the image of the workers' paradise (Robertson 1974). The depression also altered the composition of the nursing workforce: trainees were cheaper than the trained, so their numbers rose relative to the number of trained nurses. The number of private duty nurses declined, partly because of the growth of fee-paying beds in public hospitals (Bessant & Bessant 1991:3), and as a result of the decline in infectious diseases. A Victorian nurse found private nursing at this time even harder than a trainee's life:

> My training was a hard, slogging job at the Alfred. After that I did private nursing for a while, but not for very long. I could not cope with it because I was shut up with a family, and you might be expected to work for 24 hours a day because nobody was going to get a second nurse—if the patient was ill you just did it. [MC/88]

The depression also brought a renewed interest among nurses and their associations in improving their conditions of work, and they took further steps in the inevitable if reluctant move towards unionism.

The ATNA secretary, Evelyn Evans, reported in 1931 that 'some misguided members' of the profession, including 'some of the leading lights of the ATNA' had decided to form a union. She seemed to think this would not succeed since the Hospital Employees' Association (HEA), a general union which covered some nurses, would fight its registration 'tooth and nail'. The new body was the New South Wales Nurses' Association (NSWNA). Its Secretary, the Scottish-trained Georgina Johnstone (Mrs McCready), pointed out in a letter to Evans that it was essential for nurses to have a nursing–controlled union to promote their pay and conditions and to protect them from having to join the HEA, a union which she considered gave inadequate representation to nurses on its governing body and, further, was affiliated with the Trades Hall.

Johnstone's fears were justified: the HEA had applied the previous year to cover all hospital employees, and the New South Wales Labor Premier, Jack Lang (dismissed by the state governor in 1932 for unconstitutional actions), had introduced an Arbitration Bill which included a provision for compulsory unionism—nurses could be 'engulfed' by the HEA, she thought. Undaunted by the ATNA's half-hearted support and a ballot of its members with a small majority against the new body, Johnstone affirmed that the NSWNA was 'for professional women only and governed by trained nurses' (*The Lamp* 1980 December:34-5; 1981 May:9-12).

In spite of difficult early years, the NSWNA fought successfully to establish itself, gaining an award for nurses in 1936 from the industrial commission. In 1945-46 it absorbed the Trained Mental Nurses Association, whose Secretary, Les Hart, became NSWNA Secretary. This increased its membership and made it more widely representative of nurses than the ATNA was. But the Nurses' Association had a significance to Australian nursing far beyond its immediate founding. Its separate presence deprived national nursing of a valuable counterweight to the Victorians who, with their largely professional focus, dominated the ANF and later obstructed the formation of a united nursing organisation. More constructively, the NSWNA maintained its professional concerns, if not always consistently, and thus showed that it was possible to combine these effectively with industrial activity. Criticism from other nursing associations suggests that their members did not immediately appreciate this NSWNA achievement (*The Lamp*, 1981 May:9-12).

In Queensland, a Labor government had legislated for a 44 hour week in 1924, and the industrial QNA had achieved an 88 hour fortnight for nurses, but at the start of the depression this was raised to 96 hours at the same time as salaries were reduced. Both the Queensland and federal ATNA consistently supported the longer hours against the QNA claim, on the grounds that fewer hours would endanger both trainee proficiency and patient care (Law 1980). It was during the depression that pay awards, especially the component for skill, came increasingly to be determined by the principle of national economic 'capacity to pay', rather than by the original 'needs' principle applied to the basic wage (Deery & Plowman 1991:389-90)

Nurses in South Australia seem to have been industrially subdued during the 1930s, but in the West they were spurred on by the formation of a Hospital Officers' Association in 1934 to seek registration with the Arbitration Court. The result was the formation of the Western Australian Nurses' Association (WANA). Neither the ATNA Council in Sydney nor some local nurses approved, fearing a lowering of professional status, but the WANA went on to gain an award the following year.

In 1934 the RVTNA became the Royal Victorian College of Nursing (RVCN), aiming to promote postgraduate education for trained nurses. Given some medical opposition, only tepid interest from the University of Melbourne, and nurses' long hours of work and low pay, this hope was never fulfilled. The RVCN in fact became a professional association with some limited industrial goals. Faced with a threat from the Hospital Employees' Federation (HEF) in 1936 it had no choice but to push for a wages board for nurses—like Tasmania, the state had kept its wages board based industrial system. A similar threat loomed in 1943, so the RVCN had to create an employees' association to conduct its industrial affairs (Armstrong 1951; Hobbs 1980:90; Bessant & Bessant 1991:4-5).

The trend to industrial interests disturbed Jane Bell, Matron of the Melbourne Hospital, who became President of the RVCN in 1938. Like many of her peers she saw such activity as opposed to a professionalism which still embodied duty and service. Of all the nursing bodies, the RVCN seems especially to have regarded unionism as something better avoided if possible (the taint of proletarianism threatened nursing's ladylike status) and contemplated only when there was no alternative. Yet Australia's industrial system with its high level of state intervention and legal regulation forced nurses to act intermittently as a group of workers (Williams & Goodman 1988:101-103; Bessant & Bessant 1991:2-3, 7-13).

A boost to professionalism came with the ICN's acceptance of Australia as a member in 1937. To achieve this, the ANF had to reconstitute itself hastily as a national association: following a two-year 'stalemate' there was an alliance between it and the always independently-minded RVCN (Armstrong 1951; Hobbs 1980:80-82, 92-96, 114-115; Durdin 1991:95, 107-8, 121).

Another gain, for trainees this time, was the setting up of Preliminary Training Schools (PTSs) during the 1930s in many of the major hospitals, led by Jane Bell in 1927 at the Melbourne Hospital. The PTS saved the young (and getting younger) trainee from a brutal introduction to the ward routine on her first day, although as a South Australian nurse educator comments,

> ...in South Australia we had no such provision. It was a case of being thrown to the wolves the day you set foot in the hospital. We didn't get our first PTS until 1948. [JD/88]

Australian nursing ended the 'long weekend' of the interwar period with its organisations fragmented, divided into separate professional and industrial associations in some states, and with a weak national body. The associations still tended to be dominated by the matrons, but the medical presence had diminished—perhaps Australian nursing, like Canadian, was beginning to include in its ideology the 'separate but equal to medicine' doctrine (Coburn 1988). Little had happened in nurse education beyond the advent of the PTS, and the size and composition of the workforce, or 'manpower', depended mostly on ad hoc needs rather than on rational planning.

Nursing as a job still had some of its 19th century characteristics. The work was heavy, with patients kept in bed for long periods including post partum and post-operative, so that nurses often had to lift them. Medical work was becoming more differentiated and doctors delegated more tasks to them, but nurses still often acted as dietitians, physiotherapists, social workers, even radiographers—with little protection against the new radium—and the trainees retained a large number of domestic tasks. Nurses handed out a limited range of medicines, mostly as liquids, to patients who might have malaria, diphtheria or septicaemia. Infectious diseases were still common, though less so than in the 19th century owing to public health measures, but for those who had infections like 'septic' (backyard) abortion or pneumonia there were no curative drugs until the advent of sulphonamides, as one veteran nurse recalls:

> ...we didn't have anything. If you had a serious infection—I have seen so many people die in my time. Where today you would think how dreadful that someone died of appendicitis, it is very rare. In those days it was not rare. [GB/88]

Nursing discipline remained strict but those imposing it faced a tougher task: since the 1920s young women had become less willingly ladylike, more inclined to be found 'drinking, smoking and associating with young men...' to the consternation of their elders like Jane Bell. There were changes in the hospitals, with the growth of country institutions and of private hospitals where middle class patients paid fees instead of having to qualify for admission to public hospitals as objects of charity. A change which ultimately reduced the power of the matrons was the rise of the lay manager. Mental health or psychiatric nursing remained a Cinderella occupation with a very limited training, treatment consisting of sedatives and occupational therapy. In spite of the expansion of psychiatry during this period, general nurses still looked down on their psychiatric nurse colleagues, often because they knew nothing of psychiatric work but wanted to remain aloof from people they saw as mere custodians of a stigmatised clientele (Minchin 1977:37-9; Hobbs 1980:106-18, 122-3; Williams & Goodman 1988:84-5; Durdin 1991:104, 113, 120).

Nurses at war again

When the Second World War began in 1939 the army nursing services were much less well organised than the medical, since army nurses had received less support from their own associations than had the doctors. The Army Nursing Service was listed as a subordinate part of the medical services, with Grace Wilson, of the Alfred Hospital in Melbourne, as Matron-in-Chief. There was confusion about the precise status of army nurses—they did not hold military rank but were 'entitled to the courtesies extended to an officer'. The extent of their authority over military hospital staff was not clear until they received commissioned rank in 1943 following a similar benefit for physiotherapists (Goodman 1988:119-121, 185). The army men were apparently reluctant to accept women as officers with some authority, but male double standards precluded nurses from 'roughing it' with other ranks.

The war produced significant changes for nursing. The accelerating revolution in medical treatment and technology which began with the introduction of sulphonamides and of blood transfusions in the 1930s, proceeded to the rapid development of antibiotics and new surgical techniques during the war, changes which led eventually to demands for improved nurse education. Some things remained the same, such as the equipment, much of which before the age of plastic and disposables was made of metal or rubber; and a Victorian nurse remembered wartime shortages: 'Have you ever tried to insert a flaccid catheter which has been boiled a hundred times?' (Jennings 1976). Within nursing, the war exacerbated the staff shortages of the 1930s—the absolute number of nurses was growing, but not enough to keep up with demand. In 1942 the Directorate of Manpower assumed control of nursing womanpower and tackled the urgent job of recruiting more nurses for the depleted home hospitals. This turned the interest of the authorities to nurses' poor conditions of work and pay. A federal committee of enquiry realised that the low pay and often shabby accommodation could not attract the 'right kind of girl' to nursing, that more congenial jobs were now open to women, and that in any case many possibly suitable women had married during the war. Against this, senior nurses and some politicians apparently still saw nursing as a vocation—the privilege of caring for the sick did not demand a high material reward (Armstrong 1951; Minchin 1977:48, 54; Bessant & Bessant 1991:63-6).

Reconstruction

Australia after the war experienced an era of reconstruction, led by a reformist federal Labor Government. The government's use of central power included attempts to set up a national health service, based on a limited version of the British scheme which began in 1948, but this was defeated by organised medicine. President Truman's attempt to legislate for national health insurance in the US was similarly dismissed, the doctors accusing the Bill of being 'communistic'—or worse, 'un-American'. US nurses were divided on its merits and did not want to be seen as a pressure group (Kalisch & Kalisch 1978:512-14, 538). Australian nurses seem to have remained silent on the Chifley Government's health legislation. Despite their numerical importance in health services, their traditional deference to doctors carried over to public debate, inhibiting them from developing their own views even on those matters of policy which affected them (Dickenson & Law 1974). Nurses' determination to remain apolitical seems to have led them to avoid any public comment which could be interpreted as political even where their own interests were concerned.

The demographic impact of the low depression birth rate had produced a general shortage of labour. Nursing shortages (and feared shortages) in

Britain during the war had led to the demand for a second level nurse or nursing aide. The RCN accepted the second level nurse but favoured limiting and defining her activities to protect the status of the registered nurse, especially as some nursing aides had achieved better pay than trained nurses. The RCN preferred this option to lowering the standards of entry into nursing so as to admit larger numbers. The now aged Ethel Fenwick foretold disaster for her profession as a result of this 'second portal' of entry (Abel-Smith 1960:162-75). In the US the number of second level nurses expanded by 35% between 1940 and 1950, bringing 'some bitterness among registered nurses' (Kalisch & Kalisch 1978:505-6).

In New South Wales failure to recruit trainees and retain qualified nurses in adequate numbers forced the use of 'many thousands' of nursing assistants to supplement the usual staffing arrangements in the expanding health services. In 1953 they were recognised in the Nurses Act, and in 1958 training schools were set up in selected hospitals. These 'nursing assistants' became 'nursing aides' in 1958, but the authorities retained the careful distinction between their function as assistants, and that of the registered nurse (Sullivan 1990:6-7). Yet R. K. Merton described the distinction in the US between the 'professional' nurse and the licensed practical nurse (LPN) as one not of different functions, but of degree of responsibility for a similar function. The proximity of the two in the workplace, he thought, would stimulate a desire for higher status in *both* groups (Merton 1962).

South Australia also was 'desperate for nurses' and many migrant women became nursing aides after a one year training and separate registration—though a group of Aboriginal women was excluded (Durdin 1991:158, 167). In Victoria both Grace Wilson and Gwen Burbidge (Matron of Fairfield Hospital) supported the aides, but in spite of the British precedent:

> There was a lot of opposition among the nurses, led by Miss Bell and [her successor] Miss Grey...they said we were trying to introduce the Sairey Gamps back into nursing! They hadn't moved with the times...[GB/90]

The new Victorian Hospitals and Charities Commission nevertheless gave its official approval to the training of the second level nurse and set up two schools, one for the migrant women who were arriving in large numbers as part of the postwar influx, and the Melbourne school for local girls. Given the acute shortage of labour, there was little the authorities could do but establish the second category of nurse. Registered nurses, or their leaders, feared 'dilution of standards' with a consequent threat to professionalism if anyone could be a nurse after only a brief training; and they disliked the aides taking over patient care tasks considered fundamental to nursing while registered nurses became more technically specialised. In Victoria the registration of the aides was taken over in 1956 by the Victorian Nursing Council, a move requested by the RVCN (Bessant & Bessant 1991:73, 158). The RVCN refused however to admit them as members, with the result that in Victoria most joined the Hospital Employees' Federation (HEF).

The threat to nursing posed by the aides can be seen in two ways, using Parkin's theory (adapted from Weber) of social closure, 'the process by which social collectivities seek to maximise rewards by restricting access to resources and opportunities to a limited circle of eligibles' (Parkin 1979:44). Professional (registered) nursing wished to achieve social closure by means of exclusion, the closing of social and economic opportunities to a group considered for whatever reason as outsiders. In the case of the aides, the reason put forward in Victoria was their limited education, yet at the same time the RVCN later opposed raising the educational level of aides so that they could become recognised members of the nursing team (Bessant & Bessant 1991:158). Alternatively, those nurses who accepted the aides perhaps saw them as contributing to the professional image of nursing by providing a subordinate category under the control of the registered nurse—a control always insisted on by organised nursing.

Organising for reconstruction...

Joining in the spirit of reconstruction, leading nurses now established three significant organisations. The ANF set up the National Florence Nightingale Committee (NFNC) in 1946 to promote postgraduate nursing education. Victorian Edith Hughes-Jones was its first National Secretary. The NFNC and its state branches awarded a small number of scholarships for study at the RCN in London, though the lucky recipients had to pay many of their own expenses. This was obviously not enough to meet the need, and the ANF '...agreed that reconstruction is essential in every sphere of nursing...' (*ANJ* 1948 March:48-51).

In 1947, the NFNC had asked one of its Vice-Presidents, Muriel Doherty, to report on educational needs. Doherty's report shows that nursing education retained its apprenticeship style and low entry standards, but that there was a trend to 'a modified studentship' with more PTSs and a wish to introduce the block system of study. The need for postgraduate education was obvious: fewer than 36 training schools had sister tutors, and of these 'only six or seven' held university qualifications or had educational training. Matrons and ward sisters, with the medical staff, still did most of the teaching.

Australian nursing had to improve these standards to maintain reciprocity (co-registration) with the British General Nursing Council. The ANF wished to follow the example of the RCN by setting up a unified national association, the Australian College of Nursing, to 'overhaul all aspects of nursing education and work for a Federal Nursing Services Act'. The federal government's scholarship scheme for ex-service men and women which led the way to the later expansion of tertiary education may have influenced nurses' thinking, even if they did not immediately benefit from it. Doherty recognised however that educational improvements alone could not accomplish this professional reconstruction. Most 'forward-looking nurses', she said, recognised two essential characteristics of their profession: its cultural and educational obligations, *and* its economic aspects—the need to have conditions of work comparable with those of other occupations (*ANJ* 1948 March:48-51; Schultz 1974). There seem to have been few of her senior colleagues who agreed with her elevation of the economic aspects.

...through professionalism...

The College of Nursing, Australia and the New South Wales College of Nursing were together the second and more significant step towards raising nursing's status, though not one taken in a spirit of unity. In 1948 the New South Wales branch of the NFNC at the instigation of Muriel Doherty devised a plan for autonomous state colleges linked by a federal council. The federal Minister for Health offered some funding to a national postgraduate school of nursing but the RVCN rejected this as removing control from nurses. Gwen Burbidge remembers disagreeing:

> I thought we were strong enough to have checked any intervention by the government...I'd be prepared to get their money as long as we got the education going...However, four or five influential nurses were influenced by the medical people, who were having a big fight with the federal government at the time over controls, and who thought that for the nurses to accept federal government money would weaken the doctors' case. [GB/90]

The continuing push by both state and federal governments for greater control of health services, then becoming a major budget item, was a trend that would eventually bring further confrontation with the medical profession. Nurses again did not speak out publicly, but in this case they seem to have given at least tacit support to the doctors.

Early in 1949 a mass meeting of nurses in Sydney recommended that postgraduate courses should start immediately. The NSWNA, the ATNA and the Matrons' Institute then established the New South Wales College of Nursing, which began teaching in March 1949 with voluntary staff in the absence of government funding. This New South Wales pre-empting of the college idea caused 'surprise and dismay' to the other associations, but it stimulated them to action. The RVCN had shown no enthusiasm for the Doherty national plan, but Edith Hughes-Jones of the NFNC, with the help of Major-General Norris, succeeded in getting Victorian state government funding. With the headquarters of the College of Nursing, Australia in Melbourne, the traditional rivalry between the two major states was maintained. New South Wales decided not to support the Victorian venture, but other states were represented on its council (Zepps 1975; Schultz 1989; Bessant & Bessant 1991:68-71; Durdin 1991:244). All states apparently shared the view, however, that educational enhancement was the way forward for professional nursing, and education rather than clinical improvement became the major focus of attention of the leadership.

...and unionism

In the late 1940s the nursing associations endured a turbulent period. Much of this came from interstate rivalries, but even more important was the division between those whose major interest was upholding nursing professionalism as they saw it, and those who thought that industrial affairs must have a comparable place and who thus wanted to build on the modest gains of the interwar period. Conditions favouring industrial activity included low unemployment and the shortage of nurses, which could have allowed nurses to agitate successfully for better pay and conditions. Against a burst of industrial enthusiasm was the communist presence in some unions, then alarming moderate unionists, and the 'red menace' fears propagated by the non-Labor opposition parties (Bolton 1974).

Internally, enough of the Nightingale spirit remained to make it difficult for nurses to demand purely economic gains. Their organisations were dominated by the attitude expressed in an often quoted statement made by the president of the Queensland ATNA in 1947: 'I have never liked trade unionism as applied to the profession of nursing' (Eunice Paten quoted Dickenson 1975). Even the NSWNA was inhibited by members' belief that low pay and long hours testified to nurses' vocation and devotion to their patients—they were not 'in it for the money' (Castle 1987). Yet at least one future leader had begun to question this. The NSWNA secretary of the 1970s recalls her industrial initiation in 1940 at a small rally of student nurses in Sydney:

> ...there were about 15 or 20 others from various hospitals and a couple of the fellows from Parliament, they were Ministers actually...and they said to one of the girls who led the crew: 'Now now now, you wouldn't *really* go on strike?' I reckon her words should have been, 'Yes, if we are forced to, we will'. Instead of that she said 'Oh, well, no'...I really felt like giving her a jolly good hit on the head for that. [MH/89]

In a series of meetings between 1947 and 1949 the form of the nursing organisations for the next 20 years took shape. The federal ANF was anxious especially for unity, which it hoped would give nurses some control over their affairs and keep out other unions which were not primarily concerned with nursing—there were 'scares' from time to time about unions which admitted 'all classes of workers in hospitals', especially when they advocated compulsory unionism. The RVCN secretary recalled:

> In those days it was straight out warfare, and you had to send people around the hospitals telling nurses not to belong to that crowd because...we were the body that professed to look after all aspects of nursing and we were affiliated both nationally and internationally. So you had to keep carrying the flag very high. [MC/88]

Myrtle Lindsay and Jane Muntz of Victoria, who had revived the old TNG, pointed out to the ANF the advantages of amalgamating the two, since the TNG had registration with the Commonwealth Arbitration Court. Two conferences of all the nursing organisations took place in 1947 and 1948 but failed to achieve the desired unity: professionally, the ANF feared losing its ICN affiliation if it joined with an industrial body, the TNG; and industrially, the NSWNA and the nursing unions in Western Australia and Tasmania included nursing aides as members and could not agree to excluding them from a united organisation, as the RVCN wanted. The NSWNA even thought it might lose its state industrial registration if it could not cover the aides. The three unions therefore withdrew from negotiations. There were also concerns about loss of autonomy and about property ownership (Shield 1964).

The ANF and the TNG decided to form the Australian United Nurses' Association (AUNA) hoping that they could then merge into the AUNA provided the resulting organisation could maintain both the ICN affiliation of the ANF and the TNG's industrial registration. The TNG did this in 1949, but the ANF found it more difficult, partly because it included nurses who were both employers and non-employed. This made it ineligible for registration with the Arbitration Court which recognised only associations of employees. In May 1950 representatives of both organisations considered a plan for the two bodies to join in such a way that professional and union interests could remain separate, but Queensland, Western Australian and New South Wales failed to approve it, the last two because they wished to include all ancillary staff as full members (Shield 1964) in a show of worker solidarity. Behind the unfortunate disunity, at least some leaders were urging that nurses must take charge of their own affairs (Anon. 1965; Schultz 1974; Bessant & Bessant 1991:24-7).

A conference in October 1950 decided to move the ANF headquarters to Melbourne, thus consolidating Victorian dominance of the federation—perhaps a doubtful benefit, a New South Wales nurse thinks:

> My view about Victoria is that the Victorian Branch has always suffered from having a federal office right beside it—or almost—which we never had here. [JC/89]

The following year Mavis Avery as General Secretary became its first full time officer. The new President, Doris Bardsley, commented in 1952 on the advantages to the ANF of acquiring a permanent office and a full time secretary but recognised the obstacles which the Australian federal system placed in the way of nursing unity. In 1952-53 AUNA became ANFES (Australian Nursing Federation Employees' Section) and ANF branches in most states became in effect also branches of ANFES with the same staff. Victoria retained its own Employees' Section till 1960, when it was taken over by the ANFES, and it was in that state that the professional-union distinction was most fervently upheld (Schultz 1974; Bessant & Bessant 1991:116). A Victorian nurse, prominent in both ANFES and ANF, remembers the local attitude:

> Members of the ANFES tended to be more militant union types. *They* were fighting for wages, and the professionals, so-called professional people, in the RANF rather looked down on that crowd, because '*They* just wanted money'. They didn't at all, but that was the attitude...and there was this big barrier between the amalgamation of the two. [BS/90]

A reference to its British equivalent would have shown the RVCN that the indisputably professional RCN was well represented on the pay-negotiating body in the new National Health Service, the Nurses' and Midwives' Whitley Council, which gave British nurses substantially improved pay and conditions in the 1950s (Abel-Smith 1960:193, 206).

The ANF acquired the 'Royal' appellation in 1956, and planned a national journal, but its quest for unity was still unsatisfied. There was some progress in 1958 when the Arbitration Court accepted ANFES's revised constitution making it a section of RANF, with the ANFES federal council to consist of equal members of both bodies (Shield 1964). But in 1960 the RANF, the third significant postwar organisation, was still weakened by its dual structure. As a Victorian nurse observes:

> ...it was an amalgamation almost in name only, because it didn't really achieve anything. It was very difficult, because that was a federal registration, and wages were state matters...so it was a very messy arrangement, and it really was pretty powerless...but I think that, really, it was the beginning of RANF changing from a purely professional body to a more unionised type of organisation. [PO/90]

The NSWNA meanwhile remained separate, outside the national arena as far as nursing was concerned, though it affiliated in 1956 with the 'peak' white collar body, the Australian Council of Salaried and Professional Associations (ACSPA). A New South Wales nurse reflects on her training in the 1950s:

> It was learn on the job as you went...you had broken shifts and all that sort of thing. It was a manpower—cheap manpower—thing. Then of course there'd be a push for salaries etc., so the union would come in. The union movement in nursing was very quiet. [CH/89]

Relatively quiet: in 1957 the NSWNA lodged a claim for a new award for nurses, and in 1959 it campaigned for equal pay. The Commonwealth had set the female rate at 75% of the male basic wage in 1949-50, but the New South Wales Cahill (Labor) Government legislated for the gradual introduction of equal pay in 1958, the first state to do so. The association also approached the federal Menzies (Coalition) Government about its decision to introduce a 'special account' for long term patients as part of the voluntary health insurance scheme—apparently the only nursing organisation to lobby on a health policy matter. At the end of the year the association criticised state tribunals for reducing a proposed increase in margins for skill to the 28% level awarded by the federal Arbitration Commission (*The Lamp* 1959 October:14; 1960 January:1).

The quiet '50s: learning

In 1959 the RVCN Sister Tutors' Section summarised the faults of the student nurse's education as 'shortage of teaching hours, facilities, tutors, the type of experience and the teaching she is receiving' (*UNA* 1959 May:135). The system left the student nurse torn between her education needs and the more urgent demands of her job as an essential member of the hospital workforce. This status produced most of the deficiencies in her education, such as the lectures she attended in her own time, and the constant repetition of tasks 'well beyond the point at which skills have been acquired, because there is work to be done and somebody has got to do it' (Jayawardena 1961). The result of this education, the New South Wales Matrons' Institute concluded in 1967, was a nurse who was 'restricted in outlook, resistant to change, and unable to cope confidently with the scientific and technical advances in medicine and the social problems of nurses' (quoted Sax 1978:9). It was also a tough life for students, a Victorian nurse educator remembers:

> The conditions for student nurses were intolerable. They had to get up, having been on night duty, and write exams or come to lectures...they were frightful conditions. Nobody who had any humanity could be happy with them. [GBa/90]

Though some local nurses were aware of trends elsewhere, the British influence was still dominant, and British nursing had shown by its rejection of the progressive Wood Report of 1948 that nurse training had 'less to do with a complex content of work, and more to do with fulfilling the service needs of the hospital and creating a humble and disciplined character in the nurse'. The Wood Committee had found that first-year student nurses were still spending a third of their time in domestic work (Abel-Smith 1960:183; Davies 1977). An Australian nurse reflected:

> It was during my stay in London that I realised how similar were our patterns of nursing education...[Nursing] has trained in skills by precept and example; it has not, in general, sought to enliven the mind and stimulate intellectual curiosity (Pilkington 1966).

Australia's federal structure meant that although a nurse registered in one state could register in any other, the hours of theoretical content in her course, and the length of the course itself, could vary between states from three to four years, and from 300 to 1000 hours or more. There were separate registrations in all states for general nursing and midwifery, and in most for other specialties. Since nursing education remained within the purview of ministers for health and health was a constitutional responsibility of state governments, this variety is not surprising. A disadvantage everywhere was the number of small nursing schools, many of doubtful quality but defended by their hospitals which valued both the student labour and the status the school gave them (Gillam 1969).

A promising experiment which might have helped to solve some of these problems started in 1951 with the aim of raising the standard of nurse training and giving students more breadth of experience. By 1960 the Melbourne School of Nursing was already doomed, owing to the combined pressures of the participating hospitals' labour requirements (especially those of the Royal Melbourne) and the school's declining number of recruits. There was also medical and nursing resistance to raising educational and entry standards (Marshall 1985). Gwen Burbidge, who had taken a leading part in promoting the school, saw another obstacle:

> The Royal Melbourne was very traditionally minded, and it had a matron who believed in the divine right of matrons, and she didn't like the change...It certainly made the running of the School extraordinarily difficult, when you know that the underlying cause was typified by...one of the doctors saying to the Chairman of the School, Sir Alan Ramsay, 'The nurses these days don't even know if we take sugar in our coffee'! [GB/90]

Traditionalists objected to the student nurse losing her customary identification with one particular hospital, often a source of pride. The Dean, Jean Headberry, believed however that the school had had a stimulating effect on nursing education in Victoria (Marshall 1985:24). A future RANF federal secretary was one of its early students and describes its effect in raising her own political awareness:

> From the time we walked in the door at the Melbourne School of Nursing we were quite clearly in the middle of a political upheaval, a lot of which was about power between institutions, a lot was about issues of staffing hospitals, and a lot of it was about people's perceptions of nursing education. So that probably set me off down the track of taking some interest in the politics of nursing. [MP/91]

The programs inaugurated by the two colleges of nursing were for postregistration qualifications only, similar to those conducted at the RCN in London. Like preregistration and psychiatric nursing, post-basic clinical specialties such as midwifery remained in the hospitals. The college programs were based on the assumption that the registered nurse needed no further education in nursing practice, while some of her seniors should study teaching and administration (Slater 1982). But the establishment of the colleges was significant far beyond these initial gains. First, they showed a generation of leaders the value of education, as in South Australia:

> People like Zelma Huppatz, who went from the Adelaide Hospital...and Irene Kennedy, who was her successor...I'm sure their leadership was influenced very much by the confidence that came from that post-basic experience at the college. [JD/88]

Second, they would become the means of getting a foothold for nursing in higher education after years of exclusion, which would provide in turn the foundation for the later preregistration tertiary nursing courses.

The quiet '50s: working

Australian nursing retained its British characteristics of obedience and conformity, and 'a stress on *doing*, on *doing things for people*, rather than working with people and assisting them to do things for themselves...' (Place 1985). Keeping up the numbers in the workforce was a perennial problem. Nursing authorities usually addressed it by trying to recruit trainees instead of trying to keep those already trained. The doctrine of scientific management provided the rationale for a task based, routine method of work and, as in Britain, the hierarchy subordinated the junior nurse to her seniors, giving her limited job satisfaction (Davies 1977; Bolton 1981; Parker 1988).

There was confusion over what constituted the 'nursing role', the actual job of the nurse, and this affected the public image and thus recruitment and conditions: why should educated women train as nurses to do menial tasks, and why should governments give nurses higher pay for doing such work? The aide could perform basic patient care tasks more cheaply than the trained nurse, yet leading nurses who wanted professional status considered direct patient care intrinsic to the nurse's job, and therefore clung to tasks which government and hospital authorities considered relatively unskilled (Bessant & Bessant 1991:97-9). British nursing was told that this was unrealistic: 'Either the profession had to delegate part of the care of the patient to less skilled persons...or else it had to alter the requirements for state registration' (Abel-Smith 1960:239). Jane Muntz, President of the RVCN, argued that since the nurse had to expand her technical skills to keep pace with medical advances, it was 'not reasonable' to expect her also to undertake all the simple procedures (1954). Here were the effects of the accelerating technological revolution in medicine which led to the increasing delegation of ever more complex medical tasks to nurses. Nurses in turn accepted these technical tasks with apparent willingness, yet some of their leaders continued to hold sacred the 'caring' bedside role which for them embodied professionalism. Behind this, at least in the US, lay a nursing paradox: the leadership's demand for greater power and autonomy, as befitted a profession, was based on the belief in the nurse's 'duty to care'. It was thus self-contradictory, since the duty to care in a women's occupation was translated more readily into obedience to doctors than into the nurse's right to determine that duty (Reverby 1987:201-3).

Medical advances were also changing the mental health field. Attendants were legally styled 'nurses' after 1950. The impact of the major tranquillisers enabled the relationship with the patient to change from a custodial and task-oriented to a more therapeutic and less restrictive one. These nurses remained however in their education and in their work isolated from general nursing. A general nurse who did psychiatric training remembers:

> Psych in those days was regarded as at the same level probably as the prison officers...fairly low status. There were a lot of migrants doing it...you've got to hand it to them, they had to learn English and *then* train, which they did...The

> standard of the lectures was bloody dreadful...at that stage the standard of acceptance of trainees wasn't high either. [AC/90]

The isolation of psychiatric nurses remained: first, because the community still attached a stigma to their patients; second, they retained the status of public servants (Keane 1987:4-5), a legacy of the direct control of mental hospitals by government; and third, they usually belonged to unions not exclusive to nurses, such as the HEF. Exceptions were Queensland where the RANF had covered them since 1916, and New South Wales where they belonged to the NSWNA.

In 1960 these problems, such as the ambiguities and tensions of the 'nursing role', the strains and inadequacies of the education system, and the student and trained nurse 'wastage' which followed, were disturbing senior nurses. They had seldom taken political initiatives in the past even in matters which concerned them (Muntz 1954), and they faced many obstacles including the conventionally 'feminine' image of nurses, their own confusion about what the nurse's job should consist of, and their limited view of professionalism. These leaders had shown in setting up the colleges that education was central to their idea of professional status:

> ...those battles were absolutely necessary, not only because nurses felt, or began to feel that they needed a better education, but [also] they would never get any improvement in status until they could prove that they had a reasonable educational foundation. [JD/88]

In this arena at least, events were starting to move slowly in their direction.

REFERENCES

Abel-Smith B 1960 A history of the nursing profession. Heinemann, London

Anon. 1965 Australian Nursing Federation (Employees' Section). What is the ANFES? Australian Nurses' Journal, November:277-278

Anon. 1968 The professional organisation and its influence on nursing. Queensland Nurses' Journal, October:5-19

Armstrong M G 1951 A brief history of the first 50 years of the Royal Victorian College of Nursing 1901-1951. UNA Nursing Journal (jubilee issue):186-215

Ashley J A 1975 Nursing and early feminism. American Journal of Nursing 75 (9):1465-1467

ATNA 1950 Nursing in early Australia II. The Australasian Nurses' Journal, July:120-121

Baly M E 1985 The Nightingale nurses: the myth and the reality. In: Maggs C (ed) Nursing history: the state of the art. Croom Helm, London

Beaton L 1982 The importance of women's paid labour: women at work in World War II. In: Bevege M, James M, Shute C (eds) Worth her salt: women at work in Australia. Hale and Iremonger, Sydney

Bessant J, Bessant B 1991 The growth of a profession: nursing in Victoria 1930s–1980s. La Trobe University Press, Melbourne

Bolton G 1981 A training in discipline and conformity? Australian Nurses' Journal, October:34-36

Bolton G C 1974 1939-1951. In: Crowley F K (ed) A new history of Australia. Heinemann, Melbourne

Brodsky I 1968 Sydney's nurse crusaders. Old Sydney Free Press, Sydney (sponsored by the New South Wales Nurses' Association)

Brothers C R D nd Early Victorian psychiatry 1835-1905. Government Printer, Melbourne
Buxton G L 1974 1870-90. In: Crowley F K (ed) A new history of Australia. Heinemann, Melbourne
Carpenter M 1977 The new managerialism and professionalism in nursing. In: Stacey M, Reid M, Heath C, Dingwall R (eds) Health and the division of labour. Croom Helm, London
Castle J 1987 The development of professional nursing in New South Wales, Australia. In: Maggs C (ed) Nursing history: the state of the art. Croom Helm, London
Coburn D 1988 The development of Canadian nursing: professionalisation and proletarianisation. International Journal of Health Services 18 (3):437-456
Davies C 1977 Continuities in the development of hospital nursing in Britain. Journal of Advanced Nursing 2:479-491
Davies C 1980 Where next for nursing history? Nursing Times 22 May:920-922
Davies C 1983 Professionalising strategies as time- and culture-bound: American and British nursing circa 1893. In: Lagemann E C (ed) Nursing history: new perspectives, new possiblities. Teachers' College Press, New York
Deery S, Plowman D 1991 Australian industrial relations, 3rd edn. McGraw-Hill, Sydney
Dickenson M 1971 The nursing organisation at work: international—national—state. RANF Review, October:3-7
Dickenson M, Law G 1974 Nurses in the national health scheme. The Australian Quarterly 46 (1) March:29-41 (reprinted in The Lamp, March 1976:30-36)
Dickenson M 1975 The anatomy of an attitude. Australian Nurses' Journal, July:23-27
Durdin J 1991 They became nurses: the history of nursing in South Australia 1836-1980. Allen & Unwin, Sydney
Encel S, MacKenzie N, Tebbutt M 1974 Women and society: an Australian study. Cheshire, Melbourne
Gamarnikow E 1978 The sexual division of labour: the case of nursing. In: Kuhn A, Wolpe A-M (eds) Feminism and materialism. Women and modes of production, Routledge & Kegan Paul, London
Goodman R D 1988 Our war nurses. Boolarong, Brisbane
Hagan J 1981 The history of the ACTU. Longman Cheshire, Melbourne
Hamilton D G 1979 Hand in hand. The story of the Royal Alexandra Hospital for Children. Ferguson, Sydney
Hobbs V 1980 But westward look: nursing in Western Australia 1829-1979. University of Western Australia Press for the Royal Australian Nursing Federation (WA Branch), Perth
Hughes J E 1967 A history of the Royal Adelaide Hospital. RAH, Adelaide
Inglis K S 1958 Hospital and community. A history of the Royal Melbourne Hospital. Melbourne University Press, Melbourne
Jayawardena Y 1961 Whither nursing? The Australian Nurses' Journal, November: 264-269; December: 290-296
Jennings S 1976 An old objective in the jet age. Australian Nurses' Journal, June:35-36
Jones H 1986 South Australian women and politics. In: Jaensch D (ed) The Flinders history of South Australia: political history. Wakefield Press, Adelaide, Ch. 13
Kalisch P A, Kalisch B J 1978 The advance of American nursing. Little, Brown, Boston
Keane B 1987 Study of mental health nursing in Australia. Report to the Nursing and Health Services Workforce Branch, Commonwealth Department of Health, Canberra
Kelly G B 1977 A background to the history of nursing in Tasmania. Davies, Hobart
Keneley M 1988 Handmaidens of medicine: working conditions for nurses in late nineteenth century Victoria. Journal of Australian Studies, 22, May:57-68
Kessler-Harris A 1976 Women, work, and the social order. In: Carroll B A (ed) Liberating women's history: theoretical and critical essays. University of Illinois Press, Urbana:330-343
Kiddle M 1951 History of nursing in Australia (with special reference to Victoria). Lecture given at the College of Nursing, Australia, Melbourne (typescript)
Kingston B 1977 My wife, my daughter, and poor Mary Ann. Nelson, Melbourne
Law G 1980 'I have never liked trade unionism': the development of the Royal Australian Nursing Federation, Queensland Branch, 1904-45. In: Windschuttle E (ed) Women, class and history: feminist perspectives on Australia 1788-1978. Fontana, Melbourne
Marshall N 1985 The Melbourne School of Nursing 1950-1963. Melbourne School of Nursing Past Trainees' Association, Melbourne

Melosh B 1982 'The physician's hand': work, culture and conflict in American nursing. Temple University Press, Philadelphia
Merton R K 1962 Status orientations in nursing. American Journal of Nursing, October:70-73
Minchin M K 1977 Revolutions and rosewater: the evolution of nurse registration in Victoria 1923-1973. Victorian Nursing Council, Melbourne
Mitchell A M 1977 The hospital south of the Yarra. Alfred Hospital, Melbourne
Muntz J 1954 Nursing—professional responsibility. UNA Nursing Journal, November:336-343
Murgatroyd L 1982 Gender and occupational stratification. The Sociological Review 30(4):574-602
Parker J 1988 Theoretical perspectives in nursing: from microphysics to hermeneutics. In: Pittman E (ed) Shaping nursing theory and practice: the Australian context. La Trobe University Department of Nursing, Melbourne
Parkin F 1979 Marxism and class theory: a bourgeois critique. Tavistock, London
Pilkington M P 1968 Student status for nurses. UNA Nursing Journal, February: 44-47
Place B 1985 Nursing education—Australian made. Seventeenth Florence Nightingale Oration, National Florence Nightingale Committee, Melbourne
Reverby S H 1987 Ordered to care: the dilemma of American nursing 1850-1945. Cambridge University Press, Cambridge
Robertson J R 1974 1930-39. In: Crowley F K (ed) A new history of Australia. Heinemann, Melbourne
Rowley CD 1972 The destruction of Aboriginal society. Penguin, Melbourne
Sax S 1978 Report of the committee of inquiry into nurse education and training to the Tertiary Education Commission. TEC, Canberra
Schultz B 1974 Along the way. Australian Nurses' Journal, October:10-35
Schultz B 1989 Founders of the College. 17th Patricia Chomley Oration (1983), 2nd edn, College of Nursing, Australia, Melbourne
Schultz B 1991 A tapestry of service. The evolution of nursing in Australia. Vol. I foundation to federation 1788-1900. Churchill Livingstone, Melbourne
Shield B 1964 Outline of 'historical background'—presented as introduction to discussion on integration, to RANF SA Branch subcommittee formed to discuss the subject. December (typescript)
Showalter E 1981 Florence Nightingale's feminist complaint: women, religion and 'Suggestions for thought'. Signs: Journal of Women in Culture and Society, 6 Spring:394-412
Shyrock RH 1968 Nursing emerges as a profession: the American experience. In: Leavitt J W, Numbers R L (eds) 1978 Sickness and health in America: readings in the history of medicine and public health. University of Wisconsin Press, Madison
Slater P V 1963 The origins of nursing in Australia and the effect of changing economic, political and social conditions on nursing (mimeo). College of Nursing, Australia, Melbourne
Smith FB 1982 Florence Nightingale: reputation and power. Croom Helm, London
Sullivan M 1990 The emergence of the second level nurse in New South Wales: a profile of the TAFE-educated enrolled nurse, employment outcomes, course relevance and education needs. Unpublished BEd thesis, Sydney CAE
Templeton J 1969 Prince Henry's: the evolution of a Melbourne hospital. Robertson & Mullen, Melbourne
Thornton A 1972 The past in midwifery services. Australian Nurses' Journal March:19-23, 26
Trembath R, Hellier D 1987 All care and responsibility. A history of nursing in Victoria 1850-1934. Florence Nightingale Committee, Australia, Victorian Branch, Melbourne
Whittaker E, Olesen V L 1978 The faces of Florence Nightingale: functions of the heroine legend in an occupational sub-culture. In: Dingwall R, McIntosh J (eds) Readings in the sociology of nursing. Churchill Livingstone, Edinburgh
Williams J A, Goodman R D 1988 Jane Bell OBE. Royal Melbourne Hospital Graduates Association, Melbourne
Williams K 1978 Ideologies of nursing: their meanings and implications. In: Dingwall R, McIntosh J (eds) Readings in the sociology of nursing. Churchill Livingstone, Edinburgh

Williamson N 1982 'She walked...with great purpose': Mary Kirkpatrick and the history of midwifery in New South Wales. In: Bevege M, James M, Shute C (eds) Worth her salt: women at work in Australia. Hale and Iremonger, Sydney

Willis E 1983 Medical dominance. The division of labour in Australian health care. George Allen & Unwin, Sydney

Zepps K 1975 The role of the NSW college of nursing regarding the educational and professional development of nursing in NSW. The Lamp, December:3-7, 34

2. Nursing: a professional obsession

'...though a man may work for wealth or fame, a woman must labour for love—if not that of a husband and children, at least that of a profession'. (Alison Lurie, *Foreign Affairs*, 1986)

Nursing in Australia, as elsewhere, has styled itself unambiguously as a profession in spite of having enjoyed neither the social status and political influence nor the pay and conditions of occupations such as law, medicine or dentistry. This apparent contradiction can be illuminated by two interconnected themes: the debate outside nursing, mostly in academic circles, on the professions; and the developing ideas within nursing (especially in the United States) about the occupation and its standing. That is, nursing assessed from outside and nursing seen by its own members in an insider view, at times enlightened by outsiders' findings, at other times ignoring them. In nursing, professionalism has been something assumed but often misunderstood. It has held out a false promise and it has been a distraction from more productive activity; but as a British nurse says, 'Understanding the urge to win recognition of nursing as a profession is crucial to any understanding of nursing today...' (Salvage 1985:86).

From Flexner...

The emergence of the professions as a major characteristic of modern industrial societies has been a subject of considerable interest for the last 60 years, an interest which has produced an extensive literature. The accepted view of professions in the 1950s emerged from functionalist sociology: professions were a special category of occupation in which experts carried out work of a socially important kind for individual clients. Professions were therefore a valuable and necessary asset in any society. The authority of professionals was legitimately based on their possession of a unique body of knowledge, and clients could trust them because professions had an ideal of service, an ethical code, state licensure, and recognised associations. This rather flattering account often included a reference to the celebrated 'Flexner criteria', applied in 1915 to American social work (and nursing), and it led directly to the trait or attribute model of professions in which supposedly essential attributes were identified and then used to test an occupation to see if it was in Flexner's words an 'unmistakable' profession.

Everett Hughes and his colleagues studied a large number of US nurses in the 1950s and concluded that nursing was a 'semi-profession' at best, which 'largely because of the limitations of authority and independent action, cannot meet the criteria of a full profession' (Hughes et al 1958:249). Hughes himself said later (1963) that a better way to understand professions might be to observe how occupations tried to change themselves in the course of a movement to become 'professionalised'.

The attribute model implied that professionalism, taken to be the inherent nature of a profession, was a matter of degree: there were 'full' or complete professions, like medicine and law, and there were other occupations which, while not mere trades, exhibited fewer of the desirable attributes, or possessed them to a lesser degree. These were the semi-professions, whose members were really 'subordinate grades placed in the middle of the hierarchy', in contrast to the professional at the top who 'admits no superiors' (Marshall, quoted Hughes et al 1958:249). Much of the academic debate in the 1960s revolved around the observation that the semi-professions, such as nursing was held to be, were engaged in a continuous quest for professional status (the process of professionalisation) based on the attributes exhibited by the 'true' professions, attributes taken to be the source of their prestige and authority.

This attribute model inevitably influenced nursing since it was regularly applied to it and as regularly found it wanting. A study of US registered nurses, for example, found that nursing failed to meet several 'crucial criteria' of professionalism, such as the authority to make independent judgements and a high level of membership of the professional association. Still, the authors concluded that nursing was capable of making 'further strides' in the future towards professionalism (Kurtz & Flaming 1963). In Australia the chairman of the College of Nursing, Australia Council (a male non-nurse educationist) recommended the attribute model to Victorian members of the Florence Nightingale Committee:

> It is only by placing ourselves against accepted criteria or measuring devices that we are able to obtain an objective assessment of our present position and ascertain possible progress in this matter of obtaining professional status (Shears 1964).

Out of his seven traits (service, knowledge, careful initial selection, comprehensive preparation, standards, self-evaluation, and commensurate rewards), Dr Shears was able to acknowledge nursing's 'full status' only in the first (service). He tactfully stopped short of outright criticism of the profession's shortcomings in the other six, pointing out instead that the College of Nursing had a significant part to play in furthering their attainment.

American nurses experienced more academic interest in their occupation than did their British and Australian colleagues, but some academic observers were critical of nursing's attempt to pursue professional status. One scholar noted that the professionalising drive in the US was led by the academic nurse educators. This produced one of the weaknesses of US nursing: the quest for professional status was led by those who had removed themselves from the hospital, where most nurses worked. Despite all the efforts of this academic leadership, working nurses remained relatively untouched by the idea of professionalism and apathetic about pursuing it: 'The leaders of nursing have wanted their followers to become successful professionals, but instead American nurses seem to have become successful and satisfied American *women*' (Glaser 1966:25-6).

This was an early signal from a (male) academic that it was difficult to become both. In sum, sociologists found nursing wanting as a profession because it had not gained the required number of marks: it had relatively open recruitment, lacked an extensive period of university education, had failed to develop a body of knowledge and research, and accepted delegated medical tasks (and thus a subordinate position) in the workplace. They recognised the problems facing the leadership of a largely female occupation, seeing this mostly as a serious obstacle to (presumably male) 'career-mindedness'. Compared with whatever constituted a 'true' profession, nursing seemed sadly deficient.

Concentrating on the nurse in her workplace, Fred Katz thought that she had to accept a lowly position because her function was to offer socially devalued 'non-scientific, nurturant care' to help overcome inadequacies in the application of scientific (highly valued) medical knowledge. Nurses accepted their position as 'distinct underlings' and their 'caste-like separation' from the more powerful medical staff because in return they exercised in practice quite a high degree of autonomy in many of their functions, including bedside care and the co-ordination of ward activities. Katz offered little guidance to nurses seeking professional status beyond suggesting that they should develop their body of knowledge relevant to caring for patients (1969:56, 70-1, 75). An English nurse pointed out that in Britain the powerful matrons held the nursing hierarchy together and thus 'helped establish a sphere of autonomy and not just submission' (Carpenter 1977). What autonomy nursing had thus depended on the hierarchy, not on the perceived professional standing of individual nurses.

...to Roy and Rogers...

In the US, where some nursing education was already in universities, nurse academics reacted by initiating research in order to develop the required body of knowledge. They welcomed the new journal *Nursing Research* in 1952 by referring to research as a Flexner criterion and looked forward to critical analyses of nursing's professional status. In the 1960s, some leading nurses also began to pursue theories and models of nursing to establish research directions, while research in turn they hoped would validate their theories.

Some of these were based on systems theory, such as the Roy adaptation model which viewed the person/patient as a set of related subsystems tending towards homeostasis. The Riehl interaction model differed in seeing the person as behaving according to a specific system of meaning. Martha Rogers developed her 'holistic unitary field' model which put Man [sic] at the centre of the nursing universe. 'Holistic' nursing viewed people as 'unitary fields of energy who interact as a whole with other energy fields within their environments'. Orem's self-care model combined the systems approach of Roy with the Rogers holistic view, and had some similarities to Henderson's model which emphasised patient participation, though Henderson was alone in acknowledging the close alignment of *medical* with nursing care (Aggleton & Chalmers 1984). An attraction of theory building was perhaps that it came under direct nursing control, unlike workplace practice.

This spirit of inquiry spread to England from the mid 1970s. Professor (later Baroness) Jean McFarlane, head of the first British university course in nursing, described the search for theory as 'an expression of professional need'—the development of a coherent discipline was closely associated with achieving professional status (1976a). Nursing theory did not develop quickly in Britain, possibly because the matrons still dominated the scene and education remained almost wholly in the hospitals, but there was an early start to nursing research with the establishment in 1971 of the Nursing Research Unit at the University of Edinburgh. The unit emphasised 'usefulness to the profession' (Hockey 1976), perhaps because of its reliance on government funding and the close integration (compared with the US) of British nursing education with practice.

The search for a theory of nursing and the encouragement of nursing research were not just part of a professionalising strategy. Nurses argued persuasively that a more theoretical education would enable practitioners to give care that was securely based in knowledge tested through research, rather than derived from the conventional wisdom of the past, which as McFarlane said, could mean 'ritual, superstition, speculation, unsystematised experience' (1977). Expertise which had hitherto been merely 'intuition' now could be articulated (McCloskey 1981). Apart from these benefits, many nurses must have felt a genuine interest in seeking knowledge, given the dearth of intellectual excitement in hospital courses.

Yet this quest for a body of knowledge identifiably nursing was inevitably informed also by the professionalising ideology of the leadership. An Australian nurse accepted the necessity for theory because nurses, she believed, needed to examine the theories which supported their practice; but she was critical of the 'obscure' and 'patronising' way in which some theorists expressed themselves which, she said, left the feeling that the nurse theorist was 'an apologist for a vocation which will never gain professional acceptance unless The Theory is "discovered"...' (James 1976). A Swedish nurse judged the jargon–prone prose of some theorists as 'an unusually complicated way of saying that nurses and patients meet because the latter are not feeling very well' (Lundh et al 1988). Research had become a sacred cow which threatened to displace practice as 'the essence of a profession', a

US nurse considered, and some of it lacked clinical relevance (Baer 1986)—not surprising since the ideology owed more to beliefs about professionalism than to the medically ordered reality of nursing work (Dingwall 1974). An Australian nurse academic appreciates what the theorists were trying to do, but is also critical:

> I think nursing has been trying for many years, probably since the Sixties, to say, 'If we are a profession, this means we have to have a discrete body of knowledge, and therefore we've got to rush around constructing nursing models which delineate the boundaries of what nursing is and identify us as having a unique body of knowledge.' I've never liked that idea. I've always seen it as essentially a political strategy in order to justify professional status. [JP/90]

If theory building and research were in part a means of demonstrating nursing's credentials as a profession, a closely related purpose was to establish its independence from medicine (Dachelet 1978). A British nurse hoped that theory would establish nursing's independent identity as more than a collection of medically ordered tasks, which would be 'a tremendous leap forward' in its development as a profession (Clark 1982). Nurses did not blame their position directly on the medical superpower, but sought rather to get nursing out from under it, to circumvent it—not to challenge it. Medicine was not so much the 'glass ceiling' barrier of today's feminists as a brick wall.

A concomitant of the research and theory focus was the leaders' belief in education, and the conviction, chiefly in the US, that nurse education should be in universities like that of the 'real' professions. US nursing was ahead in this enterprise, but one sociologist thought that its academic leaders had made a 'fateful partnership' with university schools of education, with the result that, like the education faculties which were perceived as presenting watered down versions of other disciplines, nursing departments had low academic status. This isolated them from the major intellectual currents fostered by the post Second World War acceleration of science and research in higher education. Nurses were therefore influenced by only two professions, education and medicine—nurse educators mostly by the former, practising nurses by the doctors they looked up to metaphorically, or saw in less romantic reality across the patient's bed (Strauss 1966:84).

Given the emphasis on education as the major way to achieve professional status, one US academic was critical of educational practice which, she found, discouraged the assertive, inquiring student. The 'ghost of the Crimea' stalked the nursing school corridors, perpetuating a culture of subservience (Cohen 1981:5-8, 69, 141). Australian nursing was also influenced by this preoccupation with education, though at least one nurse thought the local variety produced graduates who connived at their own oppression, seeing it in fact as virtuous behaviour (Bolton 1981). A Victorian nurse also had doubts:

> Education for what? That was the question I asked. If education is just being tied purely ideologically to the notion of professional status, to notions of equality with other health professionals, then it seemed to me that we were building a house of cards, because we weren't building it on any substantial intellectual work to underpin it. [SMcM/91]

Still, higher education remained a symbol of professional status, and it is not surprising that in the early 1970s Australian nursing leaders decided to concentrate on getting nurse education into the tertiary sector.

...to Freidson

In their writing on nursing, sociologists in the 1960s seem to have been influenced by the image of medicine as the very model of a modern profession, so that its internal contradictions often remained unexamined and the attempts of other occupations to achieve comparable status became the focus of attention.

Then in 1970 Eliot Freidson, also a sociologist, analysed the medical profession itself, and in doing so demonstrated that a profession was distinguished not by a collection of attributes, but by its special position in an occupational hierarchy. Knowledge was a necessary condition of professional status, but it was not a sufficient one. Rather than a set of desirable qualities, professionalism was 'a deliberate rhetoric in the political process' which a profession used to attain a desirable end: full control over its work. That was the 'irreducible criterion'. Nurses and others were not only subservient to medicine now, they had little chance of ever being anything else. Only medicine could be truly autonomous. Like other aspiring professions, nursing did have a prolonged training but this did not constitute a valid claim to professional status; rather, the occupation had deliberately created such training to further its claim to such status. Training was merely a face-saving ploy to mask an embarrassing subordination (Freidson 1970a:79-80). Nursing's female composition also told against its chance of success since the leaders were '...a small proportion of policy makers, supervisors and teaching nurses dedicated to professionalisation, striving to mobilise a heterogeneous and shifting corps of often casual and transient skilled workers' (Freidson 1970b:21).

An English sociologist, Terence Johnson, also condemned the attribute model. It was both culture bound—confined to Anglo-American societies—and lacking historical perspective in that it laid down a single path for aspiring occupations to follow in the process of professionalisation regardless of changing circumstances. It was also unscientific in that it was derived from the professions' own self-image: the attributes reveal only what the established professions want us to see. In contrast to the functionalist model, professions achieve and maintain their position in the same way that any élite does, through 'arrogation by groups with the power to secure their claims and create their own system of legitimation'. Johnson also distinguished between the actual work an occupation performs (its technical function) which changes over time, and the way in which it has used its power (based on social class position) to establish control of that work, which is a product of prevailing social conditions at a particular time and place (1972:24-7, 37; Willis 1983:13).

Polite professionalising

This 'power and control' analysis had a considerable impact on subsequent sociological thinking about the professions. It helped to reverse the tendency to take the major professions at their own word and assume that professionalism was a wholly benign social phenomenon. However, perhaps because of the development of received nursing theory in the 1960s in which nurse academics now had a vested interest, compounded by academic isolation, nursing seems not to have noticed immediately the implications of Freidson's analysis. In 1971 a US nurse could still write of 'the major crisis facing the profession today—that of defining the body of professional knowledge' (Kovacs 1971). The deceptive simplicity of the attribute model was probably attractive in specifying both the qualities necessary for professional status and an identifiable path towards them.

With their emphasis on knowledge/education as the desirable attribute, the assessment by leading nurses of the professionalising effort missed some of the pointers to a change of strategy that might have helped to make that effort more effective. Freidson's critique exploded nursing's professionalising ideology but it contained a valuable message: a degree of autonomy in nursing work was critical, but the way to achieve it was through political and social means, 'a process in which power and persuasive rhetoric are of greater importance than the objective character of knowledge, training and work' (Freidson 1970a:79-80; 1970b:134).

The stricken attribute model was further weakened by Roth (1974) who described the attributes as a decoy, as 'largely mixtures of unproved—indeed unexamined—claims for professional control and autonomy'. The past preoccupation with attributes, he thought, had deflected attention from some of the less benign effects of professionalisation, such as the use of political power to achieve monopolistic control. As an example, Roth cites a study of the successful use of political power by US medicine to gain state supported monopolistic control over another occupation, midwifery, which was unable to mobilise adequate countervailing power. Though cogently argued, perhaps this overtly political message was too alien to the education centred world of the nursing leadership.

The power of theory...

Nursing thus continued to emphasise academic progress as the key to professional recognition. Not only did this strategy rule out what might have been more successful alternatives, it was not even effective in its own terms. Theories tended to be 'grand' and so difficult to test empirically. Nurse academics had not followed sociologists in establishing 'theories of the middle range' which might have been more useful in practice (Bullough & Bullough 1984:78-80). The development of nursing theory was influenced most by logical empiricism for 10 years after that tradition had first come under serious challenge so that the various conceptual frameworks developed for nursing in the early 1970s were 'essentially devoid of any explicit linkage to the philosophy of science' and separated from the work of scientific theorists. By the early 1980s some nurse theorists were showing the newer historicist influences, but those such as Orem, King, and Rogers who updated their conceptual models, did so within the logical empiricist tradition (Silva & Rothbart 1984).

A major weakness of nursing theory was that for most nurse theorists, nursing was a mentally constructed world which could not provide a useful guide to deciding what nursing was or was not since it was not based on the observed reality of nursing practice (Stevens 1979:7). A British psychiatric nurse cautioned that 'the fashionable thing to do is to design or to adopt models able to account for whatever it is nurses are found to be doing', but such models were susceptible of being seen as real in themselves, rather than as representations of a more complex reality (Altschul 1979). Theories 'fail to say anything of interest about the social reality in which nursing takes place', a Swedish nurse thought, and their reliance on systems theory led to a view of nursing as a closed system (Lundh et al 1988). An Australian nurse also doubts their usefulness:

> I've never thought that it's got very far, and I think the implications for practice, when people have tried to implement a lot of these theories, or conceptual models, have been very difficult...a lot of that early stuff in nursing, like Martha Rogers, it's not concrete enough. [JP/90]

Asking the two questions which preoccupied much nursing discussion (Is nursing a profession? What is nursing?) shows the dominance of positivist science, with its belief that any entity, including an occupation, has an essential character and is made up of atom-like constituents, so that breaking it down into its constituent parts will bring understanding. Such an approach to elucidation does not work with ideas like 'profession' or 'nursing' which are subject to many shifting and subjective meanings and cannot be pinned down for dissection like a laboratory specimen. Those who tried to answer the question, 'What is nursing?' usually ended up with a vague all-embracing definition of little help to the practitioner.

Such definitions did not dispel doubts about the role of the nurse, what work she did or should do. The wide range of tasks that comprised nursing, the many kinds of jobs that nurses did, the various places where they did them, became a source of embarrassment to those who continued to ask 'What is nursing?' Australian nurses also tried to devise workable definitions, though with little success (Russell 1991). Some saw the absence of one as risky for the profession (e.g. Garratt 1987), yet a South Australian nurse perceives the irony that

> ...people say to you 'Well, what is nursing?' and, you know, you're almost mute. But on the other hand, if someone said 'What is medicine...?' Is it because that is a male dominated profession that no one questions it? [EP/88]

A paradox of this adherence to the older scientific tradition was that while nursing leaders and theorists were emphasising the wholeness of nursing practice, its caring and subjective aspects, nurse researchers insisted on objectivity and measurement because they followed what they perceived as accepted methods, usually those developed by other disciplines which were not necessarily suitable for their own (Watson 1981). This retarded nursing's progress as a professional discipline, Barbara Stevens thought, because the methods dictated the subject matter, rather than the reverse, so 'trivial answers will be found because trivial questions are asked'. The fixation on 'acceptable' research methods was 'an outgrowth of nursing's attempt to convert itself, overnight, into a full-blown profession' (Stevens 1979:93, 187-8). The popular nursing process Stevens branded as a 'mimicry of medicine' and ascribed to nursing's unresolved relations with its great and powerful colleague.

An Australian nurse criticises the nursing process as part of this attempt to 'scientise' nursing which started in the 1960s, and agrees that nurses were handicapped in that their education kept them separated from major currents of thought. They therefore adopted the scientistic modes of thinking of other disciplines, forcing nursing into a Procrustean bed of reductive reasoning with the result that whole fields of nursing experience and feeling were omitted (Lawler 1991a:34-8). Some Australian nurses took up the nursing process with enthusiasm, though Lawler considers it an example of imported (mostly US) notions associated with 'alleged universal and proto-scientific aspects of nursing' which were imposed on local clinicians (Lawler 1991b). As she says:

> We need to be selective about who has the expertise and who does not...The North American doctrine is brought in—cultural imperialism—which is damaging because North American nursing is extremely ethnocentric, middle class and incestuous. [JL/88]

A US nurse did however condemn the ideology of professionalism for producing terms such as 'nursing diagnosis' which tortured language to avoid medical terminology (Gamer 1979). An Australian nurse is also critical of this import:

> The doctors were saying that [the patient] hadn't had adequate fluid intake, but [nursing diagnosis] took a paragraph to say they were dehydrated. I think this is questionable. Do we have to be 'pure'? Why can't we perhaps look at some of the medical things, which is what we've been taught, and what [nurses] are still saying—not throw them all out? I think that's where we've gone to the extreme...[BA/90]

And a nurse academic makes a further point:

> I hate 'medical diagnosis', 'nursing diagnosis'. I think it's all a lot of nonsense. I'd much rather see it be more person centred too. We have medical notes, and nursing notes—shouldn't they be the *patient's* notes? It's terrible. It's all this 'we own the patients'...[JP/90]

...or the power of nurses

If most leading nurses in the 1960s and 1970s took the power of the medical profession for granted without analysing its sources or modes of exercise, and assumed that nursing's goal should remain the acquisition of a body of knowledge to confirm its professional status, a few nurses in the US began to examine nurses' power. Medicine had maintained its élite position as the hospital workforce expanded partly because it could restrict its numbers by delegating routine tasks to the more numerous nurses (Strauss 1966). Nursing therefore always had the burden of maintaining a large workforce, making such élite status impossible. But this did give it the potential power of numbers. Jo Ann Ashley (1973, 1975) was adamant that nurses used their power not to promote nursing, but to 'maintain the very system that has oppressed them', often to the detriment of the patient. Medicine, she said, 'would not now be so powerful if the medical profession had not managed to control, limit, and use the power of others—notably nursing—to strengthen its own', and to obscure the vital contribution of nursing in the process. Ashley did not blame doctors for nursing's predicament but accused nurses of having made themselves into a proletariat dominated by the medical ruling class. An Australian nurse also exonerates medicine (and nursing's First Lady):

> A lot of people blame the medical profession—and I don't. I say *we* pushed ourselves back, and *we* did stupid things like holding doors open for doctors, jumping to our feet when they walked into the ward. What a lot of garbage! They all blame Flo. I don't see any reason to blame her. [PP/89]

Two US nurses ascribed nursing's powerlessness and docility to its female composition which militated against aggressive behaviour, and like Ashley blamed the nursing hierarchy for enabling nurses to escape direct responsibility to the public for their competence. Nurses, they thought, must respond to two contemporary movements: consumerism (patients' rights) and feminism (women's rights) and they extended Ashley's position by advocating the mobilisation of nursing's power, especially its numbers, through organisation (Bowman & Culpepper 1974).

An Australian nurse took a similar stand, criticising midwifery for its ideological claim to a 'unique vocational essence' while at the same time its practice was dominated by medical technology. Midwives in the labour ward acted as 'face-savers' for late or absent obstetricians, denying their own power and expertise. They had failed to challenge the interventionist consequences of medical control over normal childbirth—the 'alternative' birth movement had come from patients themselves, not from midwives (Shoebridge 1979).

Statements such as those by Ashley and Shoebridge imply an expansion of the boundary of the nurse-patient relationship well beyond the enclosed unit of study chosen by the nurse-theorists, to include its social and political dimensions. They recognise the necessity for expertise in practice, but see such characteristics as group consciousness, group action, competition for resources in the workplace and skilful use of numbers, as critical for maximising power. Such ideas were not immediately or widely accepted. A veteran of American nursing, Ada Jacox, regretted that her colleagues 'were collectively unable or unwilling to place a moratorium on our internal fighting so that we might redirect our energies to deal positively and constructively with the promotion of health and prevention of disease...' (1978). This lack of colleague solidarity, or 'horizontal violence', has also worried Australian nurses, who have linked it to 'oppressed group' behaviour (Speedy 1988, 1991). A South Australian nurse observes the irony that:

> We are very harsh to one another, we don't rush to give support...Ironic, belonging to a caring profession, our whole philosophy is to provide care, and then we don't demonstrate caring to one another. [CE/88]

Ruling class...

Those nurses who took up Freidson's critique of medicine used it to attack the power disparity between doctors and nurses and the effects of medical dominance on health care provision, rather than to reconstruct nursing's similar version of professionalism (e.g. Leininger 1973, Donaghue 1977, Labelle 1978), though one US nurse did say that gaining influence to expand the 'caring' in the health system was more important than deciding whether or not nursing was a profession (McCloskey 1981).

Nursing's professionalising strategy has not been one of creating a 'dependency advantage' (non-substitutability) in the workplace. Rather, the work incorporates both delegated medical and basic nursing tasks, and the nursing hierarchy routinises it. Despite the rhetoric of the leadership, this contrasts with the more usual strategy followed by those seeking professional status who stress the complexity and uncertainty of what they do and the consequent need for independent judgement (Davies 1976). Professional work has a dual composition: on the one hand much of the work is susceptible to technical rules which can be learned and routinely applied, while on the other there appears to be a quality of indetermination—some part of work content which appears not so readily defined and learned and which is therefore often attributed to particular qualities of the individual practitioner. Professionals gain by emphasising this indetermination, the things only they can know, but they have to stress also that their knowledge is scientific, therefore readily codifiable. They are thus forever, and often at the same time, trying to make their work more of a technical process, and parading its indetermination in the attempt to keep exclusive control over it (Jamous & Peloille 1970:112-17). It is not surprising that the tasks which doctors delegated to nurses were those belonging to the technical rules or more routine aspect of their work. The apprenticeship style nursing education also perpetuated the hierarchy through its emphasis on tasks, from simple for beginners to more complicated tasks as they progressed. This had unfortunate results for both student and patient, a New South Wales nurse found:

> ...if you start off and you're going to take so many TPRs and make so many beds, if any patient asks you anything—well, 'Sister'll be along soon.' You've got no commitment to anyone' [MR/89]

A Victorian nurse observed another effect of this hierarchy of tasks:

> I remember student nurses who wouldn't touch a bedpan—because they were no longer the most junior one. There was another [nursing school intake] coming behind them. I can remember them saying 'I've done my service. I'm not doing bedpans any more'. [GBa/90]

The hierarchy also made work an unrewarding experience for the skilled RN, a New South Wales nurse decided in the 1960s:

> I moved out from hospitals because I was disenchanted with the institution, the hierarchical systems, entrenched attitudes, and an overwhelming feeling of exploitation. Where I was working, in theatres, it was very unreasonable, with broken shifts and so on. I could see that I was contributing to the work of a number of surgeons and anaesthetists, but...[RMcK/90]

Shirley Donaghue, quoting a New Zealand nurse, observed that much of the task orientation in nursing which fragmented patient care was actually a product of the nursing hierarchy. It could not be blamed on doctors (Donaghue 1977:40). For the individual nurse a sphere of autonomy for the nursing division as a whole meant in practice managerial submission to the matron and clinical submission to the doctor. Her professional autonomy was frustrated specifically at the bedside, the locus of care. She could not be fully responsible for the care of a particular patient because, as well as being subject to medical orders, patient care was assigned to a group of nurses with little authority for those giving direct care to take independent action (Labelle 1978). A stalwart of American nursing, Virginia Henderson, talked of the paradox that her own open-ended concept of nursing, which had helped to form 'holistic' theory (though she avoided the word herself), was now linked to individual patient care plans, yet patients were unable to point to 'my nurse' in the same way they could say 'my doctor' (Henderson 1978, 1982). Professionalism was thus seen as a quality of the individual nurse. From this interpretation of professionalism (with medicine still the paradigm profession) the collective nature of nursing service was a handicap. From a different perspective, senior nurses could have seen it as a potential power-base and the nursing numbers as an asset to be mobilised—perhaps by establishing more equal relations with their clinical staff and seeing them as possible supporters (Barratt 1989).

Instead, British nursing embraced managerialism in the late 1960s as a result of the Salmon Committee's recommendations for the health service. This was an alternative to professionalism rather than a means of achieving it, Carpenter thought (1977), since the new structure benefited only the senior levels whose power depended on their domination of the rest. Similarly, American nursing since 1965 has tried to impose a clear division between professional (based on a bachelor's degree qualification) and technical nursing (associate degree or diploma), though the technical nurses saw themselves as no less professional than their colleagues and resisted this division (Dachelet 1978). In Australia one academic considered that the nursing élite had pushed for managerial functions which had produced an 'internal split' within nursing, since the nurse giving direct care felt no common interest with the nurse manager (Hicks 1985). Another saw the 'vocabulary of complaint' of ward-level nurses as their covert resistance to the dominant medical/hospital hierarchy, and thought that it engendered a degree of solidarity (Turner 1987:153-4).

Senior nurses thus maintained the hierarchy (or at least failed to attack it) despite its contravention of what they themselves defined as professionalism: 'a true professional who is an independent practitioner accountable to patients and peers for her practice has no need of any army-style structure to keep her in line' (Salvage 1985:85). Following their own model of professionalism to its logical conclusion would have entailed collaborative relations between nurses, which the hierarchy denied—and still does, a West Australian nurse thinks:

> The problem is that we've still got a very centralised management structure which isn't prepared to devolve down to [ward] level...[We've still got] the reluctance of nursing generally to devolve decision making back down to where it really should be. [HA/90]

And a Victorian nurse links this with professional status:

> If you make the assumption that you have a professional staff, then you don't need line management above them really—you have peer review etc.—which means that you don't really need that [hierarchy of] graduate nurse, associate charge nurse, charge nurse, assistant director of nursing...then a deputy director of nursing...[AH/92]

The hierarchy implied also that nursing was like other oppressed groups, for example African-Americans, in that leaders exercised power only over their own kind (Cleland 1971). An Australian nurse saw one result of this when she joined a women's network:

> I was part of that, but...although...I had a senior position, I always felt I hadn't had to fight for it, because I worked with women. I felt that I wasn't *really* part of it, that it was a natural progression for a woman, a nurse. I hadn't had to fight the men...[RB/91]

...and the nursing proletariat

The theoretical approach to professionalism in the later 1970s moved towards a more structural analysis, often informed by the work of Max Weber and by Marxism (Larson 1977:209-240). Today's dominant professions arose during the period of competitive capitalism, of free markets, but more recent professions developed during and after the rise of 'organisation' society which brought the large bureaucratic organisations of both private and public sectors and the expansion of state activity into social welfare. This gave the newer professions quite different conditions for their development, and at the same time enabled the older 'market' professions to consolidate their privileges by organising and by gaining state support. Medicine was then able to dominate other occupations in its division of labour, using in the case of nursing and midwifery the strategy of subordination. It kept some features of its free-market past, such as its attachment to an individual entrepreneurial style of practice with, as in Australia, a 'fee for service' pay structure. Nursing, as one of the more recent arrivals, developed predominantly in organisations, but influenced by the self-serving ideology of the older professions, it continued to use them as a model although it had much less potential for their independent practice.

An ideology is a system of beliefs, a structure of consciousness or mental framework through which the social world becomes understandable. Social groups can use an ideology either to criticise or justify the present state of affairs or suggest a more hopeful alternative. An ideology therefore has descriptive qualities, it explains social phenomena; and it has a normative function, a group can use it to criticise other beliefs or justify its own from the standpoint of its particular interests.

The ideology of professionalism, for Marxists, derives from the dominant bourgeois ideology, that of laissez faire capitalism with its individualistic creed. The professional ideology of medicine shares in the dominant ideology of the bourgeois ruling class, the ideology of expertise, which legitimates the monopoly of certain spheres of competence and thus allows élitism in the use of expertise. Nurses as cheap wage labour are members of the proletariat, so are the victims of 'false class consciousness' in accepting the ruling ideology (Larson 1977: 241-43). This ideology perpetuates the self-serving myth that there is a rational link between education and the labour market: more education, more effort, will bring the rewards of a higher position in the occupational hierarchy. The conclusion to be drawn from this analysis is again, that superior knowledge may be a necessary condition for professional status, but it is not enough. A profession also needs a powerful position in the class hierarchy of the bourgeois state. Professionalism is not a set of desirable qualities but, in the case of medicine, it is 'an occupational ideology which legitimates autonomy for the doctors themselves' (Willis 1983:16).

Like Freidson's analysis, the Marxist critique had a clear if harsh message for nursing: professional status and its attendant rewards are not gained through educational credentials or dedicated service; they are ultimately the spoils of battle for that occupation which is willing to exert political power in its own interest, however elaborately that interest is decked out in the dignified dress of professional prestige. Yet nurses have been reluctant to act politically, equating it with partisanship and failing to connect it with achieving professional status (Najman 1974); or from idealism, a New South Wales nurse thinks:

> ...very often you have to rely on the political process to achieve what you are looking for. But it is very difficult, and many, many nurses are simply not realistic enough. They go into nursing because they are idealists...[YJ/90]

The professional ideology of nursing also created a proletariat within nursing itself—the nursing aides and assistants, who by the 1980s had become state enrolled nurses (SENs). Like the doctors from whom they sought to distinguish themselves, nurses used exclusionary tactics such as an emphasis on credentials against the SENs to protect their own privileges, meagre as they were. A British nurse observed that while registered nurses tended to denigrate the performance of aides and others whose work overlapped with their own, in fact they depended on such workers to maintain services (Altschul 1979). An Australian nurse (originally from New Zealand) agrees:

> A lot of general nurses don't *want* to do basic nursing care. I don't care what people say, they just *don't* want to do it. So I believe there's always going to be a place for state enrolled nurses...they're very valuable, because their basic skills are tremendous. [IK/91]

The fallacy of caring

If nursing is divided into higher and lower ranks, the work of the clinical nurse also has disparate components. Sociologists in the 1950s and 1960s (e.g. Johnson & Martin 1958, Corwin 1961) divided the nurse's job into two parts: the technical or instrumental tasks, and a caring or expressive role, often aligned with bureaucratic versus professional nursing. Another categorisation comprised basic nursing or looking after the patient's daily needs, and technical nursing, made up of those tasks deriving from his/her illness. An English sociologist preferred to group the technical and basic skills together as both were part of direct patient care, and delineated a further group of tasks which the nurse used in 'coping with the environment', tasks which she considered required skill of a higher order than specific production tasks (Melia 1979). It was these environmental tasks, such as organising the nursing team and co-ordinating patient care (bureaucratic/managerial skills), that were often overlooked by the nurse theorists, though Melia did not go as far as Ashley or Bowman and Culpepper (above) in seeing their political implications. In Australia the authors of a nursing study said that if nurses wanted to attain professional status they would have to display technical as well as nurturant skills. The acquisition of technical functions increased the area of overlapping responsibilities between nurses and doctors so that some nursing tasks would have to be delegated to aides, but the caring function esteemed within nursing was not judged to lend it a professional aura outside (Katz et al 1976:10-11).

Nursing theory's preoccupation with the nurse-patient relationship to the exclusion of the political dimensions of the workplace, together with the 'separate from medicine' doctrine of the professional ideology, probably made it inevitable that the nursing leadership should elevate caring into a foundation for professional status and a central part of the professional ideology. In Britain, the Briggs Committee on Nursing in its 1972 report referred to nursing as 'the major caring profession', and leaders such as McFarlane obviously saw caring as more central than the medically–derived tasks. Nurses should give primacy to caring, she thought, and it should be practised predominantly by those skilled in it as a result of education. She feared however that the 'essential tension' between the technical and the caring work could in future 'crowd out' caring and that nurses would give this function to others (students or SENs) 'whilst we become technicians' (McFarlane 1976b, 1981). Melia's environmental tasks also failed to win a place in the professional pantheon.

Caring was however a difficult basis for professionalism because it was carried out also by family members and other unqualified or lay members of the public: 'Caring is devalued and the primacy of care is culturally invisible because caring is associated with "women's work"' (Benner & Wrubel 1989:368). Caring therefore was not seen as professional work (above). In the United States, Dachelet reported that staff nurses were puzzled by the nursing leadership's insistence that they forego the technical tasks in order to develop the caring and comforting role with the aim of establishing a distinct and independent professional identity. The caring side was of doubtful value, she thought, as a foundation for professional status; such functions were not as highly rewarded as active interventions, even in medicine (Dachelet 1978). A British nurse argues that the appropriation and elevation of care, 'a word made meaningful by its dubious distinction from an overvalued concept' (cure), will not help nursing in its quest for a professional identity (Phillips 1993). In Australia caring has become fashionable, a Victorian nurse believes:

> You get the buzz words: 'care' is very big at the moment, and as someone... was saying, every performance appraisal she'd read (she's a senior person) had that the person had a caring attitude, and...yet we don't even really know—when you start reading the care literature it's just dreadful, you have no

> idea of what it means. It's all sort of amorphous and unmanageable and not particularly helpful. [AH/92]

Caring is also too indiscriminate in its demands on nurses:

> If the nurse is to be responsible for the growth in a holistic sense of the client as a total person...then the practical professional life of the nurse will become impossible. And this is not just because there will not be time enough; it's just not going to be psychologically possible either. A manageable professional life will need to have limited and attainable goals (van Hooft 1987).

Since medicine controlled diagnosis and prescription, nursing leaders may have opted for the expressive or caring role because they could be reasonably certain that doctors would not challenge their claim. Those tasks concerned with attending to the patient's comfort have usually been seen as the basic role of the registered nurse—as in Australia (White 1972:6). In practice she has often delegated them to the student or to the enrolled nurse, while she has preferred the medically delegated or technical tasks. Student nurses, as Melia (1983) found, had the same idea of professionalism, identifying it with 'injections and dressings and giving out medicines'. Australian nurses also have accepted medical tasks:

> I think nurses have tended to pick up a lot of medical work because they have seen it as being that they've learnt something. That's been exciting...The medical staff moved on to other things, and we've ended up with a lot of the responsibility for machinery...[MS/91]

Gamer (1979), a US director of nursing, believed that in their quest for the holy grail of professional status—'so keenly desired, so long sought, and still so elusive'—the leadership's emphasis on independence as part of its professional ideology meant that it could not acknowledge the expanding work of the clinical nurse since it included the delegated medical tasks with their connotations of dependence. For Gamer, these medical functions contributed to nursing's professional status rather than negating it, as the leadership feared. An Australian nurse also sees the expansion as an asset:

> It's really like a lot of things that nurses do, we do it as treatment and it is organised and prescribed by the medical person. It doesn't mean that we're subservient to them, and that's where I think people get this mixed up... [doctors] give it to us and we do it well, and then it becomes part of our role. [VC-W/91]

US nursing in fact rejected the 'physician's assistant' as part of an expanded job for nurses. Martha Rogers called it 'the obliteration of nursing', and showed a hostility to the medical profession which was 'professionally self-defeating', thought Robin Parsons (1975). The American Medical Association went ahead to create the new occupation, in contrast to Canadian developments, where the two organisations representing doctors and nurses jointly decided not to do so (Henderson 1982). In Australia, the Karmel Committee on medical education held discussions in 1973 with the RANF among other bodies, and rejected the separate 'physician's assistant', saying that nurses could receive postgraduate training, as Canadian nurses did, to work in health centres or group medical practices. Commenting on this decision, Pat Slater (then head of the College of Nursing, Australia) supported the interdependence of health team members as preferable to 'wasting energy fighting for independence', as US nursing seemed to be doing. Statements about nurses providing a different kind of health care from that of the doctor, she thought, were 'beating the drum of seeking an independent professional status', instead of accepting that nurses could take on additional functions in order to meet consumer needs (Slater 1974). A British nurse also deplores

> ...this bull about 'autonomy' and 'uniqueness' and 'independence of role'. How can we actually work in a health care setting, meet health needs, and go on perpetuating these kinds of things? We're *interdependent*. There are times when one can define our role, but these in fact seem to be so fluid'. [JS/90]

While the emphasis on nursing theory and research has the reasonable aim of providing a sound foundation for practice, the direction it has taken has been influenced by the political aim of gaining occupational autonomy—hence the dichotomous claims of 'holism', of the person orientation in nursing as opposed to the alleged reductionist and disease orientation of medicine, and on caring as unique to nursing (Savage 1987:122). Labelling orthodox medicine this way as scientifically outmoded also accentuates the acceptability of holistic and caring alternatives (O'Neill 1991:34)—in this case 'new wave' nursing. As Robin Parsons asserted (1975): 'Nursing and medicine are two arms on the one body and should always develop together—because each needs the other and the client needs both'.

Unmasking the masculine mystique

The Marxist and other power/class analyses were a useful base for feminist attacks on what came to be seen as male as well as bourgeois bastions of power and privilege. Nurses were ultimately, though belatedly, the beneficiaries of this two-pronged assault since in the medical division of labour they were in the lower ranks of a structure based on both class and gender. Sociologists had always linked nursing's low status with its female composition (Glaser 1966), but nurses seemed unaware that Friedan's 'feminine mystique' disguised their oppression by making what then passed for femininity seem both natural and inevitable, even desirable. An Australian nurse observed that this oppression led to nurses accepting and supporting 'an ideology which made curing the exclusive province of the doctor, while caring was relegated to the nurse', with consequent inequalities of social prestige and income (Bolton 1981). And in the 1950s and 1960s the feminine mystique persuaded many women to see their work as a transient phase and to make a career out of domesticity, as a South Australian nurse recalls:

> I think women in those days had such limited horizons. So many of the nurses that I trained with in the 1950s, our one aim was to have a row of white nappies on the line and this lovely collection of children in smocked dresses! [SMcC/88]

As women, nurses contributed to the production of human labour and as mothers to its reproduction—at cut rate prices (Turner 1987:151).

It is difficult to disentangle the effects of the work that nurses do from social perceptions of their status as women: that expressive part of nurses' work which is usually thought of as especially theirs is seen as 'women's work', work that is often carried out in the private sphere in contrast to 'men's work', which is publicly visible. Status and economic reward depend on public recognition, so that those who do this 'unseen' work, like nurses (or housewives, child care workers, prostitutes) cannot achieve social status from it (Richards 1980:197-9). Medical and other hospital staff subject nurses to 'a process of selective visibility', seeing only those such as charge nurses (Street 1992:150-6). Nurses' work also remains partly invisible because it includes 'dirty' and potentially embarrassing tasks not often openly discussed (Lawler 1991a). As Lawler says:

> If there is no discourse then there is no power vested in the occupation which deals with those things. We have to look at nurses in much the same way that we look at undertakers. [JL/88]

British sociologist Jeff Hearn describes the sex role socialisation in nursing and similar occupations as 'the patriarchal feminine': feminine in that it conforms to the feminine caring stereotype, and patriarchal because in doing so it complements and thereby reinforces the masculine stereotype. The ideology of femininity is thus central to patriarchy, which divides the emotional or expressive from the instrumental or rational. Emotions are inconvenient for capitalism, so they must be controlled. Women (as nurses, midwives, social workers,) serve men as their agents of social control over the poor, the sick, the outcast (Hearn 1985:195-205). What they formerly did at home (comfort the sick, distressed and dying) women now do in the public sphere for male superiors whom they protect from the emotional impact of birth, sickness and death. Thus in health care a planetary array of semi-professions spins around the medical sun to serve and protect the established profession, which can then treat the most painful events with professional detachment. A medical school dean acknowledged this impersonal quality of medical practice in Australian hospitals where nurses carry the burden of trying to compensate for it—for example, with the families of dying patients (Maddison 1977).

If the new feminism of the 1970s did not influence nursing immediately, it did influence some nurses. US nurses were the first to see its relevance to their own predicament. Virginia Cleland, who had herself combined family and career, had no doubt that 'our most fundamental problem in nursing is that we are members of a woman's occupation in a male-dominated culture'. The consequence of nursing's infatuation with the feminine mystique, she thought, is a generation of ineffective nursing leaders, nurses whose femininity let them abrogate the rights of nurses in hospitals and in universities, and who thus failed to make nursing a more financially rewarding occupation. Instead they showed 'wife-like' submission to male doctors and administrators (Cleland 1971). Another US nurse thought that nursing should aim for the separate status necessary for 'full identification as an autonomous, prestigious profession' (Lamb 1973). Lamb's kind of liberal feminism tends to accept the male constructed world and challenges only women's exclusion from it.

A prominent nurse-feminist saw the problems of nursing as symptoms of the oppression of women. Her solution however was not that of liberal feminism—women to compete in a man's world—but to widen the common range of thinking and behaviour between the sexes, so that women—and nurses—could take part with more confidence in 'male' activities such as making decisions and thinking independently, while men—and doctors—could acknowledge their hitherto suppressed 'female' qualities of compassion and caring. This could lead, she concluded, to a humanised health service (Heide 1973). Given this kind of feminism which acknowledges the differences between the sexes, Heide's rejection of subservience for nurses does not lead her to advocate for nursing an autonomous professional identity separate from medicine; rather, she sees the two occupations as complementary in their work. Following from this, nurses can challenge, not their own medical tasks, but the perceived inferiority of 'female' work (Pringle 1988). An Australian nurse agrees:

> Women in nursing have been in powerful positions for a long time. That's never been acknowledged by the women's movement. It's as though if you don't succeed in a male world, women don't succeed...I think we need both sexes' values in society, and that women happen to represent the more nurturant, affective sorts of values—but that doesn't mean they can't be powerful. [MP/91]

The attempt to polarise the talents of doctors and nurses, as with those of men and women, ignores the many common capacities they share. The significance of medically delegated tasks was that doctors delegated the responsibility for carrying out those tasks, while nurses did not at the same time acquire the power to decide to initiate them (Tellis-Nayak & Tellis-Nayak 1984). Nurses therefore allied themselves with those who criticised medical dominance in health care with some justification, but the rejection by some nurses of the medical components of their own role led not just to an artificial avoidance of medical terminology but to a failure to examine medical practice in all its diversity, and a reluctance therefore to analyse nursing's proper relations with its powerful colleague—hence the development of an ideology which became less and less useful as an explanation of reality and as a guide to action to change it.

The essentially 'feminine' elevation of the caring functions of nursing above the technical or medically derived tasks in fact perpetuates the gender based division of labour in health care. To argue that nursing's special sphere is caring is merely to argue that its special sphere is to be 'womanly' in a traditional sense—that is, to be something which is culturally and historically established. Through contemporary feminism women learned that sex role stereotyping as much as (if not more than) biological difference accounted for much of what they did, for what they earned, and even for what they thought. Through the ideology of expertise (male defined) professionalism legitimates a largely male domination of the well paid tasks in the health division of labour, and thus mystifies what is actually a class interest (Willis 1983:25).

'Doing good and feeling bad'

'Nurses have struggled not only to create a profession but to be a profession of women' (Brand & Glass 1975)—a double whammy. In continuing to seek a separate identity for nursing by distinguishing medicine's 'curing' role from nursing's province of 'caring'—roles that are male and female stereotypes—nursing leaders were in fact using sexist ideas in a quixotic attempt to elevate the prestige of a female profession. They sought to blend two 'conflicting and irreconcilable' ideologies of (female) domesticity and (male) professionalism (Hughes 1990). Nursing was not and could not be a profession since nurses were women and professionalism itself was patriarchal. The professional ideology espoused by the nursing leaders in fact undermined their own claim to professional status: if the centrepiece of the professional ideology was expertise, which elevated the leaders above other nurses, then that same expertise left nurses for ever below medicine. Nurses could not challenge that position without challenging also their professional ideology (Melosh 1982). Nor as 'feminine' women could they challenge the system: 'real women are not supposed to be revolutionaries. If we complain about our situation, or the system, we are liable to be called ill, neurotic, menopausal, premenstrual, or in need of some curative relationship with a man' (Oakley 1984).

The feminist ferment had a limited impact on US nurses through the work of Ashley and others (e.g. Chinn & Wheeler 1985). Some proposed the depressingly sexist solution of recruiting more men to raise nursing's status (Dachelet 1978). Growing opportunities in the workplace for middle class women put nursing at a disadvantage as a quintessentially women's occupation. The new interpretations of professionalism, the 'power and control' and the Marxist, were less explored, except as they implied a need to develop nursing's own power. British and Australian nurses for some time shunned both these doctrines. In Britain they continued to discuss professional attributes and to ignore or make only fleeting references to the implications of nursing's female composition (e.g. Chapman 1977).

Australian nursing in the 1970s seems to have taken little notice of the arrival of feminism's 'second wave' in spite of the local origin of one of its most celebrated prophets, who described the plight of nurses as 'the most depressing phenomenon in the pattern of women's work' (Greer 1971:126). A local nurse comments:

> That powerful second wave of the women's movement—they stayed away from it...here was nursing on its steady conservative path...It was still operationalising its old ideologies...premised on the bloody *private* world, the women's world of domestic work, of domestic labour, of the moral order, of the good woman. They were still defining modern nursing as being started by goddamn Florence Nightingale, though the whole world was changing around them! [SMcM/91]

Another Australian nurse thinks the movement alienated her colleagues:

> Feminism put nursing down! Put us back years...A paper in [a 1970s book on women in Australia] said it was time that women were able to do better for themselves rather than just doing nursing or teaching. Boom! Down to the bottom it went!...the women's movement I don't think has really done any good for nursing...[MP/91]

A woman's work is never...unionised

One strategy for increasing the power of nursing which many nursing leaders did not favour until recently is trade unionism, often viewed as an alternative process for a group seeking upward mobility (Summers 1985; Short & Sharman 1987). Larson (1977:185) thought that 'since no amount of externally sanctioned expertise can compensate for the subordination of auxiliary medical professions to the physician, unionisation remains a choice at least as effective as further professionalisation'. Unionism however tended to be seen as distinct from professionalism since it was a class ideology most likely to be adopted by subordinate employees, whereas professionalism was a status ideology characteristic of those exercising their skills with some degree of autonomy.

Parkin's use of the idea of 'social closure' can be applied in this connection to nurses as a social group. Social closure can be applied through a strategy of exclusion: the process by which members of a social collectivity seek to maximise their own rewards by restricting access to resources and opportunities to a limited circle of eligible persons. Exclusion commonly leads to action taken by the 'negatively privileged' themselves, who respond to this use of downward directed power by exerting in turn upward pressure to attack the privileges of their legally defined superiors and win more rewards for themselves—the process of usurpation. Nurses could see themselves both as usurpers (towards doctors) and as excluders (towards SENs). The collective action associated with unionism is usual for usurpers, though by its nature usurpatory activity is more severely punished than exclusionary, since it challenges the prevailing system of distributive justice (Parkin 1979:43-5, 73-4).

Nursing has been described as one of the bureaucratic professions, since nurses work in organisations rather than in independent practice like doctors and lawyers—who themselves have increasingly come to be salaried and organisation based. An irony of this is that many of these occupations cling, like nursing, to an outmoded ideology of professionalism:

> In short, professionalism has become an occupational ideal in a society in which its attainment becomes less and less likely as more and more work is routinised through technological advances, and occupational practice increasingly finds its typical setting within bureaucratic organisations of various kinds (Johnson 1984).

Occupations which at the time of their expansion lacked an established place in the occupational structure (like nursing in the 19th century) were likely to adopt professionalism, but when their place is securely established they tend to adopt unionism, especially if professionalism is failing to achieve benefits for occupational members (Black 1981). An Australian researcher has shown that many professionals, especially those working in large organisations, increasingly regard membership of a professional association and of a trade union as 'complementary rather than contradictory' (Lansbury 1978:133, 151). Nurses have had the advantage, like doctors, of associations which combined professional and union functions, though they have usually put less value on the latter. This may reflect the traditional separation between professional nursing as a vocation which sanctified the performance of menial and even dirty tasks, and nursing as work which earned a low financial reward (Ch. 1).

In the United States nurses in the 1970s were demonstrating more support for unions, and more militancy. A survey of public health nurses in California showed that younger nurses, who tended to have higher status parents and were more likely to have been educated in degree programs than older nurses, had more favourable attitudes to union tactics and were more militant than their elders. Younger nurses 'seemed to find that unionism and militancy are compatible with professionalism', and images of professionalism were changing (Bloom et al 1979). The American Nurses' Association (ANA) implicitly rejected 19th century ideas of vocation by dropping its no strike policy in 1968 and pursuing collective bargaining for better job conditions.

In Australia the RANF (Victorian Branch) industrial relations officer was concerned to dispel both the assumed profession-union dichotomy and the confusion among nurses about the functions of a trade union, especially since some, she revealed, did not realise that the RANF *was* a union (Fox 1979). If Victorian nurses felt hostile to unions because they did not understand their functions, it was probably the result of their conventional view of professionalism. The RANF upheld at the time its 'Rule 31' forbidding nurses to take strike action in what appeared to be a linking of a union's most public action with 'unprofessional' behaviour. Those who did accept unionism were the members of the nursing proletariat, the enrolled nurses, since orthodox professionalism denied them a place in nursing.

Australian nursing in general did however show an awareness of the need to organise and to develop politically so that nurses could exercise power both on behalf of their patients and to support each other (e.g. Pratt 1980). It mostly escaped the 'education-practice gap' of the US system, and it showed less of the class–tied hierarchy of the British. Australian nursing seems to have developed during the 1970s, despite federal boundaries, a more collective orientation than its US or British equivalents. This difference perhaps arose from the then relatively high levels of unionisation in Australia, from the three years of a reform Labor Government, but especially from the collective effort of the leadership for improvements in education. Yet although nurses in Australia (as elsewhere) became more politically conscious in the early 1980s, they continued to be regaled by their colleagues with the moribund attributes of professionalism (e.g. Roberts 1980; Tiffany 1982). They had not yet linked political awareness with the professionalism debate. A Victorian nurse explains:

> I just think nursing has held on to so many ideologies that have only served to work against it. I think their notion of professionalism has served to mask to nurses their place in the world. Nurses in their pursuit of professionalism haven't been quite sure what they're professionalising. They haven't thought it through. [SMcM/91]

Like most women, nurses were complicit in their own subordination though not in the sense that it was an intentional act. An Australian nurse observes that 'the world sets up possibilities' for what each person, male or female, can or cannot become, and thus 'constrains the ways in which the self constitutes its world' (Parker 1991). As Davies (1976) argued such a strategy may have served nurses well for a time, but its cost was an impoverished sense of professional identity and little awareness of collective power. By the 1980s some preconditions for a change were becoming apparent, yet nurses continued to base their arguments on the attribute model, and could still say, looking upwards, that doctors were supreme because they had a 'unique body of knowledge' (e.g. Sleicher 1983). Looking down, they used the inherent élitism of their professional ideology to exclude the SENs, as a rancorous exchange in the ANJ revealed. A New South Wales RN wrote that the SEN was not entitled to be called 'nurse' because of her limited education. She thought medicine had become a highly valued occupation by excluding from practice those with inferior education. The response was immediate: 'SENs are nurses', retorted a Victorian enrolled nurse. 'Obviously [the RN] has her head in the clouds', accused another; 'Delusions of grandeur', from Western Australia; and 'Just how far are some nurses going in the pursuit of professionalism!' asked a WA psychiatric nurse.

All said emphatically that SENs did care for patients and were trained to do so (*ANJ* December/January-May 1986). The 'discourse of professionalisation' which nursing has appropriated has conservative and élitist implications: it 'does not challenge the existing occupational hierarchy, but rather seeks merely to relocate nursing to a new and higher level' (Bruni 1991). A South Australian nurse also attacks élitism, and connects it with the pursuit of education as a professionalising strategy:

> Nurses have fallen into professional protectionism, professional élitism, and I think that's been the danger with striving for education. Lots of the protagonists of the education and professionalism model have been élitists... they're an élite club, apeing traditional models of power...which are principally male...the traditional academic models. They're not *suitable*'. [LS/88]

The attribute model was indeed a decoy, as Roth said. It diverted nurses from seeing (as they could have done in medicine's case) that the question, 'What is nursing?' can be answered without the trouble of finding an elusive 'unique essence'. Nursing is what nurses agree to say it is, and what definition they have the collective power to enforce.

Anstey on accountability

The fundamental issue in the struggle to upgrade nursing as a profession has been that of accountability, according to a US academic (Muyskens 1982). Allied to medical dominance has been the individual nurse's inability to be fully accountable for her practice. US nurses saw accountability as linked to professional autonomy but, influenced by the market and attribute models of professionalism, they tended to see the 'agency service' character of nursing (patients are cared for by a group of nurses) and nurses' status as employees as barriers to accountable care. Professional autonomy and accountability were closely linked to the idealised model of professionalism and thus to an individualistic notion of professional practice (e.g. Maas 1973) so that there was little appreciation of the collective as potentially accountable. Muyskens sees the crucial question as 'the interface of individual and collective responsibility'. The purely individual kind deals harshly with the nurse who cannot, for example, enforce aseptic standards with doctors—she is behaving in an understandable if regrettable way, possibly fearing retribution. But we are entitled to expect the group authorised to provide nursing services to attain a higher standard because it has a collective responsibility to the public. Collective responsibility can thus be used to upgrade nursing practice and to improve the delivery of health care (Muyskens 1982:165-7). Without this idea, the individual nurse is shackled to the oppression deplored by Ashley (1973, 1975) and others, since she sees her single action against the status quo as unprofessional. Collective accountability provides the link between political action and professionalism because it necessitates responsible organisation for that action, as nurses have demonstrated by, for example, providing a skeleton staff during a strike.

Nurses have often stopped short of making this connection. British nurses wrestled with the idea of accountability in a *Nursing Times* symposium (7 September–5 October 1983). One contributor did say that the nursing profession was accountable to society, so nurses could not ignore political issues, but other writers in the series concentrated on linking individual accountability with professionalism and with acquiring appropriate knowledge (Lisbeth Hockey) or with primary nursing (Alan Pearson). In Australia Olive Anstey gave a wide interpretation to accountability when she announced it as the watchword for the ICN, of which she was then president. Anstey (1979) recognised that accountability to the patient could bring the nurse into conflict with those farther up the hierarchy. As a director of nursing she perhaps hesitated to condemn the hierarchy for stifling professional practice, but she did emphasise the collective responsibility of nurses, to each other and to the public, which could oblige them to act politically in support of high quality health care. Yet accountability often continued to be limited to ideas of individual responsibility, such as the patient advocate role, and primary nursing was seen as embodying 'full accountability' (e.g. Gray 1982). More recently, an awareness of collective accountability (e.g. Gray & Pratt 1989), and a realisation of its complexities in practice, have emerged in Australia:

> There's obviously a central accountability to the patient, but there are circumstances when one is accountable to the doctor…there's an accountability to one's employer, to the profession, to the professional body, accountability to oneself. There's tremendous potential there for multiple accountabilities. [RP/89]

The RANF has demonstrated its commitment to public accountability by starting in 1978 to develop a set of standards for nursing practice through a national quality assurance program and a series of associated publications (Pratt 1987).

Nurses and doctors on the 'game'

Since the medical profession maintains its authority through controlling the health division of labour, 'then doctors' own professionalisation organises and requires nurses' subordination' (Melosh 1982). Medical dominance was a fact that nurses either lived with and criticised, or tried to ignore. The medical mystique and medicine's (and their own) ideology of professionalism had convinced them that doctors 'knew more' than nurses, despite occasions when this was patently not the case. This belief ignored the reality that if doctors in general know more than nurses do, it does not follow that they are at all times infallible, or that nurses therefore, because they know less (of certain things anyway), know nothing, and should thus be completely subordinate at all times on all matters. Nurses are and have been subordinate for quite different reasons, to do with gender and class and with a consequent lack of power, more than with what they knew or with what skills they had. The actual complexities of the nurse-doctor relationship have become obscured by the fictions of both professions with the aim on the medical side to minimise the extent of what nurses actually do—the 'handmaiden' syndrome—and on the nursing side to ignore the dimensions of the delegated work—the 'independent profession' ideology (Gamer 1979). An Australian nurse attacked the medical fiction about nursing skills with some style:

> [The surgeon] said to me 'Oh, you can teach a monkey to do anything, to hand up instruments'. I just looked at him and I said 'Well, if you have him for a bit longer, he could even do the operation!' But this is what they think of nurses—handmaidens, isn't it? [IK/91]

Medicine has allowed another occupation to learn at close range much of the routine and practice of medical work. In Goffman's dramaturgical scheme, nurses have been permitted to see medicine behind the scenes of its public 'on stage' persona. The dominant profession saw no risk in this proximity: first, its professional ideology said that there were skills which doctors alone possessed, indeed could possess, especially the skill of diagnosis (jealously protected); second, the ideology was backed up by state support of the medical monopoly of surgery and prescription; third, nurses (or their leaders) accepted the ideology of professionalism themselves; finally, how could nurses be seen as a threat when they usually came from a lower social stratum, had limited education, and above all were women? Still, both groups took care to preserve the superior-subordinate ranking (Speedy 1987). The 'doctor-nurse game' became a cliché of nursing circles from the late 1960s. The game showed the elaborate social rules followed by both doctors and nurses to avoid any suggestion that even occasionally a nurse might know more on any subject. In competence, skills and knowledge, doctors and nurses are in many ways complementary (Chiarella 1981), but professionally the major difference between them is one of power, a difference coloured by the gender factor. It is illustrated daily in the many routines which are symbols of a structurally unequal distribution of power, and any attempt to change things will have to tackle both these 'faces of power'—the structural and the symbolic (Tellis-Nayak & Tellis-Nayak 1984). An Australian psychiatric nurse observes doctors' reactions to such a threat:

> People that we look after have got an enduring disability...and unless we've got good continuity of care, people are going to fall into the gaps and come back into hospital. So we have to have interdisciplinary care plans. Well, medical staff have gone bananas about that...because that really impinges on their practice...Their independence is such a valued part of their professional upbringing that all they see [is] that *they* get the patient well...They see themselves, yes, as the whole rather than the actor on the stage. [EC/91]

Achieving greater autonomy for all nurses will entail by definition a degree of power sharing, or at worst a power struggle, with doctors. It will also demand proper legal recognition of nurses' responsibilities, which in turn will bring full legal liability for their actions (Chiarella 1990).

Some doctors have thought about their relationship with nurses, not all of them in doctor-nurse game terms. A Canadian nurse found that doctors thought the relationship was more satisfactory than nurses did, though they hesitated to delegate some functions to the nurses for fear of losing control. The whole relationship was suffused with the awareness on both sides of sharp status and power disparities and a wide economic gap (Devine 1978). A US doctor regretted the time spent by nurses in administration as opposed to patient care, but then acknowledged that the hospital as a complex institution 'is held together, *glued* together, enabled to function as an organism, by the nurses and by nobody else' (Thomas 1983:67)—an achievement which surely requires some time for administrative tasks.

British doctors in traditional style deplored 'a lack of true vocation' in contemporary nursing, and put their emphasis heavily on basic nursing care, on nurses who realised that 'bottoms are as important as electrocardiograms'. A nurse responded more rationally: 'Bottoms in coronary care are very important, but we have to know to stop rubbing if the monitor shows ventricular fibrillation'. Another issued a thoughtful challenge to her medical colleagues: 'Autonomy may be difficult for you to accept, but a sharing rather than a division of responsibility could be to the advantage of all'. This nurse saw that a strict separation of the two professions, whether by tasks and knowledge or by power and status disparities (bottoms vs ECGs) was unproductive (*British Medical Journal* 12 September-7 November 1981). An Australian doctor thought that the nurse was capable of independent judgement about treatment policies. The problem was that she was unable to influence those policies (Legge 1979).

Nurses may not have analysed medicine dispassionately, but they did occasionally analyse their relations with doctors—apart, that is, from intimate relations, which were unfortunately left to a sub-genre of romantic fiction. Beatrice and Philip Kalisch (1977) analysed doctor-nurse conflict with some sympathy for the pressures on doctors—such as the fear of making mistakes—as well as for nurses' subordination. The nurse's deference they thought led to impaired communication, often to the detriment of patient care, and fears on both sides of 'role erosion'. Nurses must have more power if they want to remedy this situation, even if it means strikes and protests, they concluded.

A group of Canadian nurses thought that doctors had always protected their status and power 'long the hallmarks of the medical profession', and that nurses also 'unknowingly or inadvertently' had perpetuated this (Keddy et al 1986). The power difference, daily reinforced by their professional ideology with its aggrandisement of medicine, has led nurses to undervalue their own contribution. This may explain the impact of Patricia Benner's

(1984) analysis of nurses' complex work and responsibilities, as an Australian nurse recognises:

> Nurses I think want to understand the human condition...the suffering, the pain, the despair, the hurt, the disturbance that they deal with...They want ways of understanding that and working with it...A lot of this is what they currently do in intuitive ways, and I think this is sometimes what Benner's trying to do when she's getting them to lay open their practice so that they can turn it into words, because it has been silent. It's been this unspoken dimension. [JP/90]

Another Australian nurse shows that much nursing work, however skilled and complex, is such that it cannot be publicly discussed and so creates for nursing 'a problem of power/knowledge' (Lawler 1991a:219). Benner may want to uncover and value nursing practice, but in the process of doing so she 'disregards the politics of power at work in nursing' (Street 1992:74).

Doctors have become more aware of nurses, of their work and of their views, during the 1980s. If this was the result of the women's movement making women in general more visible, and of encouraging nurses to speak out, it confirms gender as a major reason for nurses' past subjection, fostering both that subjection and their acceptance of it. The new medical awareness does not always go with greater understanding, nor has it changed the relationship. An Australian nurse found that local doctors did not think nurses needed to have decision making skills, while nurses said they did (Partridge 1984). Such an underestimation of nurses' work may originate in part in the medical fear of 'role erosion', together with the usual low value put on women's work—the handmaiden stereotype. Nurses are doing a great job as long as it is a woman's job.

The publication of the Marles Report in Victoria in 1988 brought into the open what nurses had been saying for years about doctors as colleagues. What had changed was that some senior medical practitioners now accepted that a 'team' approach to health care was the appropriate model, though this was a view 'more often put forward as a solution to current problems than as a description of present practice'. Doctors as well as nurses recognised that better relations between the two groups were 'an urgent priority' since each felt frustration and resentment towards the other. Even so, the poor medical response to the Marles Committee suggests that this concern was confined to a minority of doctors. The report also reinforced impressions that the new independence being encouraged in nursing education still came up against the entrenched power structure of the hospital which excluded nurses from decision making even in those instances where they had the obvious expertise to contribute. Particularly vexatious were doctors (especially the older, more senior ones) tending to subsume all nursing under their professional authority: 'In reality, the practice at the workface is often consultative but no avenue exists to distinguish nursing's contribution; within the medical model it remains informal and undifferentiated' (Marles 1988:249, from the Austin Hospital nursing division).

Freidson's medically dominated division of labour was alive and thriving in Australian hospitals and nurses were well aware of its effects on their work and on their professional status. Doctors often valued the nurse's medically delegated tasks but took her caring tasks for granted (women's work) and denigrated her co-ordinating function (see Thomas 1983) as paper work which removed her from—by implication more useful, perhaps more 'feminine'—tasks at the bedside. Doctors, like many men, found it hard to assimilate the effect of feminism on nurses—'namely, the drive for recognition and equality'—in contrast to their former submissiveness (Marles 198:246-7, 255-9). Some medical criticism of the transfer of nurse education to colleges was clearly ideological rather than rational, using 'unsubstantiated claims of incompetence in both educators and graduates (Hazelton 1990). Some doctors have conceded however that the roles of doctor and nurse in individual patient care 'are not mutually exclusive' (Jones & Lawrence 1988). An Australian academic sums up:

> It can't be an accident that nursing as a profession has stayed as low status as it has all this time. It's got something to do, I suppose, with the way the older leaders saw the profession, but it's also got to have a lot to do with the way the doctors saw it. It's always been within the power of the doctors to do something about it, had they ever wished to—but I'm sure they never wished to. [JL/90]

The Marles Report showed that many nurses were sharply aware that professionalism was not compatible with a lack of power, with subservience to any group: co-operation and collaboration, yes; unquestioning obedience to orders, no. Perhaps Victorian nurses, having recently defied the government and hospital managements, could see this with special clarity:

> I think that's part of the burden we bear, because of...the stereotypes and the roles we've played in the past, inasmuch as we've always been people who have gone 'Yes, no, three bags full', and whatever people have told us. It's all to do with women in society and how nurses are perceived generally—that's the doctor's handmaiden, and 'Who are you to question?' [HV/88]

Professionalism as 'professionhood'...

Ironic then that when US professor of nursing Margretta Styles spoke to Australian nurses on professionalism, she concluded that 'the core of the nursing universe' is the individual nurse and her beliefs. As the then President of the American Nurses' Association, Styles did advocate power, professional unity, political astuteness, and colleague relations between nurses, but her major emphasis was on the individual nurse, for whom she coined the word 'professionhood'. Nursing is 'an art and science fusing the attitude and the act of caring'; and 'Our beliefs are the essence of nursing', she says (in capitals). Her new professionalism consists in empowering those beliefs, though on how this will be engineered she is vague (Styles 1987).

Styles's 'beliefs' are redolent of the normative in nursing theory and reflect the dominant individualist professional ideology. She seemed unaware that Australian nursing had progressed with some recent success along the path to collective power. One local nurse reminded her audience on the same occasion that 'nurses are rapidly gaining industrial strength, and because of this, salary parity with other health care providers' (Garratt 1987); and another that prestige attaches to high incomes, so if nurses want prestige they should attend to industrial matters (Woodruff 1987). Australian nurses seem more alert than some of their US colleagues to nursing as a collective force. They have promoted nursing research through joint setting of research targets, for example. Ideas about both research and nursing theory are reported to be open minded and eclectic: nurses welcome overseas ideas and influences, but are discriminating borrowers in addition to developing the home product (Emden & Young 1987). Yet in spite of their political awakening (Ch. 3) some have not yet accepted the idea that nursing theory is itself political. Not to acknowledge this openly 'is itself a political act, substantiating and perpetuating the status quo, and repeating all the mistakes that have sustained nursing's oppression in the past' (Holmes 1991:443).

...professionalism as space...

An Australian sociologist combines the 'power and control' theory with the 'technicality-indeterminacy' thesis (pp. 47–8) and cites three features of 'the professional situation' as especially important:

1. a body of knowledge accepted as relevant and effective for client needs, which practitioners can expand through research;
2. wide scope for the interpretation of this knowledge, that is, a 'range and necessity' for professional judgement, so that the knowledge cannot be codified into a set of routine rules which are automatically applied;
3. direct access to people and to the interests of the client 'as a whole' (Turner 1985).

Provided the state supports its exclusive use, this 'space' for the use of professional judgement in the application of knowledge to particular cases is vital. Anyone can read a medical text, but only a licensed medical practitioner has the legal right to use professional judgement in applying the knowledge it contains. A 'space for judgement' has considerable importance for the way a profession works, because it is in this area of freedom to move that the ideological aspects of professional work are joined to the scientific content, and this ideology is always culturally and politically defined. For example, doctors have applied the (neutral, objective) scientific properties of tranquillisers to reduce a social problem (ideological, subjective) to the level of individual illness – 'suburban neurosis' (Willis 1983: 20). In a different example, doctors have long known how to procure an abortion, though not with today's safety, but most have complied with prevailing legal, cultural and political norms by refusing to carry out the procedure. The knowledge of abortion possessed by all doctors could not be applied legitimately, even though it was no less valid as science. As some feminist scholars are now pointing out, scientific truth is socially constructed (Dugdale 1990).

Nursing has always had a body of knowledge, even if it is not unique since much of it is based on the same scientific disciplines as that of medicine (also not unique), and on the social sciences. It has lacked control over its access to clients since they are usually available through the agency of doctors, and it has seemed to have a very small space for the use of nurses' own judgement if most activities are assumed to derive from medical orders. But this seeming restriction often does not operate in practice. Observers over at least the last 30 years have noticed that doctors claim more authority than they can actually exercise, and nurses have more authority than others acknowledge (Hughes et al 1958; Gamer 1979).

The professional ideology as defined by medicine has created and maintained a complex division of labour in health care, often on the apparent grounds of technological determinism. That is, the evolution of medical technology appears to dictate the evolution of the division of labour, so that it is technically 'rational' that nurses carry out certain tasks (giving injections, taking out stitches) but are barred from others (inserting stitches, setting up IV drips), except in unusual circumstances—and even if a nurse carries out what is normally a medical task she will not get a medical rate of pay. Technological determinism functions as a screen to disguise what is actually a social arrangement. It is an ideological representation of the capitalist division of labour, designed to keep wealth accumulation in the hands of dominant groups (Willis 1983:33-5). Nursing's space for professional judgement exists, but it is unofficial. The powerful influence of the professional ideology will keep doctors opposed to any attempt to make it formal, as a psychiatric nurse observes:

> We've always had a much more colleague relationship in psych than in general [nursing]...there's certainly always been an acceptance that there would be a lot of independent decision making...However, the problem is [now] it's being articulated, and because it's being articulated, the hackles go up. As nurses are feeling threatened, so are psychiatrists—absolutely threatened. And they've lost an enormous amount of power because of this articulation of the position. [EC/91]

...and professionalism as struggle

A recent analysis of professions sees them as forming an unfolding and interdependent system: control of knowledge and its application is essential, but the ineluctable accompaniment to that control is competition with other professions. Each profession's jurisdiction or territory contains certain activities. Over some it has complete control, with others it may be subordinated to another group, and 'jurisdictional boundaries are perpetually in dispute' (Abbott 1988:2). These jurisdictional disputes, Abbott believes, explain much professional behaviour. The threat of challenges from other professions encourages groups to define rigidly those tasks they see as within their own jurisdiction. Such definitions hold publicly in law but they are often impossible to implement exactly as intended in the workplace, with the result that in practice actual divisions of labour may be established through negotiation and custom. This in turn may have repercussions later on the boundaries of the professional jurisdiction. In the workplace subordinates learn, on the job, a craft version of the dominant profession's knowledge system, partly because members of the superior and subordinate groups vary in their degree of talent: the more talented nurses will excel in capacity the less gifted doctors, though the legal formalities hold otherwise. Dominant professions maintain in public that members of the subordinate group lack the theoretical education necessary to understand what they have learnt in the workplace, so: 'The public fiction survives that only doctors can do certain kinds of things, when nurses and others are in fact doing them all over the professional world' (Abbott 1988:68).

The ideal for a profession is to have 'a heartland of work over which it has complete, legally established control', which it can defend and expand. But the number of such jurisdictions is limited, so some groups have to settle for alternatives, the most common of which is subordination. Nursing is the classic case, but the settlement is inherently uneasy, partly because of what nurses learn on the job, and partly because they have become essential to medical practice. The public fiction is part of maintaining formal subordination, so that the public believes 'that all nurses know less than all doctors about all medical things', something most nurses know to be untrue. To maintain this in the midst of workplace realities requires constant reinforcement, hence the familiar 'Don't ask questions, just follow my orders.'

A further example of jurisdictional settlement also relevant to nurses is that by workplace, or client differentiation. So, nurses have more autonomy outside the hospital, in remote places, or in serving less desirable clients (Abbott 1988: 61-77). The nurse practitioner movement in America began in the 1960s because there were few doctors practising, for example, among the poor. Nurse practitioners functioned as doctor 'extenders', though they redefined their work as promoting health or wellness. Does such a movement give nurses genuine autonomy, or are they just filling a gap which medicine willingly leaves? (Zadorosnyj 1988). Australia's remote area nurses are in this position, but their independence allows them to stress a way of practising which is as much a contrast with hospital nursing as it is with medicine:

> We use a community development approach to allow Aborigines to develop their own priorities and programs, but...most nurses are prepared in a hospital training system which doesn't foster development of that approach, because they act on people as 'captive clients'...[HB/90]

Abbott's account of professions redirects attention to the work of professionals, rather than to their organisational structure, and it shows how professions have in the past and are now continually defending their territory. He too rejects the attribute model: what has to be explained is not whether a particular occupation is or is not a profession, but 'how expertise is structured in society, the division of expert labour'. Like the 'power and control' theorists, he argues that dominant professions use state backing and class power to uphold the legitimacy of their jurisdictions.

In seeing all professions as part of a system Abbott makes the encouraging claim that this system is dynamic, its constituent groups are always defending their positions, contending for better ones and fighting off attackers. To demand an absolute and enduring definition of what nursing is or to lament the hard-to-define territory and the disagreement about the nurse's 'role' is not the central point. That role, that territory, are always in flux, subject to continual pressure from other groups and to forces outside the professional system altogether, such as technological and social change. True, boundaries tend to be defined from the top and the impetus for changing them is likely to come from the most powerful profession (Oakley 1984), but this dynamic system does at least allow nurses to play an active part in negotiating for their own desired place, even if they have to reconcile themselves to perpetual struggle.

Or, should nurses adopt an alternative model of professionalism, since the one they have pursued with such energy and persistence fits neither the character of nursing work nor the sex of those doing it? Another kind of professionalism entails 'integrity' in work related to 'setting one's own goals and parameters, and one's own standards and methods of achieving these' (Bessant & Bessant 1991: 223). This 'in-group' professionalism, which depends on a shared belief in upholding standards rather than on competing with others for power, is appealing. It is akin to a British alternative professionalism, in which nurses share knowledge and skills with patients, and which sees the quality of nursing care as more important than professional status (Webb 1987). Though less individualistic than the Styles professionhood and much less élitist than the orthodox blueprint, these versions would disengage nursing from Abbott's system, thus reducing nurses' influence within it. But if they are to challenge the less acceptable face of professionalism in health care, such as the tendency to élitism, male domination, and the relative neglect of less favoured clients, then nurses must remain in the system to 'balance the scale with a focus on women's experiences, attitudes, views and needs' (Speedy 1988). For this, the size of the nursing workforce is a potential asset rather than a handicap. A South Australian nurse reflects that,

> ...no one listens to nurses, unlike the AMA [Australian Medical Association]. The nurses have got to play the numbers game, the AMA doesn't, and this is why I don't think we've come very far. I don't think we'll ever achieve the kind of professionalism that says that one doesn't have to play the numbers game...[EC/88]

Nurses may have directed their energies to achieving a kind of professionalism that put them at a disadvantage (Pittman 1985), but their pursuit was further hindered by their interpretation of it, so that they overlooked the advantages of collective power. Such power will be a political asset they will need if they are to help transform health care—perhaps through using the radical feminist analysis of caring with its wider, social (rather than individualistic) perspective (Moloney 1986: 28; Beaumont 1987; Speedy 1991). A British nurse describes her own vision:

> I think we have a great opportunity to create a new kind of occupational identity which doesn't, for me, go down the bad old professional road, but actually picks up the bits about professionalism which are good, which are about having high ideals about what you want to achieve. And they are about service to society; they are about self-esteem; and also about having other people's respect—not the kind of respect that comes from a class position but a genuine respect for someone's skills and contribution...a newer king of occupational strategy that isn't old style professionalism. [JSa/90]

Nursing leaders were not mistaken in fighting for tertiary education, but in tending to rely on it exclusively as the path to orthodox (male) professionalism. An Australian nurse saw this clearly at a time when she and her colleagues were questioning their traditional quiescence: 'I see professionalism as a "lure", and education is part of this. The bid for professional status has *not* helped improve nurses' working conditions, and without that (if they remain overworked, rushed etc.) they can't achieve professional status. Therefore I see industrial action as important' (Wiesel 1985).

Another confirms the value of having more power: 'I would never say now "I'm just a nurse"'. [AH/92]

REFERENCES

Abbott A 1988 The system of professions: an essay on the division of expert labour. University of Chicago Press, Chicago

Aggleton P, Chalmers H 1984 Models and theories (series of articles). Nursing Times, 5 September-6 March 1985

Altschul A T 1979 Commitment to nursing. Journal of Advanced Nursing 4:123-135

Anstey O 1979 The watchword 'Accountability'—international and national implications for nursing. Australian Nurses' Journal, March:28-31

Ashley J A 1973 This I believe about power in nursing. Nursing Outlook, October:637-641

Ashley J A 1975 Power, freedom and professional practice in nursing. Supervisor Nurse, January:12-29

Baer C L 1986 Nursing research: sacred cow or fatted calf?. Holistic Nursing Practice, November:8-20

Barratt Y 1989 Personal communication

Beaumont M K 1987 The nursing struggle. Australian Nurses' Journal, September: 48-51

Benner P 1984 From novice to expert: excellence and power in clinical nursing practice. Addison-Wesley, Menlo Park

Benner P, Wrubel J 1989 The primacy of caring: stress and coping in health and illness. Addison-Wesley, Menlo Park

Bessant J, Bessant B 1991 The growth of a profession: nursing in Victoria 1930s-1980s. La Trobe University Press, Melbourne
Black A W 1981 Professional associations: part of the problem or part of the solution? Australian Journal of Social Issues 16(2):149-161
Bloom J R, O'Reilley C A, Parlette G N 1979 Changing images of professionalism: the case of public health nurses. American Journal of Public Health, January:43-46
Bolton G 1981 A training in discipline and conformity? Australian Nurses' Journal, October:34-36
Bowman R A, Culpepper R C 1974 Power: Rx for change. American Journal of Nursing, June:1053-1056
Brand K L, Glass L K 1975 Perils and parallels of women and nursing. Nursing Forum XIV (2):160-174
Bruni N 1991 Nursing knowledge: processes of production. In: Gray G, Pratt R (eds) Towards a discipline of nursing. Churchill Livingstone, Melbourne
Bullough V L, Bullough B 1984 History, trends and politics of nursing. Appleton-Century-Crofts, East Norwalk
Carpenter M 1977 The new managerialism and professionalism in nursing. In: Stacey M, Reid M, Heath C, Dingwall R (eds) Health and the division of labour. Croom Helm, London
Chapman C M 1977 Concepts of professionalism. Journal of Advanced Nursing 2:51-55
Chiarella M 1981 The relationship between the bodies of knowledge of medicine and nursing. Australian Nurses, Journal, March:48-49
Chiarella M 1990 Trends in expectations of nursing responsibilities—professional and legal perspectives. In: Nursing in the nineties. Conference papers, Royal College of Nursing Australia, Sydney, May
Chinn P L, Wheeler C E 1985 Feminism and nursing. Nursing Outlook 33(2):74-77
Clark M J 1982 Development of models and theories on the concept of nursing. Journal of Advanced Nursing 7:129-134
Cleland V S 1971 Sex discrimination: nursing's most pervasive problem. American Journal of Nursing August:1542-1547
Cohen H A 1981 The nurse's quest for a professional identity. Addison-Wesley, Menlo Park
Corwin R G 1961 The professional employee: a study of conflict in nursing roles. In: Skipper J K, Leonard R C (eds) 1965 Social interaction and patient care. Lippincott, Philadelphia
Dachelet C Z 1978 Nursing's bid for increased status. Nursing Forum XVII(1):18-45
Davies C 1976 Experience of dependency and control in work: the case of nurses. Journal of Advanced Nursing 1:273-282
Devine B A 1978 Nurse-physician interaction: status and social structure within two hospital wards. Journal of Advanced Nursing 3:287-295
Dingwall R 1974 Some sociological aspects of 'nursing research'. Sociological Review 22(1):45-55
Donaghue S 1977 Goals in nursing practice. RANF, Melbourne
Dugdale A 1990 Beyond relativism: moving on—feminist struggles with scientific/medical knowledge. Australian Feminist Studies 12, Summer: 51-63
Emden C, Young W 1987 Theory development in nursing: a delphi study. In: Professionalism...what is it? College of Nursing, Australia, Proceedings of 9th National Conference, Hobart, May
Flexner A 1915 Is social work a Profession? School and society, 1(26):902-911
Fox C 1979 RANF: professional association or trade union? Australian Nurses' Journal, April:17-20
Freidson E 1970a Profession of medicine. Random House, New York
Freidson E 1970b Professional dominance: the social structure of medical care. Aldine, New York
Gamer M 1979 The ideology of professionalism. Nursing Outlook, February: 108-111
Garratt S A 1987 Practice—a challenge. In: College of Nursing, Australia, Proceedings of 9th National Conference, Hobart, May
Glaser W A 1966 Nursing leadership and policy: some cross-national comparisons. In: Davis F (ed) The nursing profession. Five sociological essays. Wiley, New York
Gray G 1982 Accountability. In: Jenkins E, King B, Gray G (eds) Issues in Australasian nursing. Churchill Livingstone, Melbourne

Gray G, Pratt R 1989 Accountability: pivot of professionalism. In: Gray G, Pratt R (eds) Issues in Australian nursing 2. Churchill Livingstone, Melbourne

Greer G 1971 The female eunuch. Paladin, London

Hazelton M 1990 Medical discourse on contemporary nurse education: an ideological analysis. Australian and New Zealand Journal of Sociology 26(1):107-125

Hearn J 1985 Patriarchy, professionalisation and the semi-professions. In: Ungerson C (ed) Women and social policy: a reader. Macmillan, London

Heide W S 1973 Nursing and women's liberation: a parallel. American Journal of Nursing, May:824-827

Henderson V 1978 The concept of nursing. Journal of Advanced Nursing 3:113-130

Henderson V 1982 Issues and trends in nursing. Royal Prince Alfred Centenary Conference (conference papers) Sydney

Hicks N 1985 The history and politics of legislation for nursing status. Australian Journal of Advanced Nursing, March-May:46-54

Hockey L 1976 Edinburgh University's Nursing Research Unit: the first four years. Journal of Advanced Nursing 1:437-442

Holmes C 1991 Theory: where are we going and what have we missed along the way? In: Gray G, Pratt R (eds) Towards a discipline of nursing. Churchill Livingstone, Melbourne

Hughes E C 1963 Professions. Daedalus 92 (4):647-653

Hughes E C, Hughes H MacG, Deutscher I 1958 Twenty thousand nurses tell their story. Lippincott, Philadelphia

Hughes L 1990 Professionalising domesticity: a synthesis of selected nursing historiography. Advances in Nursing Science 12 (4):25-31

Jacox A 1978 Address to the next generation. Nursing Outlook, January:38-41

James J 1976 Activating theory. The Lamp, May:23-25

Jamous J, Peloille B 1970 Professions or self-perpetuating systems? Changes in the French university hospital system. In: Jackson J (ed) Professions and professionalization. Cambridge University Press, Cambridge

Johnson M M, Martin H W 1958 A sociological analysis of the nurse role. American Journal of Nursing, March:373-377

Johnson T J 1972 Professions and power. Macmillan, London

Johnson T J 1984 Professionalism: occupation or ideology? In: Goodlad S (ed) Education for the professions. Nelson, Guildford

Jones D B, Lawrence J R 1988 Change and professional interactions between nurses and physicians (conference report), Medical Journal of Australia, 4 April:364-365

Kalisch B J, Kalisch P A 1977 An analysis of the sources of physician-nurse conflict. Journal of Nursing Administration, January:51-57

Katz F 1969 Nurses. In: Etzioni A (ed) The semi-professions and their organization. Macmillan, New York

Katz F, Mathews K, Pepe T, White R 1976 Stepping out: nurses and their new roles. University of New South Wales Press, Sydney

Keddy B, Gillis M J, Jacobs P, Burton H, Rogers M 1986 The doctor-nurse relationship: an historical perspective. Journal of Advanced Nursing II:745-753

Kovacs A R 1971 Towards professionalization of nurses. International Nursing Review 18(3):272-279

Kurtz R A, Flaming K H 1963 Professionalism. The case of nurses. American Journal of Nursing, January:75-79

Labelle H 1978 Nursing authority. Journal of Advanced Nursing 3:145-154

Lamb K 1973 Freedom for our sisters, freedom for ourselves: nursing confronts social change. Nursing Forum XII (4):328-352

Lansbury R D 1978 Professionals and management. University of Queensland Press, St Lucia

Larson M S 1977 The rise of professionalism: a sociological analysis. University of California Press, Berkeley

Lawler J 1991a Behind the screens. Churchill Livingstone, Melbourne

Lawler J 1991b In search of an Australian identity. In: Gray G, Pratt R (eds) Towards a discipline of nursing. Churchill Livingstone, Melbourne

Legge D 1979 Nurse education: a contribution to discussion. Australian Nurses Journal, June:42-45

Leininger M 1973 An open health care system model. Nursing Outlook, March:171-175
Lundh U, Soder M, Waerness K 1988 Nursing theories: a critical view. Image. Journal of Nursing Scholarship. Spring 20(1):36-40
Lurie A 1986 Foreign affairs. Abacus, London
Maas M L 1973 Nurse autonomy and accountability in organized nursing services. Nursing Forum XII (3):237-259
McCloskey J C 1981 The professionalisation of nursing: United States and England. International Nursing Review 28(2):40-47
McFarlane J K 1976a The role of research and the develoment of nursing theory. Journal of Advanced Nursing 1:443-451
McFarlane J K 1976b A charter for caring. Journal of Advanced Nursing 1:187-196
McFarlane J K 1977 Developing a theory of nursing: the relation of theory to practice, education and research. Journal of Advanced Nursing 2:261-270
McFarlane J K 1981 Changes in the nature of nursing. Australian Nurses' Journal, November:39-40,44
Maddison D 1977 Coping with crisis: a challenge for the health professions. 11th Patricia Chomley Oration, College of Nursing, Australia, Melbourne
Marles F 1988 Report of the study of professional issues in nursing (F Marles, chairperson). HDV, Melbourne
Melia K 1979 Sociological approach to nursing work. Journal of Advanced Nursing 4:57-67
Melia K 1983 Doing nursing and being professional. Nursing Times 1 June:28-30
Melosh B 1982 'The physician's hand': work, culture and conflict in American nursing. Temple University Press, Philadelphia
Moloney M M 1986 Professionalization of nursing. Lippincott, Philadelphia
Muyskens J L 1982 Moral problems in nursing: a philosophical investigation. Rowman & Littlefield, Totowa, NJ
Najman J A 1974 Asking the unanswerable. (Where is nursing going?). Australian Nurses' Journal, January:35-37
O'Neill A 1991 Enemies within and without: educating chiropractors, osteopaths and traditional acupuncturists. Unpublished PhD thesis, University of New England, Armidale
Oakley A 1984 The importance of being a nurse. Nursing Times, 12 December:24-27
Parker J M 1991 An interpretation of person and environment. In: Gray G, Pratt R (eds) Towards a discipline of nursing. Churchill Livingstone, Melbourne
Parkin F 1979 Marxism and class theory: a bourgeois critique. Tavistock, London
Parsons R 1975 Nurse practitioner as medical assistant. The Lamp, December:15-24
Partridge B 1984 The swinging pendulum of nurse-doctor relationships. Australian Nurses' Journal, February:50-52
Phillips P 1993 A deconstruction of caring. Journal of Advanced Nursing 18:1554-1558
Pittman E 1985 Goodbye Florence. Australian Society, February:8-10
Pratt R 1980 A time to every purpose. 14th Patricia Chomley Oration, College of Nursing Australia, Melbourne
Pratt R 1987 A case study of setting professional standards. Paper given at Royal College of Nursing International Conference: In pursuit of excellence. London, November
Pringle R 1988 Feminist theory and the professions. In: Pittman E (ed) Shaping nursing theory and practice: the Australian context. La Trobe University, Melbourne
Richards J R 1980 The sceptical feminist. Penguin, Harmondsworth
Roberts K L 1980 Nursing: profession or pretender? Australian Nurses' Journal, May: 33-35, 51
Roth J A 1974 Professionalism: the sociologist's decoy. Sociology of work and occupations 1(1):6-23
Russell R L 1991 Are we asking the right questions? In: Gray G, Pratt R (eds) Towards a discipline of nursing. Churchill Livingstone, Melbourne
Salvage J 1985 The politics of nursing. Heinemann, London
Savage J 1987 Nurses, gender and sexuality. Heinemann, London
Shears L W 1964 The characteristics of a profession. UNA Nursing Journal, December:388-391
Shoebridge J 1979 Questioning current attitudes in nursing midwifery. Australian Nurses' Journal, September:44-49

Short S D, Sharman E 1987 The nursing struggle in Australia. Image: journal of nursing scholarship, Winter:197-300

Silva M C, Rothbart D 1984 An analysis of changing trends in philosophies of science on nursing theory development and testing. Advances in nursing science, January:1-13

Slater P V 1974 Nurse practitioner, family practice nurse or physician's assistant. Australian Nurses' Journal, January:31-34

Sleicher M N 1983 Nursing is *not* a profession. In: Duespohl T A (ed) Nursing in transition. Aspen, Maryland

Speedy S 1987 Feminism and the professionalisation of nursing. Australian Journal of Advanced Nursing, 4 (2):20-26

Speedy S 1988 Feminism and nursing: from theory to practice. In: Pittman E (ed) Shaping nursing theory and practice: the Australian context. La Trobe University, Melbourne

Speedy S 1991 The contribution of feminist research. In: Gray G, Pratt R (eds) Towards a discipline of nursing. Churchill Livingstone, Melbourne

Stevens B J 1979 Nursing theory: analysis, application, evaluation. Little, Brown, Boston

Strauss A 1966 The structure and ideology of American nursing: an interpretation. In: Davis F (ed) The nursing profession. Five sociological essays, Wiley, New York

Street A F 1992 Inside nursing: a critical ethnography of clinical nursing practice. State University of New York Press, Albany

Styles M M 1982 On nursing: toward a new endowment. Mosby, St Louis

Styles M M 1987 Professionalism—what is it? In: College of Nursing, Australia, Proceedings of 9th National Conference, Hobart

Summers A 1985 Twin drives for twin needs. Australian Nurses' Journal, May: 37-39

Tellis-Nayak M, Tellis-Nayak V 1984 Games that professionals play: the social psychology of physician-nurse interaction. Social Science and Medicine, 18(12):1063-1069

Thomas L 1983 The youngest science. Viking Press, New York

Tiffany R 1982 Nursing: industry or profession? Australian Nurses' Journal, May:43-45

Turner B S 1985 Knowledge, skill and occupational strategy: the professionalisation of paramedical groups. Community Health Studies IX(1):38-47

Turner B S 1987 Medical power and social knowledge. Sage, London

van Hooft S 1987 Caring and professional commitment. Australian Journal of Advanced Nursing 4 (4):29-3

Watson J 1981 Nursing's scientific quest. Nursing Outlook, July:413-416

Webb C 1987 Professionalism revisited. Nursing Times, 2 September:39-41

White R 1972 The role of the nurse in Australia (Report to the National Health and Medical Research Council). University of New South Wales, Sydney

Wiesel E 1985 Personal communication

Willis E 1983 Medical dominance. The division of labour in Australian health care. George Allen & Unwin, Sydney

Woodruff A 1987 Professionalism—ethics—the basis. In: College of Nursing, Australia, Proceedings of 9th National Conference, Hobart

Zadorosnyj M 1988 Collective mobility strategies in US nursing. Paper given to Medical Sociology Group, La Trobe University, Melbourne, 8 July

3. Nursing education: apprentices to students

> ...the fundamental problem in nursing today is an educational one (Powell 1963).

The 13 000 student nurses in Australia in 1960 were probably unaware of the stirrings for change that were about to affect the education system which had lasted for 100 years since the inauguration of the first Nightingale school in London. A survey carried out around that time of views on nursing, including those of preliminary training school (PTS) nurses, showed that almost half the PTS group still believed that the nurse was born rather than made, and more than half thought personal understanding was a more important quality for the ideal nurse than technical knowledge (Congalton 1962:89-90). That these students should elevate personal qualities over education reflects contemporary popular views about nursing. Inside nursing however there were some who had started to criticise the student nurse's education as inadequate for the demands of the changing hospital scene and even as brutalising for the youthful students:

> I was appalled at what we were doing to school leavers, putting them straight out there into the workforce, and into a totally unstable environment. And the vulnerability of those students, it was just appalling. We lost a lot of good students, potentially good graduates, because they simply didn't have the maturity to deal with the environment of practice plus the student role...[SMcC/88]

Innovative ideas about nursing education had emerged elsewhere by 1960 and were to influence Australian thinking. Some nurses in North America and a very small number in Britain had been educated in universities. The American Nurses' Association (ANA) in 1965 declared its educational standard for professional nursing as a bachelor's degree, with an associate degree for the second level or 'practical' nurse, though most student nurses were still in hospital schools (Olesen & Whittaker 1968:57). A major influence in the 1950s was a series of reports from the World Health Organization (WHO) (Creighton & Lopez 1982:27-32). The implications of these reports for nursing education were that it should be comprehensive (programs should include mental health, paediatric, maternity and community health nursing); that it should incorporate a wide range of subjects including social and behavioural sciences; and that it should take place independently of the service needs of hospitals, preferably in educational institutions such as universities. The nurse who graduated at the end of such an education would be an intellectually and socially aware professional with a wide range of skills.

The holding of the International Council of Nurses (ICN) Congress in Melbourne in 1961 gave a further impetus to change (Russell 1990:150), though not one immediately accepted by Australian nursing. The proposal to alter the rules for membership of ICN by restricting it to countries which provided a 'generalised' (comprehensive) basic course was controversial, inducing 'lengthy and sometimes emotional discussions' (Jayawardena 1962). Although the proposal was defeated at the congress, some prominent Australian nurse educators later supported the idea of comprehensive training.

Even preliminary discussion of such training accentuated the restricted requirements of current nursing courses in Australia, not only in their dearth of such broad experience, but also in the no more than minimal attention they still gave to the psychological and social aspects of illness (Slater 1963). Another profound change implied in the idea was the inclusion of psychiatric nursing, thus bringing it closer to, even integrating it with the higher status general nursing programs. Psychiatric or mental health nursing remained isolated from the mainstream. Mental health and mental retardation nurses still suffered from the general stigma attaching to mental illness and subnormality (Keane 1987:5).

More fundamentally, leading nurses were becoming aware that the present nurse training, as well as lacking breadth, did not even equip nurses for the work they would have to do, given the already noticeable growth in the numbers and complexity of medical specialties in hospitals. As the matron of the Canberra Hospital said,

> At this moment, when every aspect of our hospital service requires well-prepared nursing specialists in each of the diversified fields, the nursing is, in the main, semi-skilled apprentice labour (Guy 1964:114).

In South Australia the Secretary of the Royal Australian Nursing Federation (RANF) branch, Marjorie Ladkin, used the occasion of a College of Nursing, Australia conference in Adelaide to speak out bluntly about the need for higher education standards. The present low standards in her view would 'increasingly repel intelligent girls who are vocationally drawn to [nursing], but unwilling to waste their abilities on a low-status occupation' (Cockburn 1966).

These statements contain both stated and unspoken motives for improving nurse education. One of the effects of the growth of scientific medicine and of its associated technology was that doctors increased their domination of the other (usually female) occupations in the medical division of labour (Willis 1983:202). Nursing's low status was of direct concern to Ladkin who linked it to poor education, while in Guy's case the low status was rather implied by her reference to 'semi-skilled' labour. Nurses needed more education not just to keep up with workplace changes but also to raise the status of their profession if they were to challenge medical supremacy.

There was clearly a case for improvement, but the diversity of nursing conditions between the states and the fragmentation of their organisations made it difficult for nurses to achieve a concerted national effort. Much of the activity over the next 20 years was conditioned by the growth of central (Commonwealth) control of education, and by nurses' realisation that they had to create a national focus to pursue their educational goals since education itself was increasingly a Commonwealth responsibility. Tertiary education in Australia was itself changing in 1960, its function about to be transformed 'from the specialised preparation of intellectual élites to the provision of general education for the middle classes' (Treyvaud & McLaren 1976:25).

Rehearsals for reform

In perhaps the first significant step, the RANF set up in 1959 (with the National Florence Nightingale Committee) the National Nursing Education Division (NNED) headed by Yvonne Jayawardena, an experienced nurse researcher. The federation was thus able to respond effectively when in 1961 the Martin Committee invited it to make a submission. The Prime Minister, R. G. Menzies, had set up this committee to examine the future development of tertiary education in Australia.

The RANF-College of Nursing, Australia submission to the Martin Committee commented on the unsatisfactory nature of the preregistration courses and recommended higher entrance standards, a curriculum of 1500 hours of study to include a much broader range of subjects, a separate budget for nurse education, a nursing program in a university for a select few, and the extension of postregistration education to augment the desperately short supply of qualified nurse teachers (Creighton & Lopez 1982:46-51).

The report that emerged in 1965 did not accept all these recommendations. The Martin Committee, describing the nurse training available in Australia, noted the lack of uniformity between the states, the generally low admission requirements (only 1.6% of entrants to Victorian schools of nursing in 1961 had matriculated), and classified preregistration nurse education (accurately) as 'of a sub-tertiary standard'. The Committee had no hesitation in recommending that undergraduate courses in the various paramedical disciplines such as physiotherapy should be 'of a tertiary status'—not in the universities, whose standards it considered would be too high, but in the colleges of advanced education it was recommending as part of a new 'binary' system of education.

The committee was more encouraging towards post-registration nursing education though its benevolence was limited: the courses at the Colleges of Nursing had 'a particular value', but, in spite of a reported shortage of places to meet demand, the committee did not think that additional colleges should be set up. It did however recommend that the colleges should become 'constituent members of the appropriate Institutes of Colleges', that is, part of tertiary education. It was 'firmly of the opinion that the need for training in vocational nursing should not be met by the universities' (Martin 1964-

65:121-3). The College of Nursing, Australia in Melbourne was approved as an independent college of advanced education in 1965 though it did not become a full member of the Victoria Institute of Colleges until 1970.

Although the RANF submission did not succeed in its immediate aim, the educational system that developed from the Martin Report was crucial for nursing since it created the college or advanced education sector within tertiary education, and it was this sector that accepted nursing, something that even now some universities are reluctant to do except when forced by the demise of the binary system.

The Martin Committee was itself the Menzies (Coalition) Government's response to continuing pressure for the expansion of tertiary education. It recommended that although such an expansion was desirable for continued economic growth by producing enough trained manpower, it should not be confined to the universities but should take place also through existing institutions such as senior technical and teachers' colleges. The Commonwealth government welcomed this suggestion, partly because it promised funding economies. But this expansion through diversity led to continuing confusion and overlap of function between the two kinds of institution in spite of efforts to maintain a distinction by claiming that colleges were more vocationally oriented, had an applied emphasis, and that their staff regarded teaching rather than research as their major priority. A similar overlap existed in England where a binary system was also developing after the 1965 Robbins Report, but Robbins had rejected British nursing in spite of its small presence in higher education.

A leading Queensland nurse educator later observed that the diversification which had occurred in tertiary education was 'intimately related to the aspirations of the nursing profession' (Godfrey 1978). The creation of the college sector widened the opportunities for occupational training programs in higher education, but it did so by adding another kind of institution ('equal but cheaper') which in effect left the universities at the apex of the system. The distinction between the university and college sectors was in fact one of status and difference in the social background of their students (Treyvaud & McLaren 1976:7-13). It was this actual as well as the claimed vocational distinction which enabled nursing to establish itself in the college sector. This left it still in a structurally inferior position to medicine which of course continued exclusively in the universities.

The RANF-College of Nursing, Australia submission to the Martin Committee, while not acted on as they wanted, was widely circulated and thus helped leading nurses to become more aware of the problems and possible solutions in nursing education (Creighton & Lopez 1982:57). After this disappointment nurses in most states began work on new curricula with more hours of theory. They thus accepted for the moment that although postregistration education would eventually be eligible for the tertiary sector, preregistration training would remain in the hospitals. Yet as the NNED Director remembers,

> ...they were never really discouraged. They just got up, dusted themselves off, and got into battle again. Of course, in the meantime you had all the schools in the hospitals getting fairly well educated tutors from the college, and they took up the battle...[YJ/90]

Further support for improved standards in nurse education came during the 1960s from conferences held jointly by the various state nurse registration boards. These encouraged common standards, broader course content, a lower teacher-student ratio, and a year 11 entry level. Another WHO Report, from the Fifth Expert Committee on Nursing, was published in 1966. Again, WHO provided a vision of the benefits higher standards of nursing education could bring both in the workplace and to nursing at large: a much broader education to include preventive and rehabilitative aspects of care, and to cover patients' psychosocial as well as physical needs; and a welcome (if optimistic) assertion that nurses were no longer subservient but complementary to the doctor, that they should be educated for creative and critical thinking, and have the same education as other professionals—that is, in tertiary institutions free from the service pressures of the hospital (Creighton & Lopez 1982:52-6).

It was at this time that the decade of reports began. For the next 10 years leading nurses in the various states were constantly either sitting on committees of inquiry into aspects of nursing, including education, or digesting the subsequent reports and recommendations of those committees and commenting on them to their colleagues. The numerous reports that appeared from 1967-78 especially in New South Wales were initiated and conducted by a variety of state government bodies and nursing organisations, and finally by the federal government. It is clear from the analyses of Russell (1990), Creighton and Lopez (1982), and Wood (1990) that these reports agreed about the problems in nursing education, but that there were important differences between them in the solutions they proposed.

Many of the problems discussed had their origin in the so-called apprenticeship system, the 'earn while you learn' training that went back to the days of Florence Nightingale, though Nightingale herself had wanted autonomous schools of nursing with education taking precedence over service. The problems were by now familiar. Australian research confirmed that the result of this training was that the newly graduated nurse did not function as effectively as she could have in her work (Pilkington 1972). An English study of the time found:

> The learner in the hospital is never sure whether she is a 'student' or a 'nurse' and suffers from insecurity in both roles. The registered nurse and the enrolled nurse finds that her qualification is valued, to a greater or less degree within the nursing and medical professions but has no currency in the field of higher education. The overall pattern of recruitment to nursing and withdrawal from training is closely bound up with these general considerations (MacGuire 1969:122).

Nurse training was inadequate precisely because it took place in hospitals. The student nurse was at a three-fold disadvantage: her education was effectively shorter than that for many other professions since it was subject to service demands; it was intellectually impoverished since it was isolated from education in general; and ironically, despite its hospital base, it did not even equip her for the demands of her own expanding job within acute care. Even less did it prepare her for the developing field of community health.

Nurses themselves were becoming frustrated. In 1966 in New South Wales they were reported to be threatening strike action, and the Deputy Leader of the Opposition in state parliament called for a select committee to inquire into nurses' conditions of work and training, and into 'the shortage of young women applying to be trained in hospitals'. This proposal was defeated by the Askin (Liberal) State Government, although the Premier, like many politicians of the time, went through the usual ritual of claiming to have 'a great deal of sympathy and admiration for nurses and for the dedicated work they perform' (*NSWPD* 10 August 1967:361-4).

At the federal level unrest among Canberra nurses in 1970 precipitated a debate in the House of Representatives which demonstrated that at least some MPs were aware of the current issues. Labor (Opposition) member Bill Hayden (who actually used the then daring word 'womanpower') criticised the Gorton (Coalition) Government for 'only now getting round to' some of the proposals which had been made for change, and referred to the high 'wastage' (drop-out) rates in hospital programs. Labor members Gun and Reynolds supported tertiary education for nurses, linking it with professional status and recognition. The Minister for Health, Dr Forbes, while stressing the responsibility of the states for nursing, admitted that there might have to be 'a change in emphasis' from hospital training. Government member Cameron voiced a more conventional view when he attacked the Leader of the Opposition, E. G. Whitlam, for making a political speech to the nurses who had gathered outside Parliament House: far from being anything as unseemly as political, nurses were 'on the whole a bunch of very attractive women' who would inevitably get married, so that wastage from training programs was 'normal', he said (*CPD* 20 May 1970:2391-2403). The demonstration in this exchange that the Opposition Australian Labor Party (ALP) might have a more sympathetic attitude than the government to nursing problems was an intimation of future events.

If there was some agreement about the problems, disagreement about solutions revolved around the apprenticeship system itself—whether to keep it, with modifications, as the New South Wales matrons (Sax 1978:9) and the medical profession wished, or to move right away from it into tertiary institutions as a growing number of reports later recommended with varying enthusiasm. The opposing sides for and against the traditional system had already formed, as in any occupation on the eve of reform: educators conscious of new knowledge and research advocated changes; practitioners with the daily responsibility of patient care wanted to keep the system they believed reliable and effective (Olesen & Whittaker 1968:58-9).

A false dawn for tertiary nursing

University education for a few nurses had already begun. In 1967 the New South Wales Nurses' Registration Board agreed to finance a combined university and nursing course at the University of New England, followed the next year by one at the University of New South Wales. This was an experimental scheme which aimed, as the state Minister for Education said, to find out 'what can be done to attract highly educated girls into nursing...' and to recognise 'the increasing importance of the profession and the burden to be carried by the more senior people on the nursing staffs of our hospitals' (*NSWPD* 22 October 1968:1866). The scheme however admitted very small numbers and failed to integrate the two parts of the course, so that the nursing component was not taught at university level. This was unsatisfactory to leading nurses, who were already determined that nursing must be part of the academic curriculum rather than being seen as merely a set of occupational tasks (Slater 1970). The existence of such a course also led some politicans, including the New South Wales Minister for Health, to assume that a higher tier of tertiary trained nurses was being created, 'a small group of people who will provide the higher echelons' (*NSWPD* 28 March 1973:4145-53). The combined degree program was closed down in 1975 having graduated 54 students but with a wastage rate of 50% (Russell 1990:181-5).

In 1969 the College of Nursing, Australia proposed a pilot three-year preregistration program at its Melbourne headquarters, which should then become a single purpose college of advanced education (College of Nursing, Australia 1969). In the same year the authors of a Victorian study stressed the shortage of nurses as an urgent issue for the whole hospital system. They discussed the 'world wide phenomenon' of high wastage rates for trainees, and the high drop out rate of graduate nurses from the workforce. The medical author (who later co-wrote the 1970 report on nursing in Tasmania) suggested among a number of other ideas that the academically gifted student nurse could be relieved of some routine duties so that she could undertake single university subjects (Lawson 1969), a measure likely to encourage the formation of a professional élite.

This idea of an élite minority of tertiary educated nurses dates from the time when the only alternative to hospital programs was either university or technical education (Jayawardena 1961), and was perhaps encouraged by the development of the Colleges of Nursing which could educate only very small numbers. But some senior Australian nurses had decided that higher education for a minority only was not what they wanted. In 1970 Pat Slater, then Director of the College of Nursing, Australia rejected the implied élitism of a recent ACT report on nursing which recommended a higher level education for a small group of specialists. She believed this would neither 'attract and retain in the profession adequate numbers of nurses of the calibre needed, nor...enable quality nursing care to be provided' (Slater 1970). The following year she criticised the Victorian Ramsay Report for the same reason, pointing out that 'if adequate nursing services are to be maintained the first priority must be to improve the lot of the majority' (Slater 1971). In 1972 the RANF also supported an anti-élitist position (editorial, *ANJ* October:5). The leaders were to hold firmly to this principle throughout the reform process. In this they were part of an Australian egalitarian tradition which distinguishes them from their US and British colleagues.

A small step for education...

The New South Wales Truskett Committee Report of 1970, in the most radical Australian document of the time on the subject, concluded that nurse training should be re-oriented towards tertiary education, through nursing colleges of advanced education (including the NSW College of Nursing), and regional groupings of nursing schools affiliated with colleges, and that these institutions should come under an education authority, a Nurses' Education Board under the Minister for Education. The registering and educative functions of the Nurses' Registration Board would therefore become the responsibility of two separate authorities (Russell 1990:119). Over 20 years earlier a member of the English Wood Committee on nursing had commented: '...it is difficult to see why nursing should be unique among professions in dissociating control of teaching from the control of examining' (Cohen 1948:44). With the Truskett recommendations one authority would approve and examine courses, while another would register nurses. An editorial in the *Medical Journal of Australia* (13 September 1969) agreed that nursing education should move away from dominance by service needs, though it assumed that student nurses would continue to fulfil those needs. It opposed strongly as 'going to the other extreme with very unhappy results' the proposal to remove control of nursing education from the registration board, claiming that there was 'ample precedent' for registration and education being controlled by the same body—but not of course in medical education. Not all nurses were persuaded of the value of a transfer to the education portfolio, some fearing control instead by educators who would not appreciate the importance of nursing to the curriculum (Russell 1990:119-121). This was an early expression of their determination not to exchange hospital control of their education for an academic yoke.

The New South Wales Liberal Government went ahead with the Nurses' Education Board (NEB) proposal. The Minister for Health had said earlier that the government wished to see nurse education 'at a number of levels in different institutions', including universities, CAEs, regional schools, and 'for the time being', in some hospitals (Jago 1972). The Minister for Education, (later Sir) Eric Willis, commenting on the Truskett recommendations for tertiary education, said that the government had examined them closely but had concluded that while possibly desirable in the long term there was neither the money nor the personnel to implement them at the time, though like his colleagues the Minister professed his gratitude to nurses for their 'dedication to duty'. A future Labor Minister for Education, Eric Bedford, worried that the powers of the board were vague, so that other educational bodies could intrude: 'who will win', he wondered, 'when it comes to a knock-down, drag-out tussle about what the nurse education courses will be'. Willis assured members that the NEB would be superior to other bodies when it came to nurse education, with a supervisory task 'although this is not spelled out in so many words' (*NSWPD* 28 March 1973:4139-58). A future NEB executive commented at the time that the board had no effective power, and that nurses were 'angry and resentful' (McGrath 1973). She comments further on the government's intentions:

> When it was set up it's really my belief that what was intended was that it would sort of be a debating society, that it wouldn't do very much, that it wouldn't rock the boat. But I think what the politicians hadn't anticipated was that the Board would *work*. But the Board—of course it consisted of nurses—had pretty much in mind where it wanted to go, that it wanted to go into the tertiary sector...[MMcG/89]

The NSW medical profession continued its objections to the NEB and to educational change: 'while student nurses are providing service—and there is no argument that the best nurse is produced through training at the bedside—the Minister for Health should retain the responsibility for nurse education' (Larkins 1972); 'no argument' in medical circles perhaps.

In Victoria the Ramsay Committee, set up to look at the implications of the Victorian Nursing Council's proposed 1600 hour curriculum, endorsed in its 1970 report only a shortened version of that curriculum. It did not suggest that control of nursing education should move from the health portfolio, but it did take up the College of Nursing suggestion for a 'pilot' preregistration college course. The Royal Victorian College of Nursing (RVCN) concentrated on its 1600 hour curriculum and succeeded in persuading the new Minister for Health in the Bolte (Liberal) State Government to adopt it, though it was not fully implemented for some years. A Queensland committee considered that the traditional inservice education was no longer appropriate, and that CAE education should be explored (Saint 1971).

In most states nursing authorities began to lengthen the theory hours in nursing courses, which kept the old system going but at the same time made it more costly. As a Western Australian nurse pointed out, the hospital funded the school and its teaching staff and paid the student nurses for their services, but this service component was expensive since over half the students' time was spent in the classroom and 'the nursing care these students give is inexpert and requires constant supervision by instructors' (Lambert 1975).

Both the Truskett and Ramsay Committees also gave some thought to nursing aides. Courses should be extended, they said, but should remain in hospitals and the aide should be renamed the 'enrolled nurse' thus becoming a second level nurse. Mainstream nursing continued to oppose any elevation of the nursing aide to a recognised position (Slater 1971), but this was to change within a few years.

The many reports at this time, in all states and in the ACT, led to only limited progress: New South Wales set up the NEB in 1973, though effective control of nursing education remained in the health portfolio; and curriculum hours were lengthened in hospital programs. These modest gains did not satisfy the demands of the pro-tertiary nurses, but they did at least begin to shift the focus of discussion towards tertiary education so that the hospital based system now had to be defended rather than taken for granted.

...and the first step in the transfer

It was significant for nursing that the Whitlam Labor Government, elected in late 1972, a year later assumed full responsibility for the cost of higher education and considerable control over its constituent parts. In 1974 the Commonwealth government agreed to set up six preregistration nursing courses as pilot programs. The first of these, at the College of Nursing, Australia in Melbourne, had already started in that year, funded partly by the college itself (Wood 1990:165, 171).

By developing in the college sector nursing education achieved more autonomy than if it had had to battle for a university place, a goal which would have taken longer to achieve. Further, university education would have been for a minority of nurses only and an education overshadowed by proximity to more established professions. In colleges the nursing content had more chance of remaining the central focus of the programs. Yet at this time there were doubts about the feasibility of aiming right away for tertiary education for all nurses, however desirable that was as an ultimate goal. Pat Slater considered it unrealistic to think that college courses could produce the numbers required without an enormous increase in qualified nurse educators, and believed that any transfer to colleges must be done 'very, very gradually to avoid disruption of nursing services' (Slater 1970). This was a politically astute view which would help calm the fears and potential hostility of the matrons and the medical profession. Robin Parsons, of the NSW College of Nursing, believed that a 'wholesale change' from the hospital based system would eventually happen 'though probably not in my lifetime' and that a proportion should attend colleges in the meantime (Parsons 1973a). With so far still to go, it must have seemed impossible to avoid creating an élite, at least temporarily.

New South Wales now took what appeared to be a divergent path by adopting a policy of group or regional schools of nursing, as both the Matrons' and the Truskett Reports had recommended. The first school was established in the Newcastle and Hunter region, and became controversial by being part of Technical and Further Education (TAFE) (Russell 1990:175-6). Nursing objections to this were inevitable, given the NSW College of Nursing's refusal in 1967 to join the proposed Paramedical Institute, partly because it was to be responsible to TAFE and would therefore lack the autonomy of a college (Parsons 1973b). Some objections to the TAFE affiliation took on a political character, as a New South Wales nurse educator describes it:

> The TAFE Newcastle course started to get off the ground. I drew up a petition...I was trying to get everyone, all the hospitals, to run bits and pieces off, to run off this jolly petition to the Minister for Health. I think we got 4800 signatures, which was not a *bad* showing. It said 'No TAFE. Only UG2 [diploma] and in colleges'. [CH/89]

The secretary of the New South Wales Nurses' Association (NSWNA) on the contrary welcomed the Newcastle program, referring to it as 'one of various forms of training envisaged by the Minister for Education' (editorial, *The Lamp,* May 1972). This support for the TAFE policy was probably influenced by the threat to the association's membership base of a total college transfer. The controversy suggests also a degree of class distinction: at least higher education would separate nursing from all connection with merely technical occupations.

In spite of the New South Wales 'maverick' action, Australian nursing in 1973 could rely on a promising foundation for its next venture, the uniting of its senior organisations to frame the 'goals in nursing education'. The college sector was established and included postregistration nursing; a preregistration course was about to begin and others would follow; at the same time the curriculum in the hospital courses was becoming longer and the training therefore more expensive; and a national government more sympathetic to nursing aims was assuming responsibility for higher education. The Whitlam (Labor) Government was also the first in Australia to set up an office specifically to address women's issues, and the first to give official encouragement to projects designed to raise the status of women.

Among nursing leaders there was also agreement that education reform was the most significant goal to pursue. Robin Parsons, assessing the various New South Wales reports, was 'particularly impressed by the reform movement's preoccupation with the question of nurse education'. She saw the deficiencies of that education as 'without any doubt, the major weakness of our profession' and a barrier to professional status (Parsons 1971). The same year Merle Parkes of the College of Nursing, Australia challenged her colleagues to establish goals and to implement a course of action to achieve them. 'What the profession does in the next ten years may well determine its entire future', Parkes warned in a farsighted statement:

> Only by improving nursing education, do we improve the quality of nursing service, raise the public image of nursing and attract recruits to the profession. Education can no longer be regarded as a luxury, it is essential to our survival (Parkes 1971).

If improved education was the major goal, then Parkes realised that to achieve it nursing must become 'a co-ordinated profession' which would be able to develop a program for the future 'giving nurses a sense of direction and purpose'. Many of the nurses leading the education reform movement at this time were unusual in that, like Parkes, they had gained university degrees and understood higher education's potential benefits for their present and future colleagues (Parsons 1978). For many other nurses, undertaking a course at one of the colleges was a formative experience, and although there were few graduates among the total number of working nurses they formed at least a potential source of support in the coming 'reformation' (Parsons 1971).

Leading nurses were also very much aware of the continual questioning and turmoil which had come out of the many reports and inquiries going back to 1966. They wanted to take control of all this seemingly random activity 'and make it goal-directed and purposeful' (Lambert 1975). They knew also that Australian nursing was behind developments elsewhere, though this did not lead to a mere cultural cringe. Other systems were critically assessed: some university courses for nurses in the US, for example, were unsatisfactory since their nursing content was inferior; but at least the US had 'a clear plan for integrating professional nursing education into the general education stream' (Slater 1969). The final impetus to action was the 1973 report of the Commission on Advanced Education which excused government inaction on the grounds that there was confusion among nurses about what should be the future of nursing education (Patten 1980).

Grouping around the 'goals'

It was therefore a propitious time for leading nurses to direct their efforts to the national scene. To do that they had to combine some previously separate forces, both federal and state. Fortunately a major step had already been taken with the unification in 1970 of the RANF, which set up the new national Australian Nurses' Journal (ANJ), though the powerful New South Wales Nurses' Association remained an independent force, also with its own journal (Ch. 5). The then RANF federal secretary looks back at this period:

> The nurses from Canberra put a resolution on the books for a [RANF] Federal Council meeting, that we look at nursing education, where it was going...then it was really Joan Godfrey [Queensland nurse educator] who took it up and said 'It has to be the three organisations. We can't do it on our own. Let's involve College of Nursing, Australia, and the National Florries'. [MP/91]

The Canberra stimulus originated in a two-year pilot program at the Canberra Hospital which gave priority to students' learning needs so that service and education were to some degree separate (Fellows 1971). The subsequent banding together of the major organisations not only created a significant force, it also had the potential to defuse any political attempts to divide and rule, as a Northern Territory nurse saw:

> That had an awful lot to do with the strides that were made, because it meant that nursing was at last speaking with one voice...[politicians] couldn't say 'Well, *you* might say that, but the RANF doesn't'....they had solidarity there to convince politicians...[KR/90]

The 'goals in nursing education' emerged from a working party made up of nominees from four organisations: the RANF; the College of Nursing, Australia; the New South Wales College of Nursing; and the National Florence Nightingale Committee (the Florries). The Working Party (chaired by Mary Patten, RANF Federal secretary) then commissioned Tasmanian nurse Shirley Donaghue to carry out a national survey. Donaghue interviewed 60 key nurses for part one of the report, published in April 1975.

The first document to appear, in February 1975, was Goals in Nursing Education Part II. This was the working party's report. It acknowledged limitations in its scope and the need for further research but boldly set out a five stage program (1974-91) for moving nurse education out of hospitals and regional schools and into the general education system 'during the years 1975-1985'. At least one nurse educator appreciated the plan's audacity:

> The 'goals' statement was a very clever thing—putting that date on it. And yet people didn't want a date on it. Sure, you were looking that far ahead...[CH/89]

The stated aim of the plan combined improving the quality of nursing care; and seeing that nursing education was equivalent to that of other personnel in the health team. In International Women's Year, nurses were beginning to take up some of the claims of the new women's movement, so that they openly attacked the lower standard of nursing education compared with that for other health professions, by implication male-dominated medicine in particular.

Other notable recommendations in the 'goals' were that by 1986 there should be only two levels of nurse, the professional nurse educated in CAEs and universities, and the state enrolled nurse (SEN), educated in TAFE—that is, the lower level nurse was now accepted, but not the unqualified; that psychiatric and mental deficiency nursing courses should become part of the basic general course in recognition of the lessening division between the two kinds of nursing (perhaps too optimistic a view at the time); and that postgraduate education should be developed both for general nurses and for the various specialties, even to the level of 'post-master's degree programmes...by 1991', a visionary idea in 1975.

The working party presented its recommendations to the profession at a national conference in Melbourne in July 1975. This conference brought together 280 nurses from around the country. Pat Slater discussed the first aim of moving all nursing education into the general education system, in carefully planned stages, confirming that this meant colleges and perhaps universities. In a clear reference to New South Wales, Slater rejected 'sub-tertiary level programmes' in TAFE as being no more advantageous to the profession than remaining in hospitals. The working party had however seen TAFE as a suitable site for improved 'auxiliary nurse' courses: the SEN was carefully distinguished from the professional nurse by her lower level of nursing knowledge and responsibility (*ANJ* 1975 August:7-27). Nursing leaders still wished to keep the profession away from the taint of technical education, but saw it as suitable for raising the status of the second level group.

Merle Parkes related the specific proposals of the 'goals' to the wider scene, referring to contemporary changes and problems in the health system. She concluded that 'Nursing is irretrievably involved in social change and nurses are inescapably affected by political pressures', showing the profession's new awareness of the need to pursue its aims through political means. Parkes also endorsed a view of education seldom heard among nurses at that time: that it could provide 'opportunities for enrichment of life in cultural and intellectual dimensions' (*ANJ* 1975 August:7-27). Most of the educational debate concentrated in fact on what education could contribute to nursing and to nursing practice. It was seen primarily as a means to a worthy end and only rarely as an end in itself. Perhaps this was inevitable after a century of life in an educational ghetto. This instrumental view was also a necessity for the leaders of the campaign, who wanted to persuade reluctant colleagues of the benefits they would receive. A nurse present at the conference sums up:

> Everyone got a go at what they wanted. Now I went with one thing in mind: there could be nothing less than a UG2, and the nursing aides had to go...We came away—we didn't win the aides, but we won the minimum UG2...All the big ones [leaders] were there, but it really was a free-for-all. [CH/89]

The Melbourne conference was followed by a series of workshops in the states at which 'practitioners, students and auxiliaries...determined the preferred direction for the development of nursing education'. Nursing opinion at these workshops then contributed to the policy statements on the 'goals' issued by the four collaborating bodies the following year (*ANJ* 1976 April:10-14).

It is clear from the discussion of the policy statements that the diploma or UG2 was the minimum level of tertiary award nurses would accept. One controversy had however become acute: psychiatric nurses did not agree that the aim of a comprehensive course could be achieved satisfactorily in a three year program, and they would continue this stand. It had also become clear that changes in the mental handicap field had produced uncertainty, so that policies for those nurses had to be deferred. The policy statement also left out the dates which had struck such a bold if risky note in the original 'goals'—nurses at the workshops had judged the dates to be unrealistic. They had also queried the clinical competence of the tertiary graduate, a question that was to recur.

In spite of these inevitable reservations the document 'Goals in nursing education policy statements' is remarkable for its time, the product of three years of intense study and discussion and of an unprecedented degree of unity within nursing, at least in its senior ranks. The statement was remarkable also for providing the guiding principles of a campaign which eventually carried Australian nursing to a position of political consciousness and influence which would have seemed impossible to the committed pioneers of the early 1970s. Yet there was scarcely any press or medical comment on the 'goals' and no reaction from the NSWNA, then preoccupied with a pay dispute and an imminent state election (below).

The long march begins

The organisation which conducted what became eventually an active campaign for the transfer of nurse education was set up after a further national workshop in November 1976, which put forward a single goal:

> By 1985 all basic nursing programmes which prepared professional nurses to be conducted by multi-discipline institutions at a level not less than a tertiary diploma (UG2) and provide both breadth of education and comprehensive nursing preparation.

Rightly describing this statement as 'historic', an editorial reflected that it was in fact the culmination of 50 years of discussion and debate on the education question, adding with some irony that 'overnight success is invariably a lengthy and complex phenomenon' (*ANJ* February 1977).

The November conference set up a widely representative structure for implementing the 'goals' with state and territory task forces, representatives from the nursing organisations, and three from mental health nursing. There was also to be a three person National Steering Committee (NSC) with Pat Slater, Mary Patten and Sister Paulina Pilkington (for the National Florence Nightingale Committee) to keep in touch with state activities and co-ordinate the nationwide effort. The state task forces would continue the work of 'involving nurses throughout the country in the whole process of change'. The nurses at this meeting recognised that this structure would have to establish and maintain lines of communication in two major directions: with nurses at large, especially to keep them informed of the implications of the proposed change; and with state and national political bodies. Initial priorities were, first, to make submissions to the two state inquiries and one national inquiry into education which were then in train; and, second, to oppose the New South Wales regional schools/TAFE policy (*ANJ* 1977 February:12-16).

Having reached such a degree of consensus on the educational goal and having established a potentially effective organisation for achieving it (Cochrane 1989:28), nurses saw it as a setback, as Russell points out (1990:161), that the Fraser (Coalition) Government had taken over in Canberra and ushered in a period of budgetary restraint that would affect developments in both health and education. In fact, it was already clear at a Goals in Nursing Education conference held in Canberra in late November 1975, just after the dismissal of the Whitlam Government, that whatever the government in power, economic conditions would have dictated restraint. The chairmen of the Universities Commission (Karmel) and of the National Hospitals and Health Services Commission (Sax) both warned that a transfer of nurse education to colleges had serious cost implications (Duke 1975:16-17).

After the advances of the previous three years it was probably inevitable that nursing leaders would see the new government as less sympathetic to their aims than Labor had been. A task force member has referred to 'obstructive tactics' between 1977 and 1983 (Cochrane 1989:29). The Fraser Government was certainly cautious, especially about government expenditure, and reluctant to embark on any expensive changes, but the impatient task forces, like the leaders of all radical movements, would probably have seen any hesitation as deliberate obstruction.

Nurses on the attack in the states

Further illustrating the spirit of unity, a new group had become active in New South Wales. The Nursing Organisations Representative Committee (NORC), formed in December 1974 by the councils of the NSW College, the small RANF state branch, the NSWNA and the Matrons' Institute, directed its efforts to keeping a watching brief on policies affecting professional issues in nursing, and to communicating its findings to nurses and its views to government. One of the NORC activists remembers:

> We also decided that we would act as a lobbying group, and we decided we would take ourselves off to see the [Liberal state] government. We were treated like children, like kindergarten children, by Pickard who was then Minister for Education—Willis had just become Premier. We said 'Blow this!' so we took ourselves off to the [Labor] Opposition. [CH/89].

Kevin Stewart, then shadow Minister for Health, proved more receptive to NORC's demands. The ALP Health Committee agreed that if Labor won the election due in May 1976 it would implement an NEB report which the Askin Government thought too 'revolutionary' (Russell 1990:125), and increase nursing representation in the state Health Commission and on the Nurses' Registration Board. The ALP had championed nursing representation at the time the NEB was set up, though Kevin Stewart had not then been particularly enthusiastic about tertiary education for nurses (*NSWPD* 28 March 1973:4147-50), but the significance of the new unity among these organisations was not lost on the politicians:

> Kevin Stewart said, the political impact it made, getting a letter...with all those four organisations named on the top of it, and that landing on a politican's desk (he was in opposition at that stage)—the effect of that was just absolutely tremendous: 'Hullo, hullo! they've all got their act together!' [CH/89]

As another NSW nurse says: 'It was a *collective* battle'. [JH/89]

Early in 1976 NORC had another dispiriting meeting with Pickard. The minister foreshadowed 'further enquiry and research' (this after a decade of reports) and gave NORC the impression that the Liberal Government would support 'various types (levels) of nursing education programmes such as the proposed development of a technical education program in the Illawarra Region'. NORC described this as 'an insult to the NEB and to the nurses of New South Wales' (*ANJ* 1976 May:45) and intensified its activities in the weeks before the NSW election:

> We got printing done, and we ran off these papers, and we flooded them out through everyone, with a document of what the politicians said they would and they wouldn't do, when the election was called. That's how that came about, 'Vote One Nursing Education'...Kevin Stewart has admitted that it did have an effect [on the election] [CH/89].

The NSWNA Secretary, M. V. ('Ronnie') Henlen, though not always an enthusiastic supporter of NORC, did champion its cause this time. In an apparent change of heart, she attacked the latest TAFE proposal: '...the same old twenty-year-old programme, not even remotely geared for 1976...Who do the government think they are fooling?' she demanded. 'Nowadays nurses are not even given a hackneyed promise of a better deal...Let us hope that the revolt on the way will not be too long in coming'. It wasn't, and after the Wran ALP victory Henlen welcomed the new government's assurance that it would keep its pre-election promises which she considered had 'significantly influenced many nurses to vote [Labor], many for the first time in their lives'. Speaking to NSWNA members the following year, Neville Wran confirmed that his government's aim was 'to ensure that nurse education gradually becomes integrated into the education system as a whole', but he emphasised the gradual transition (*The Lamp* 1976 March:3:August:3,1977 August:11-12).

NORC's success showed that nurses could act effectively in the political arena and that New South Wales nursing was not as far away from the 'goals' as the other states sometimes feared. The NSW College of Nursing was not represented on the NSC, but its President, Judith van der Wal, continued the college's support for the 'goals' (*ANJ* 1980 November:17-18). Even the regional schools system eventually took a more acceptable direction. In 1977 the NEB's then Executive Officer, the late Betty Lyons, said that in the face of the Commonwealth (Coalition) government's 'constraints' on college education the NEB saw the regional schools as 'an interim measure' until all nursing was in CAEs, and as a measure that would 'facilitate' that eventual transfer (Lyons 1978). The lure of tertiary education being promoted nationally had obviously diminished the appeal of TAFE courses. The advent of the Wran Labor Government in 1976 when the ALP was in eclipse elsewhere in Australia gave NSW nurses' hopes a further boost, though such is the nature of the federal system that this could not last for long in isolation.

When the NSC and the state task forces set out on their campaign in 1976-77, the prospect appeared less hopeful politically than when the working party had begun its discussions a few years earlier. Still, there were five preregistration nursing diploma courses running at CAEs: two in Victoria and one each in South Australia, New South Wales and in Western Australia. All except two had been in Colleges of Nursing which transferred their educational programs to multidisciplinary CAEs, with the College in Melbourne the last to do so. Tertiary nursing was now in line with the 'goals' statement, and with the 1973 Cohen Report on teacher education which had recommended that small colleges should amalgamate with larger institutions (Godfrey 1978). A further circumstance favouring nursing was the decline in teacher education, so that some colleges opportunistically saw nursing as a possible replacement which would maintain their funding (Durdin 1991:194).

Developments in some states were disappointing: the 1976 Livingstone Committee in Queensland recommended three-year diploma programs in higher education institutions, but the Bjelke-Petersen (Liberal-Country Party) state government decided not to act on this until there was Commonwealth funding. The Minister for Health (Sir William Knox) agreed with a government member who said that 'nurse education should take place in hospitals, because they are the best place for those engaged in that caring profession to learn their duties' (*QPD* 16 October 1979:1052-5). A nurse member of the Livingstone Committee recalls the opposition:

> Nurses were a cheap form of labour...and after all you don't need [tertiary education], you need dear little girls who know how to give a bedpan and feed a patient and make them comfortable, and that was it...there was this attitude permeating the Health Department, from the Director-General down, because he said 'Over my dead body!'—the number of times that was said to me, ultimately by the Minister. [JG/91]

The Tasmanian inquiry in 1970 had recommended higher education for a minority of nurses only (Wood 1990:161-2), and in the West the Federal Commission on Advanced Education had refused to approve the innovative four-year pre-registration degree set up by Merle Parkes at the Western Australian Institute of Technology (WAIT) even when it was modified to three years. This led to a bitter dispute between the Commission and the nursing organisations (Parkes 1986; Wood 1990:172-7). Some nurses later regretted what they saw as a lost opportunity to introduce a preregistration degree: '...we nearly had a basic degree course back in 1975...Why was it that the profession, the College of Nursing Australia, and I, personally, did not support [Merle Parkes] more?' (Slater 1982). As Slater's NSC colleague, Mary Patten, recalls, one reason goes back to old rivalries which the new national unity had not entirely buried:

> I really regret that nurses in Australia weren't able to push that through at that time...I don't think they pushed it as hard as they could have...that's the way

we could have won it. But...there was no way the nurses in this country were going to get behind a course in Western Australia. That was over *there!* And if it had been in Victoria it would have been no better, because New South Wales wouldn't have supported it...*we* lost that, nurses lost that...It was a hard climate, but climates are always hard. There's no such thing as 'the right time'...[MP91]

The question of whether nurses could have succeeded in the late 1970s in 'leap frogging' over the proposed diploma to a degree is now hypothetical, but it remains as a regret for what might have been.

In New South Wales the scene was more promising. The new Wran Government provided $2.7 million for a longer (1000 hour) curriculum and Kevin Stewart, now Minister for Health, said that from 1980 the Higher School Certificate would be the entry requirement for nurse training. In 1977 the Minister for Education, Eric Bedford, announced that an interdepartmental committee would oversee the gradual transfer of responsibility for nurse education to his portfolio, but on the question of further tertiary education programs the Minister had to admit that there was a 'significant constraint' on developing further courses, since the federal government had decided not to fund any 'pending the outcome of a review it had recently initiated' (*NSWPD* 30 November 1977:1071).

The campaign goes national

The review referred to was the Sax inquiry into nurse education, set up by the federal Minister for Education, J. L. Carrick. Announcing the government's decision to set up the inquiry, Senator Carrick acknowledged 'increasing pressures from the nursing profession and from colleges of advanced education for the movement of basic nurse education and training out of hospitals into the tertiary education system'. The Minister realised however that this would have 'widespread implications' for both health and education, so the government wished to have 'detailed advice on the options for varying the present arrangements' (Sax 1978:2). Detailed advice was available in quantities after the decade of reports, but these were state reports and the federal government inevitably wanted more information before it would even consider such a major change.

The nursing organisations had taken the initiative in establishing a unified national stand, so the national government sooner or later had to respond, especially since the nursing bodies had chosen education as their focus and higher education had become federal business. Leading nurses had made a clever move in 1973 by combining the new unity with a focus on education, whether or not they realised that fully at the time. Also, in 1975 the new Medibank health insurance scheme's arrangements for funding hospitals meant that half the cost of nursing education was now a direct Commonwealth burden rather than wholly in the state budgets.

There were three senior nurses on the Sax Committee of Inquiry into Nurse Education and Training: Mary Patten for the RANF; Judy Porter from the South Australian Health Commission; and Sister Paulina Pilkington (who had made a significant contribution to the earlier New South Wales Truskett Report) from the Commonwealth Department of Health. Of the other eight members of the committee, four, including the chairman, were medical practitioners (though Dr Sidney Sax was also an experienced bureaucrat and policy adviser), two were from educational bodies, and two were public servants. The committee's deliberations took place at the same time that the 'Goals in nursing education' state task forces and the NSC were setting about their work of persuading nurses that tertiary education was the wave of the future.

The Sax inquiry had a wide brief: 'possible developments and changes in nurse education and training including whether such education should take place in hospitals or educational institutions or both' (Sax 1978:1). At the time the committee was sitting, Sister Paulina said publicly that the present hospital based education could not remain, even with some changes, since health services themselves were changing. The focus now, she argued, was not on formulating plans, since nursing had already done that, but on implementing them (Pilkington 1977).

One implementation exercise, in Western Australia, struck trouble at this time, and the subsequent dispute overshadowed the setting up of the Sax Committee. The course for registered nurses at WAIT (now Curtin University of Technology) had been approved for accreditation as a degree (UG1) in 1976 by the Australian Council on Advanced Awards in Education, but had now been refused approval by the new Tertiary Education Commission (TEC). The 30 registered nurses waiting to graduate in November 1977 were told they would not receive their degrees. The 'goals' NSC approached the federal Minister for Education (Carrick) and the Chairman of the TEC (Karmel), since the NSC was at the time trying to have a further degree course approved for registered nurses in Victoria, but it was clear that the government had decided that approval would pre-empt the Sax Committee's conclusions (*CPD*, 2 May 1978:1659). The Western Australian incident brought a forthright response from the late Olive Anstey, then President of the ICN and a well known Perth director of nursing. Nurses were being 'victimised and discriminated against', said Anstey, and she blamed in particular 'some members of the medical profession' for their opposition (Martin 1978). The RANF also responded forcefully, condemning the action of the TEC as a 'backlash' against the vulnerable, sending a copy of this ANJ editorial (November 1977) to every federal MP, and urging nurses to write to their own MPs.

Merle Parkes, Head of the WAIT nursing department and the leading figure in this dispute, believed that the degree issue did much to sharpen the conflict over nursing education, bringing about a clearer divide between the 'best at the bedside' traditionalists (who included many nurses) and the reformers who wanted higher education for its contribution to the professional and personal development of nurses. Most significant of all, she thought, the issue and the protests that followed it made nursing education 'a matter not only for public debate but also for political party competition' (Parkes 1986).

In the face of years of government delay and incidents such as the WAIT dispute, it is not surprising that the 'goals' had by this time acquired some aspects of a crusade:

> It would never have been done if we'd ever wavered—and you couldn't...One thing you can show in that 'goals' statement, it was absolute, we didn't waver from it, we just kept going...You can't keep changing your policies as you go along'. [CH/89]

Had the tertiary education goal become an unquestioned ideal? One student psychiatric nurse (with tertiary experience himself) thought this was a danger. Many nurses, he wrote, equated professionalism with tertiary qualifications rather than with the ability to perform well in providing a skilled service. They had come to idealise tertiary education, yet many tertiary institutions were actually conservative and conformist, he considered, and did not automatically produce inquiring, critical minds. Further, their élitism could engender alienation between professionals and their clients. Nurses might be more influenced by the mystique of tertiary education, he thought, than by a rational analysis of how and where nursing education could be most effectively conducted (Curry 1977).

In spite of official statements that 'a rise in status is but a small part of the profession's motivation in seeking changes to nurse education' (Patten 1979), a transfer to the tertiary sector, as well as providing a solution to the obvious and admitted problems of the hospital programs, was perceived by many nurses as a way of raising the status of their occupation. To this extent they were using credentialism: 'the inflated use of educational certificates as means of monitoring access to key positions in the division of labour', and a technique widely used by white collar occupations which wish to attain the status of professions. A comparable technique by trade unionists is that of restrictive practices, but this is more of a rearguard action to try to make up even slightly for the disadvantages that labour faces in its unequal match with capital (Parkin 1979:54-7).

To identify the educational ambitions of nurses as 'credentialism' does not necessarily invalidate them, since they accompanied a justifiable belief that nurses were excluded from higher education for reasons of educational élitism, and because they were women. This in turn was connected to their low status in the 'health team', a status confirmed by their inferior training. The former RANF federal secretary describes the difficulty at the time of pushing for professional status:

> It was not a very popular thing to be saying. People who kept on saying that—it was as though we were going for some self-seeking thing that was intrinsically

> wrong. Actually I think we probably should have played that *up* more, rather than playing it down a bit, which we tended to do…[MP/91]

The low (female) status of nursing, combined with the relatively large number of nurses, had always provided the rationale for excluding them from higher education. Now in the 1970s the second-class status of women, including their educational deprivation, was being questioned and nurses were able to use this to their advantage. What remained was the problem of their numbers: the federal government was understandably cautious about the cost of transferring such a large group to higher education.

Sax speaks…

With a budget conscious government in office (and few governments are otherwise) and with a mixed committee membership, the Sax Report was inevitably a compromise. The committee appreciated the difficulties and disadvantages of the present system as they had been discussed in the numerous previous reports, and was aware of the nursing arguments. It was also aware of the cost implications of a transfer, estimating these at $6.4 million a year just to increase the then 700 tertiary preregistration students to a proposed 2200 by 1985. The committee also referred to the 'risk of credentialism' in producing over-qualified and therefore frustrated nurses as a further reason for caution (Sax 1978:5, 97)—surely a case of shutting the educational stable door when most other health professional horses except nursing had already bolted. Nurses in any case had dismissed the supposed dangers of 'over-education' years before: such statements, especially by doctors, came from the fears of a rival profession and from doctors' failure to appreciate the value of a broad education in producing nurses ready to respond to changes in practice (Jayawardena 1961).

Nurses were disappointed that the number of CAE students was to increase only to 2200 by 1985 (the 'goals' statement's target year for a total transfer), but at least there was approval of college courses in principle. The NSC accepted these figures as a 'minimum objective' only, but the slow pace of growth for preregistration courses envisaged by the Sax Committee does not seem to have caused as much consternation at the time as other recommendations, such as the proposal to accredit hospital schools of nursing as advanced education and the barriers to registered nurses wanting entry to degree courses (Sax 1978:118-19). Later, when post-registration degrees were well established and the threat of accreditation of hospital courses had faded, the slow growth of basic courses loomed larger as a source of discontent.

The degrees for registered nurses were of special concern as two-year degree courses were under way by 1979 in Victoria and Western Australia, though with small enrolments. This concern was part of a larger problem which underlay much of the debate: the position of nurses currently in the workforce who had no higher qualifications. These nurses could be at a disadvantage when a transfer occurred, which created the potential for divisive hostility to the change. Nursing leaders thus were anxious to see as many nurses as possible gain higher qualifications, particularly nurse educators of whom only 45% in the hospital schools were qualified (Sax 1978:135).

...and nurses talk back

The Sax Report, like most such documents, was in some ways a disappointment, but in others a small step forward: at least college courses would expand, if slowly, and post-registration degrees were approved. One nurse member of the committee looks back on it with political realism:

> Well, we didn't get what we wanted...What do you do? Do you ignore the committee, or do you get the best that you can in the short term, knowing that any committee that is set up has to keep in line with what is feasible, what can be done, as against what should be done. They can be two separate things... As nurse members of that committee, we would have preferred to see a deeper commitment to change...What do you do? You can't afford to be politically naive if you want to get a position accepted. [PP/89]

The then RANF federal secretary points to the Report's advantages:

> It was I believe a very honest reflection of what was said to the committee. But we got two things in...One was that there was no reason why nurses should be educated any differently from any other health professional. I thought the whole report was worth that sentence. And it did away with the idea of UG2 diplomas...[MP/91]

The Australian press gave some serious space to the Sax Report, a change from the usual coverage of nursing events showing smiling graduates. The *Financial Review* of 25 October 1978, for example, gave a balanced summary of the problems noted in the report and a short account of the recommendations. Metropolitan papers in Victoria, Queensland, Tasmania and South Australia gave it brief coverage. In the west the press was more interested in the TEC's decision to fund the WAIT degree course, one positive result of the report and of the persistent protests of local nurses: 'most gratifying' agreed a restrained Merle Parkes (*West Australian* 13 January 1979).

In New South Wales, the NSWNA secretary said that the Sax recommendations appeared to be 'closely parallel' with the policies of the NSWNA and of the NEB (*The Lamp* 1978 November:3). The *Medical Journal of Australia*, despite earlier medical interest in nurse education, was silent on Sax though at the time the report was tabled Professor Rod Andrew, commenting on some of the previous nurse education reports, estimated that a probable '10% or so' of nurses required full tertiary education (*MJA* 4 November 1978). The doctors were probably preoccupied with changes to the health insurance system, Medibank, then in its third convulsion since 1975.

The federal Minister for Education, tabling the report, said that the government's decision would 'await the advice' of the TEC and the reactions from the states (*ANJ* 1979 February:11). Nurses continued to come out fighting: Pat Slater reflected on years of inquiries and reports—'the usual but understandable delaying tactics of governments'—and reminded nurses that '...the Sax Report is not God speaking. It is the nursing profession which must act to implement the recommendations or, if it does not support them, to implement what it believes is desirable and possible' (Slater 1979). The first thing to be done, Slater recommended, was to get the minimum numbers given in the report into colleges two or three years sooner than recommended, and to work for an earlier start for additional courses so that planned course evaluations would have some validity (Slater 1979). The RANF federal secretary went on the attack about the cost of the transfer, asserting 'in response to growing public debate on health costs' that it would actually save $80 million from the health care budget (*ANJ* 1979 July:17). This comment reflects another circumstance which ultimately helped the nursing cause—rising health service costs. The Fraser Government had just set up the Jamison Commission of Inquiry into the Efficiency and Administration of Hospitals and by 1979 it had also largely dismantled the Medibank scheme of universal health insurance as part of its continuing attempt to contain federal budget outlays on health care.

The campaign gathers momentum

By early 1980 the RANF suspected that nurses were getting the 'run around' from the government, being shunted between federal and state education and health departments and the TEC (editorial *ANJ* April 1980). Perhaps the abiding belief of leading nurses in their cause encouraged them to overestimate what were probably the normal ponderous processes of government by seeing them as deliberate obstruction. They pushed on with their task force activity and carried out a versatile variety of lobbying activities to get the federal government to come to a decision on the Sax Report. The RANF also prepared a submission to the Jamison Inquiry and continued its attack based on the financial cost of nurse education to the health budget (*ANJ* 1980 June:8).

The Fraser Government announced on 25 June 1980 that federal cabinet had decided to hold the number of nursing places in colleges at the current level and to accredit hospital schools. The NSC and the task forces rejected this 'do nothing' decision. Mary Patten was reported as saying that the decision showed the government's 'total indifference to the welfare of the sick and to the professional experience and aspirations of the largest group of women in the national workforce' (*Financial Review* 4 July 1980). The leaders planned a national campaign and they enlisted the support of the federal (Labor) Opposition.

In making its decision, the Fraser Government underestimated the force of the nurses' reaction and gave the Opposition a prime opportunity to attack it for being both élitist and sexist. Dr Neal Blewett and Senator John Button, then shadow ministers respectively for health and education, issued a press release condemning the rejection of the Sax Report. The shadow ministers accused the federal government of pandering to doctors while ignoring nurses' requests 'perhaps because they are dealing with a largely female profession'. They also declared that the ALP was committed to 'the gradual shift' towards tertiary education (*ANJ* 1980 August:12-16). This statement illustrates how the political debate about nurse education had now embedded itself in the wider debate about equal opportunity for women. The then RANF federal secretary describes one incident which encouraged this vital opening out of the nursing cause:

> [John Button] had been in [hospital] as a patient...he said to me 'I don't know why you people are wanting to change nursing education. I've been *perfectly* well looked after here'...he kept on saying 'I can't understand what you're on about'...In the end I said 'Look John, we're actually talking about a shift in power relationships in health care, and we're shifting the balance between doctors and nurses for a start, and I believe ultimately it'll help shift the power balance in relation to [patients]'. 'Oh', he said, 'why didn't you tell me that in the first place? That I could understand!' [MP/91]

Some Labor politicians were ambivalent about the transfer as a women's issue, understandably worried by the implications for women in lower income groups whose access to nursing could be reduced. The task forces and other nurses in the field had to persuade the politicians of the potential advantages, as a task force convenor recalls:

> I think people were starting to recognise discrimination and equity policies, that they could discriminate against themselves by fighting to continue with what could be seen as a program of lesser value...[SMcC/88]

At this time too, nurses mounted what became a successful defence of Sturt CAE (now part of Flinders University) in Adelaide, home of one of the earliest preregistration programs and threatened with closure. This incident enabled South Australian nurses to show that they had become effective political activists:

> It was during a Liberal administration in this state that they tried to get rid of Sturt College...In the campaign that followed...we would get people who would phone up the Minister for Health...people who would go to their local MPs with questions, and identify people who were likely to be ambivalent or slightly in our favour, and then feed them masses of information about what the impact on the various [electoral] constituencies was going to be. [AP/88]

The success of this campaign gave encouragement to South Australian nurses 'to carry on the struggle to attain their goals well into the 1980s' (Durdin 1991:198).

Nursing education had now become a public issue, no longer largely the private concern of the nursing world. Press coverage from all states described nurses as 'angry'. Politicians risking an official hospital visit had to brave a phalanx of heckling nurses, and state RANF secretaries were widely quoted on their determination to fight the decision. The move to tertiary education seemed certain, the only question was 'how soon?' (Patten 1980).

In 1980, a federal election year, nurses showed that they were ready for action: the RANF federal office mailed a questionnaire to all candidates from the two major parties and the Australian Democrats, with four questions on support for the transfer (*ANJ* 1980 October:14-15). The results give only limited information and the RANF made no direct comment on them, but they suggest that ALP candidates were more likely than those of the Liberal or National parties to support the transfer (*ANJ* 1980 November:11). The year's political activities had a tangible if modest result: in October, just before the election, the government approved a further 350 college places.

The Jamison Commission, reporting in late 1980, said little about nurse education apart from supporting the Sax recommendations. But Australian nursing had now gone beyond the Sax Report which it had always seen as a minimum only. The RANF declared that 'current activities' were directed towards the 1976 'goals' policy (*ANJ* 1981 March:10). The leaders by this time would probably have rejected anything from government short of a rousing endorsement.

The (almost) silent majority

How did 'rank and file' practising nurses, nearly all of whom had been educated in hospital programs, feel about the proposed transfer? A South Australian nurse analysed letters to the ANJ over a six-month period from August 1980. She concluded that many letters were opinions only, in the absence of systematic evaluation. They were often emotive, prompted by fears of job loss and showed a tendency to generalise from a few examples of college graduates (Boxall 1981). Most nurses did not have tertiary qualifications, partly because the number of places in post-registration programs was so limited, and the letters show that some at least were not convinced that tertiary education was what they wanted. One nurse looks back from the perspective of an enthusiast talking about those not part of the fight:

> It's very difficult to say what the rank and file were thinking about, and I really wonder how much they thought about it *at all*...I suspect that if we'd had to wait until sheer weight of numbers of the profession *forced* a decision, we would still be waiting. [RP/89]

Another remembers the doubts and fears that many must have felt:

> My recollection is that there was a perception that 'It might never happen. If we ignore it it'll go away'...I was always supportive of it, and I was delighted when it happened...but I must say that I wasn't too sure that it was ever going to be successful. [JC/89]

The dissenters failed however to mount a concerted or sustained campaign against the proposed transfer—their location in numerous separate hospitals would have told against such action, and they had no coherent alternative to offer. By 1980 the initiative and the leadership strength were with the reformers. Having commanded most of the major bodies early on, they now had a firm hold of organised nursing.

A female force

The structure which nurses built and operated throughout their struggle contributed immeasurably to its success. One of their most effective devices was the network they built, a 'sisterhood in action', which spread from the NSC to the task forces in all states, and beyond to other nurses, often in strategic positions, who were interested or engaged. In Western Australia post-registration students at WAIT set up one 'cell':

> At that time we had a group called the Nurses' Action Group (unfortunately the initials came out as NAG, but none the less it worked)...we had the NAG as an arm of our task force. It was quite an effective little system, because we were represented...by people committed at all levels. [RH/90]

Victorian nurses started SIGNAL, an RANF Special Interest Group (Nurses Action Lobby). Queensland had PANE (Political Action for Nursing Education), and in South Australia:

> ...locally we had a group of about 10 people, but each of those people had their own network...so that we knew we could get rapid support...We had a fairly intricate networking system worked out right across the state, so that if there was new information we knew where to place it so that that person would then network it through...[SMcC/88]

Over time, those in the networks developed their political skills and influence:

> The task force members divvied up the politicians...we went in twos to interview politicians, give them our views, ask for their support...On the whole I suppose it's fair to say that we were shrugged off...I think a real turning point was [in the WA state election of 1978]. Young, who had been [Liberal] Minister for Health, had one of the big seats round Stirling. We mounted quite a big campaign about the issue, and because there was a huge number of nurses living in the electorate, and we raised the issue very significantly, we feel that he probably lost his seat because of that...[RH/90]

A South Australian nurse witnessed the transformation of her colleagues into a political force:

> The task force in this state...was a collective. There was this group of senior nursing personnel who had a common goal, and that was the transfer of nurse education. And I saw that group move from a traditional 'nice nurse' committee

...to an extremely active political lobbying group. It was a *powerful revolution* that took place...[CG/88]

The revolution had to occur within nursing if nurses were to present an apparently united front to the political decision makers. The task forces and their networks were active also in educating their colleagues, as in West Australia:

If any of it was painful...it was the meetings with colleagues. We used to hold these open forums, and invite people along...We used to get a great response: 200, 250 nurses would come to talk about nursing education, and there would be quite a bit of anger. We were able to dissipate quite a bit of it...We continued those for quite a long time...we'd go down to country areas, wherever we could get an invitation, to talk to groups of nurses. [RH/90]

This internal work of persuasion and the outwardly directed political activity in fact combined to produce the necessary political influence, a South Australian nurse thinks:

The 1976 'goals' and campaign prepared the *profession*. It kept it in the politicians' view, it popped up enough for them to say 'Bloody nurses' from time to time. But in my view what it did was really to take the profession and shake it...because we couldn't then have gone on to mount the kind of political campaign we did unless we could demonstrate that we had a significant proportion of the nursing profession with us. [AP/88]

The sheer dimensions of the campaign are appreciated by another:

The transfer of nurse education, how we achieved it, has been used as a blue-print for political lobbying, because of the networks, and how it was set up...it was a major task, a major organisational task. [RB/91]

Diploma or degree...

A major event for the 'goals' task forces was Workshop '82, held in Melbourne in October with the aim of developing policy for 1983-87. The 'goals' had been widened in scope to include education *and* practice, and the discussion paper published before the conference (*ANJ* 1982 July:12-14) shows that nursing concerns had expanded to include health policy in general. This reflected the entrance into the political arena over the previous six years: once there, it was difficult to avoid realising that nursing education could not be seen as an isolated 'cause'. Events in health care such as the continual changes to health insurance had also affected nurses, as the pages of the *ANJ* show. 'Be there—be seen—be involved' nurses were exhorted, and over 250 were.

The conference, opened by the then (but not for long) Governor of Victoria, the late Sir Brian Murray, adopted ten resolutions on 'Standards for nursing practice', and two on the 'Goals in nursing education', including expediting the transfer (ANJ 1983 December-January:11-20). Disagreement erupted about the level of award to aim for, though the official account says only 'moving towards' UG1 (degree) level. Some nurses thought the 'goal' should now be definitely a degree, like the 1974-76 disputed WA program. A Western Australian nurse reflects:

> It caused such a furore that people crossed the floor to register their vote. It was almost equally divided, seems to me...and the majority—just—went for the UG2 [diploma]...I think it really taught us that we had to decide what were our principles, what we were prepared to compromise on—and that was one thing that we shouldn't have—but the profession compromised...[RH/90]

This dispute brought high emotions, such was its significance:

> We had a big division at that conference...I was screaming 'Up the ante!' and that's when we should have said UG1. If we were going to change anything, we should have gone to UG1...some of the others and I had big rows about it, we were screaming at each other across the room. It was terrible, terrible. [CH/89]

Looking back, other campaigners disagree:

> The diploma was a good credential for a vocational course at that time...[it] was in keeping with the system of the day. You have to marry the two in where you want to go, it must be compatible with current trends...[PP/89]
>
> We could have certainly had degrees, but it would have been for 20% of the workforce and 80% would have had two-year diplomas, and that we wouldn't buy. [MP/91]

This incident illustrates how the members of a movement such as the 'goals' will disagree when there is a choice to made between aims, and how those who fervently espouse one choice will see choosing another as a compromise, however rational it may seem at the time. Faced with what was possibly a choice between gaining the diploma for all or risking a degree confined to the few, nurses actually reaffirmed their principle of improving the education of all.

Shortly after this conference, the RANF National Executive met the federal Minister for Health, Jim Carlton, to lobby for the transfer, and reported that the minister was 'well briefed' on nursing matters (*ANJ* 1983 December-January:11). By this time ministers probably felt they had to be. Early in 1983 the NSC and the task forces were meeting to plan for a possible federal election. Under the slogan 'Qualified nurses for quality care', the election manifesto again had a wider scope than education alone, though the 'goals' in education were evident in much of the statement.

New South Wales to the fore...again

The advent of the Hawke Labor Government in 1983 encouraged the RANF federal secretary to think that tertiary education might be achieved more quickly. The new government in fact announced that it intended to set up more college courses as part of a plan for gradual transfer, in line with the Sax recommendations (*ANJ* 1983 June:11-14).

But it was in New South Wales, where Labor had been in office for seven years, that events surged ahead to an exhilarating climax. Apart from its desire as the self-styled 'premier state' to be in the vanguard, New South Wales had some distinct advantages: there were more nurses in New South Wales than any other state (75% of them in Sydney), and in the NSWNA they had an organisation which under the secretaryship of M. V. ('Ronnie') Henlen (1968-82) had developed an aggressive political style. New South Wales also had the active and determined NEB, as its executive secretary at the time points out:

> There were two things which meant that we moved ahead: one was that we had a *focus,* if you like, which was the Board, which had the specific task of preparing and implementing a co-ordinated system of nursing education for the state...The second thing that I think is worth looking at...is the effect in New South Wales of not having anything like the same proportion of places available to nurses in [degree] courses...so you ended up having a lot of nurses who'd had exposure to multidisciplinary tertiary institutions, and who were no longer fearful of [them] as distinct from tertiary *nursing* institutions. [MMcG/89]

The NEB's officers were able to draw on the skills and experience of these nurses around the state during the critical years 1977-82, when the board and the Interdepartmental Committee for the Implementation of Government Policy on Nurse Education were investigating the available options, and concluding that 'the retention of hospital schools of nursing and/or group regional schools of nursing could not be supported on educational or economic grounds', mainly because student nurses were employees (McGrath 1984:3). The board used these years to set up the framework for the future system based on the existing regions, as the secretary relates:

> Betty Hall was the one who did the foundation work right throughout this state...So that by the time we came to, say 1982, right throughout the country we had groups of people in senior positions in health and education, who were used to working with each other, many of whom had already started developing the kinds of preregistration nursing programs they thought would suit their areas, and most of whom had already started involving the educational institution in the ongoing hospital-based program. [MMcG/89]

There were eventually nine of these regional committees. The board also took care to report regularly to representatives of the major nursing bodies, such as the NSWNA, the Institute of Nursing Administrators, the RANF and others:

> We'd bring them in, give them the report, and then we'd all have lunch! That worked very well, so that again, they were used to coming in and meeting with us. [MMcG/89]

In this way the NEB's officers developed the co-operative structure which would underpin the future transfer, though they did not know precisely when it would occur, such are the political uncertainties which afflict rational planning. New South Wales nurses meanwhile kept up their lobbying, as one remembers:

> ...of course NSW [nurses] badgered Brereton from when he was an Opposition member...then when he came in as Minister for Health he kept on and on about saving money in health...I was constantly called in to discuss planning issues, which gave me constant access to him...I said, 'I know how to save you money', and he said 'How?' 'Move nursing education holus bolus into CAEs'. [JH/89]

The Interdepartmental Committee confirmed in 1982 that the cost of hospital programs was high, and would become even higher, so that there was a financial incentive for the transfer. By late 1982 the Wran Government had before it a working party recommendation, option 1, that the state should use the funds then spent on hospital programs to contract with CAEs for the provision of diploma level basic nurse education programs. The government next asked the working party for details of the financial and administrative implications of this option, but it did not endorse the report on these until April 1983, and then 'pending clarification' by the federal government of its position on granting student allowances.

This clarification failed to emerge during the next six months, until 'it became clear that the Commonwealth's decision would not be made in time for New South Wales to meet its planned 1985 starting date' (McGrath 1984:3-5). Then the NSW Minister for Health, Laurie Brereton, made his celebrated announcement on 7 November 1983, the day that shook the nursing world, of the state's decision to go it alone and transfer all nursing education from January 1985. There would be three-year programs incorporating extensive practical experience; and the courses would be comprehensive, that is, with community health, aged care and mental health components. The new training, said the Minister, 'should allow nurses to take a greater professional responsibility in the health care system'.

The sequence of events here suggests that the state government had already made up its mind on the transfer possibly by late 1982, or by the following April at the latest—hence the planned 1985 starting date. Some nurses certainly thought so, including a NORC activist:

> The following April [1983] we knew it had been to Cabinet...But it didn't happen...It came to September, October, I was pretty down. I made the decision it was never going to happen, because we knew unofficially that it had got through, and they'd been sitting on it all this time and nothing had happened. Then out of the blue, on 7 November...it was at a press conference, and he announced it. [CH/89]

Why did the state government delay? Federal events may have been influential. In late 1982 the Fraser Government was still in office, but by the time the working party report was before cabinet the Hawke Government was in Canberra. The NSW Cabinet would have been reluctant to get out of line with a new federal Labor Government. The immediate precipitating reason for the timing of the announcement was, in part, the large numbers of graduating nurses (unusually) seeking employment from their hospitals—the economic recession of 1981-83 had brought some unemployment among nurses. And 1982-83 had been a stormy time for Laurie Brereton with the NSWNA under its new secretary, the left-wing Jenny Haines, staging well publicised protests against reductions in hospital funding and in favour of wage rises:

> It was an orchestrated event by the Nurses' Association...and there was to be another major outbreak [of nurses demonstrating] so Brereton attempted to spike their guns by saying, 'We, the government, are going to take this decision and this will open up 1500 new positions for registered nurses, by whatever time'. So that was it. [MMcG/89]

There was also the attraction to a Minister for Health of saving his own portfolio some expense, as New South Wales nurses pointed out:

> We tried to say it wasn't cheaper, that the costs would remain the same but that...the costs of educating the nurse would right and properly move out of the health portfolio and into the education portfolio. After all, what was he spending his hard-won money on education for? [JH/89]

The state government also had pressing political reasons for trying to appease at least one fractious group. As a result of the corruption allegations then dogging the premier, four safe Labor seats in Sydney had been retained in by-elections on 27 October 1983—but with a 10.1% swing to the Liberal Opposition under its new leader, Nick Greiner (Turner 1985:206-7).

The NSWNA responded cautiously to Brereton's announcement, 'Beware Health Ministers bearing gifts' (*The Lamp* November 1983:5) but for some New South Wales nurses it was a fitting climax to their years of struggle:

> Well, all hell broke loose! We had the press out, it was really go, go, go. Canberra went off its head. *Canberra* went off its head! 'Why did New South Wales go off on a tangent like this, on their own?' Wendy Fatin [nurse and federal Labor MP] was up here a few weeks later...'What's the matter with Brereton?' They were all turning on each other. The Labor Party turned on the heat and gave him the 1-2-6! [CH/89]

Despite the NEB's careful preparation for the change, the surprise initiative came in for criticism from nurses in the other states, as well as from Canberra politicians, as the secretary found:

> So, can you see, that the step from there to the next wasn't very great. That's why, I guess, we became so *frustrated*—and I particularly did—at the reaction of some of my interstate colleagues, who said 'You're mad!...You're moving too fast, you'll put on botched-up courses...you'll destroy it for everybody because you'll do it badly'. [MMcG/89]

Those in the vanguard of a movement always run the risk of such misunderstanding, but later accounts celebrate the New South Wales nurses' victory (Cochrane 1989:30-1; Wood 1990:181). It subtracts nothing from their achievement to realise that other political circumstances influenced the NSW decision, especially the economic realities of nurse education as recent reports had revealed them. The state government could hope to transfer the cost eventually to the Commonwealth, though initially (since it was ahead of Commonwealth policy) it had to fund the new programs itself; and it wanted to win support by pacifying the local nurses. Still, the political realities of the time, though pressing, may not have been the Minister's only motive:

> Laurie had a genuine interest in women. He did do it on that basis...but what went to Cabinet was on money. He himself supports women, and furthering education...He was philosophically on our side, but you can't win Cabinets on that...[CH&KM/89]

Even so, this motive was an appropriate one given that nursing education had become part of the debate on the 'woman question', as New South Wales nurses recognised:

> We were able to say to him 'You will...use proper health money to run health services—it's a social issue. It's a women's issue...nurses are the only group not properly educated in the health system...We cited ICN, we cited women's health—but it would be cheaper for *him*. [JH/89]

Whatever his personal ideals, Laurie Brereton based his startling decision on predictably political grounds: the government would save money in the long term, and in the short term the initiative could win electoral support and the NSWNA might leave him alone. He felt able to disregard serious warnings of future shortages in the NSW nursing workforce should the transfer proceed with 'too much haste', rather than according to the measured march of the Sax recommendations.

This shortage did occur, for a number of reasons including a lower enrolment than expected in college courses. These did not reach their target figure for two years (McGrath 1987). A shortage of registered nurses also developed which had nothing to do with the transfer but went back to a possibly illusory oversupply in 1978 leading to a fall in the student nurse intake (Jayawardena 1983). A 'wild card', unforeseeable at the time, was the 1984-85 New South Wales doctors' dispute with both state and Commonwealth governments. The dispute exacerbated the shortage of nurses:

> ...because without the effect of that we would have had a shortage, but a livable-with shortage...The central teaching hospitals, they *slaved* during that period of time, the nurses did...At the end of the doctors' dispute, nurses perceived that the doctors got what they wanted and the nurses weren't even thanked. So there was an exit of nurses from the teaching hospitals as well...[MMcG/89]

The doctors' dispute had the adverse consequence for the transfer of giving it the stigma, however unjustly, of causing the shortage. But it had the advantage of distracting those doctors who opposed the transfer, so that their reaction came too late to have any weight. The doctors, while exercising their considerable power on their own behalf, had unwittingly helped introduce a nurse education system few of them wanted, as NEB officers realised:

> The doctors were so busy disputing that they didn't realise the transfer had occurred...They woke up some 12 or 15 months afterwards and said, 'Why weren't we told?...The Nurses Education Board invited them to come and discuss the matter on several occasions, but they were so busy with other business...[MMcG/89]

The major effect of the New South Wales great leap forward was to provide the 'essential impetus' to the federal government and to nursing in general (Hamilton 1986). The Commonwealth at first reacted cautiously when Wendy Fatin asked in parliament on 8 November if the government supported the 'innovative change' (*CPD* 8 November 1983:2367). A month earlier the Minister for Education (Senator Susan Ryan) had emphasised that, contrary to rumour, she had not asked the Commonwealth Tertiary Education Commission (CTEC) to 'reopen the question of the training of nurses' but 'rather to report on options for implementation of the Sax Committee's recommendations' (*ANJ* 1984 December-January:14). The Labor Government was committed to the transfer, but only at the Sax speed.

Outside New South Wales nurses were quiet about the change, perhaps because the RANF was preoccupied at the time with the 'no-strike' ballot. It was a US nurse, Dr Sarah Archer, who made the point at the 'Australian Nurses and Politics' conference in November 1983 that the Brereton announcement of two weeks earlier showed that 'political activity does pay off'. Archer went on to reassure nurses, as did Wendy Fatin and other speakers, that political power and its exercise were worthwhile aims and that the pursuit of power was not something they need feel embarrassed about. Comments from the local (Melbourne) and interstate audience showed that nurses were conscious of their handicaps as women and as nurses, and that some had begun to encourage more political awareness and action.

This conference illustrated the symbiosis that now existed in nursing between the education transfer and political action. The first had become the major stimulus for the second. In 1976 the adoption of the transfer as the official goal of the leaders had prompted them to establish the framework for a political campaign which had slowly gathered momentum. Now that campaign seemed about to succeed and the goal was within reach. Nursing was on the march—literally.

Nearing the goal

The immediate reason for the now legendary march in Adelaide was CTEC's report for the next three years in higher education. The report was tabled in federal parliament on 10 May 1984 at the same time that 400 nurses were attending the annual conference of the College of Nursing, Australia—among them many of the reformers and an august English visitor, Baroness Jean McFarlane. The commission had considered a number of options for basic nurse education including the New South Wales decision (with a reproachful reference to not having been consulted about it) but had actually gone back to the 1978 Sax recommendations (CTEC 1984:107). CTEC's reasons were that according to evaluation studies the differences between hospital and college graduates were 'not conclusive' and did not justify a preference for one kind of course over another; and it estimated the cost to the Commonwealth budget of a complete transfer at an annual minimum of $95 million, not including capital works.

When the nurses at the Adelaide conference heard about the CTEC recommendations on 11 May from the college's executive director, June Cochrane, they were so incensed that they voted overwhelmingly (on Elizabeth Pittman's suggestion) for a symbolic burning of the Sax Report and a march to the office of the federal Minister for Health. With victory in sight, they were in no mood for last minute prevarication. The Sax Report was out of date, said Judy Porter, and she and Sister Paulina, who had both been members of the original committee, led this unusual public display of senior nursing strength:

> We led it, we marched up, and I had a policeman on a bike next to me. I said 'How much farther do we have to go?' and he said 'Oh, it's not very far, just up there', very helpful. All this meant that the profession became aware of the power that it should exercise...[PP/89]

A South Australian nurse sees the march as silencing some dissent:

> We were really...becoming politically literate and we weren't about to be mucked around, and [some senior nurses] found that difficult to handle...in no way would they have marched unless the body of the hall had up and marched. It was like national fervour, it got carried along, and they wouldn't have dared not be there. [SMcC/88]

And a New South Wales nurse thinks it hastened the final result, as well as impressing Jean McFarlane:

> It was very fast, that [last] little bit. It was really the march down to Blewett [federal Minister for Health] and putting the rubbish on his front step. Actually the Baroness didn't want to get on the plane and go home—she wanted to keep walking! [CH/89]

The conference resolved also to ask nursing administrators not to process student applications for hospital programs, a resolution followed up with further threats of political action a few days later when June Cochrane and the RANF Federal Secretary, Judy Cooney, met senior officials in Canberra

(Cochrane 1989:33; Wood 1990:201). By the end of the month the federal government had set up an interdepartmental committee (IDC) to examine nursing education, with six government departments represented. The nursing organisations also had access to the ALP caucus Social Policy subcommittee through Wendy Fatin.

'Unity is the key to success', Fatin had told the RANF Federal Council in April, perhaps fearing a damaging outbreak of disunity at this critical moment. Nursing organisations kept their unity and lobbied federal and state governments unrelentingly during the life of the IDC. They threatened industrial action, attacks on the federal government in marginal seats in the 1984 election, and urged nurses to write to the ministers concerned. Many did. (*ANJ* 1984 June:14; August:15-16; Martins 1990:185; Wood 1990:202-9).

The student nurse becomes the nursing student

As Patricia Wood's account (1990:209-14) makes clear, the majority of departments represented on the IDC, after considering the implications for health services and for the nursing workforce, supported the transfer as did most health and education authorities. The IDC reported to Cabinet on 26 July, but the final decision was not made public until 24 August 1984 when Neal Blewett announced that the government had decided to transfer all basic nurse education to colleges by 1993. The one-month delay suggests that the government had hesitated to take the final step. What pushed it finally—and perhaps reluctantly—over the edge? Later the Prime Minister justified the decision to state premiers on health and education grounds and because it was 'consistent with policies on the status of women' (*ANJ* 1984 October:26) but that was just dressing sprinkled on a turbulent salad of manoeuvring, arguments and political pressure.

Governments seldom make policy decisions for entirely rational, and never for altruistic reasons. What finally tipped an uncertain balance in nursing's favour? Wendy Fatin stressed the effect of '...months of high-level negotiation during which the nursing representatives exhibited a level of political sophistication and conciliatory skill which left the Government in no doubt about the validity of the nurses' claims' (*ANJ* 1984 October:5). In fact that validity was not self-evident, as the CTEC hesitation about the performance difference between hospital and college graduates suggests. Valid educational reasons in favour of the transfer did exist, but they were not those which had finally persuaded the federal government (Lublin 1985). The government was unlikely in any case to base its decision on validity alone whatever the political skills of the advocates. Some nurses saw other more pressing reasons:

> I think [Hawke] knew that if he had another election coming up there was no way he could go into that election feeling comfortable unless he had announced the transfer. [SMcC/88]

Others were convinced financial considerations had affected the decision:

> The dollar: the Campbelltown and Camden Hospital inquiry in New South Wales that demonstrated that in fact registered nurses were cheaper...there was no point talking about better health care or better educational opportunities, what you had to do was demonstrate that ultimately it was going to be cheaper... When you look back on it, it's self-evident. The thing that speaks in cabinet is the dollar. [AP/88]

New South Wales nurses saw the effect of the federal system as it reacted to their own jump ahead:

> There was no way that the feds could continue to block the transfer of nursing education to the tertiary sector once New South Wales had made the stance. We forced the issue—at least I believe we forced the issue. [MMcG/89]

Another likely influence was that during the time the IDC was conducting its inquiry in Canberra, nurses in Victoria embarked on industrial action which lasted from 1 June to 16 August 1984. This dispute brought few unequivocal benefits to nurses but the RANF demonstrated that it could win a major financial concession from a state government (Fox 1989:85). The Hawke Cabinet thus had before it the actual transfer of nurse education in one large state and serious industrial activity among nurses in the other, with the possibility of more to come since the RANF had just rescinded its 'no-strike' clause. As far as nurses were concerned, the government was probably influenced more by what it feared they might do, with their growing tendency to lobby and demonstrate and their developing industrial militancy, than by the validity of their claims to tertiary education except as these related to the principle of equal opportunity. It was fortunate also that the transfer decision was made before the serious decline of the Australian economy became apparent in the mid 1980s. This would have reinforced the government's reluctance. Two New South Wales nurses regard it as significant that the transfer occurred despite the absence of any overt demand for it by members of the public (McMillan & Dwyer 1989). From the government's point of view the absence of any effective public opposition was probably more important.

Looking back at events over the ten years leading up to the final decision it almost seemed as if the transfer in the end became inevitable, at least to some nurses:

> It was so big you couldn't stop it, I think, in the end. [RB/91]

This impression is reinforced by the reaction in late 1985 to the New South Wales government's attempt to take a step back towards hospital training, apparently to try to deal with staff shortages. Nurses—and not just those already in colleges—took to the Sydney streets, finally forcing the Premier to meet their representatives and eventually to reverse his decision, as a Sydney nurse remembers:

> The number of clinicians who had appeared to be avowed opponents of the transfer, people I saw from North Shore [Hospital], for example, who were diehard conservatives in this respect...and there they were in uniform protesting outside the premier's office! [RP/89]

A victory for women, equity and political skill

Certain social and political changes helped the nursing cause: the expansion of higher education and the emergence of the women's movement; higher pay for nurses, including students; the federal system which enabled New South Wales to seize the high ground; and the change of government in 1983 which, as in 1972, brought to power a party more sympathetic to the principle of equity in general and to the demands of women in particular. These two issues provided a conduit through which nurses could channel their demands (Henderson 1990). The tide in the affairs of women was favourable, but nurses were ready when the time came to exploit this for their own good fortune. Wendy Fatin reminded MPs:

> ...nurses started arguing many years ago that the level on which they were being required to function had to be backed up with a tertiary education. As time went by, the nursing organisations became increasingly effective at putting their case. By 1984, we were not just talking about how to get nurse education into CAEs. The issue was couched in terms of the status of women, industrial relations and professional equity (*CPD* 20 November 1985:3290).

The transfer was not just a cause and a campaign, it was the dynamic engine that drove nurses to make themselves into a political force:

> ...we were frightfully naive politically, frightfully. But we certainly learned quickly. I'd have to say that I think that was the first big step in the politicisation of nursing, when we found out...how powerful we could be...just by the strength, the power of our vote. [RH/90]

But the power of the vote was not enough on its own, and many nurses found that governments respond especially to persistent pestering. At least one senior nurse learned how well this worked:

> Pat [Slater] and I were at some sort of soirée...at Newcastle...and [Neal Blewett, Minister for Health] turned to Pat and he said, 'You're the woman who's caused all this trouble for me'...And he was very serious, he wasn't being funny...She enjoyed that moment very much. [AD/90]

The leaders' original principle of uplift for all and not just for the few accorded with the later widening of the campaign to the general issues of equity and the status of women. This combination also gave Australian nurses the chance to move ahead of their US and British colleagues: the US still had a wide range of program provision, and in Britain the best that the new 'Project 2000' offered nurses was what appeared to be a tenuous link with higher education and a continuation of 20% of their student time within the paid workforce.

The federal government's decision did delay (till 1993) the total transfer more than some nurses would have liked (Hamilton 1986), but the Minister for Health was following a principle of the Sax Report: a planned and orderly transfer which would not disrupt health care by causing further nursing shortages, or education through the impact of the numbers of nursing students. The federal government wanted a 'co-ordinated and co-operative' approach between the two levels, so its financial assistance to the states was based on 'an element of cost-sharing'. Ironically, as Martins (1990) shows, the transfer process in those states which followed the 'planned and orderly' method was not in the end so different from the accelerated process in New South Wales.

The transfer process: a federal-state pull and push

In its States Grants (Nurse Education Transfer Assistance) Bill of 1985 the Commonwealth proposed a progressive rise in student numbers, that is beyond the 1200 already in CAEs (and wholly Commonwealth funded) and in cost (Table 3.1). The cost would arise from the indexed grant for each approved student place, and the Commonwealth faced also an additional cost of $2.5 million in 1985 for tertiary allowances for nursing students (*CPD* 15 May 1985:2419-21).

Table 3.1 Funding the transfer

	1985	1986	1987	by 1993
Student places	1000	2700	5000	18000
Cost ($m 1985 prices)	1.62	4.43	8.2	29.5

Later that year the Minister for Health told parliament that the Commonwealth would give a further $7.3 million for retraining nurses not in the workforce in 1985-87, an offer whose aim, the Opposition said, was as much to placate the state Health Ministers, who felt they had not been adequately consulted about the transfer, as to help them with their shortages of nursing staff. The Opposition did however support the transfer, though with some misgivings about access to courses and predictable misunderstandings about the amount of clinical education nursing students would have in the colleges courses (*CPD* 20 November 1985:3280-3). Neal Blewett told nurses in Melbourne on 1 October 1985 that the transfer now depended on co-operation with the states, and on their willingness to negotiate. Most states were in favour of the change and had tertiary programs, so 'things should progress pretty much as nurses want them to', the Minister thought, though he did not overlook the problems faced by the states' health services having to replace 18 000 trainee nurses by 1993 (*ANJ* 1984 November:33-4). Nurses clearly could not sit back and collect their reward without further effort.

State governments in fact hesitated to accept the Commonwealth offer of $1500 (indexed) for each nursing student, since they believed that the true cost was nearer $6000. Further, the offer did not include any provision for major capital works. The Federation of College Academics, the CAE staff union, was worried by the Commonwealth's apparent intention 'that nurse education should remain essentially a state responsibility', and by possible threats to the working conditions of the new nurse academics (Summers 1985). States would of course save some money through the attrition of hospital based programs, but this would vary depending on the numbers of students in the workforce who had to be replaced. State and territory health ministers called the Commonwealth's funding proposals 'inadequate and unfair' (*ANJ* 1984 July:41). In South Australia, for example, the Minister for Health, J. R. Cornwall, reported ruefully: 'The RANF was dancing in the streets when [the transfer] was announced, but I am not sure that it had read the fine print. From our point of view, it is far from a generous offer, although in the short term it may be an offer that we cannot refuse' (*SAPD* 25 October 1984:1490). Audrey Martins (1990:56-7) shows convincingly however that in a federal system such as Australia's, when state governments are implementing federal policy as in this case there is an inherent potential for conflict between the two levels of government because the states will inevitably perceive central funding as inadequate.

The variety engendered by a federal system had also produced diverse provisions for nursing in higher education: in 1985 Victoria, South Australia and Western Australia had well established tertiary courses and plans for setting up new ones. All had state Labor governments though only the Victorian government had allocated specific funding. The ACT had a school of nursing at Canberra CAE and a course would soon begin. The Northern Territory already had courses for registered nurses and its government supported the transfer, so the existing hospital course would move in 1987 to the Darwin Institute of Technology.

In Tasmania a course did not begin until 1988 because of a major disagreement about its location. The Liberal premier (Robin Gray) said the state could afford only one course, at Launceston, whereas the RANF wanted a second in Hobart. The government's preference would leave Hobart 'the only capital city in Australia not to have a nursing course', a former (Labor) Minister for Health, Doug Lowe, lamented. The Minister for Health (Roger Groom) declared that since his wife was a nurse he was 'a great supporter of the nursing profession', but the federal government had been arrogant, he thought, in deciding unilaterally on the transfer and then giving the states, including the Labor states, inadequate funds (*TPD* 10 July 1985:1734, 1737; 21 August 1985:2255; 16 July 1986:1915-18). The wrangle ended only when the federal Minister for Education stepped in to choose the CAE at Launceston (*ANJ* 1985 August:18).

In Queensland there was only one preregistration course, at the Queensland Institute of Technology, and a degree course for registered nurses had just begun. There were plans to increase numbers and to start four new courses, but local nurses were 'dismayed' by the apparent absence of any commitment to achieving the transfer by 1993—the state had already rejected the Canberra offer of $1500 for each student (*ANJ* September 1985:39). The Bjelke-Petersen (National Party) government thwarted Commonwealth policy with complete success for four years in spite of the well organised actions of the local nurses, including the Queensland Nurses' Union. The government saw itself as electorally secure at this time, so the Minister for Education felt able to reject offers of federal funding as a 'pathetic contribution', demanding that Canberra pay the full cost. It was only after the change in National Party leadership in late 1987, when the Premier was deposed by former Health Minister Mike Ahern, that Queensland moved to implement the transfer. The state finally signed the transfer agreement in 1988. The Queensland case shows how a state government which actually agrees with a Commonwealth policy can still act unilaterally to frustrate its implementation if it thinks such action is in its own interests (Martins 1990:153-78).

New South Wales of course was out on its own: 2300 students (fewer than the numbers expected) were enrolled in 15 colleges, and a 'significant' consequence of the transfer was an amended Nurses Registration Act which reduced seven categories of registered nurse to two, with the effect that on registration nurses would be able to practise in all areas except midwifery (*ANJ* 1985 July:28-31). Here was the other state which had defied the federal government, though from different motives. In this case the major difference between the two levels was over the implementation schedule, which entailed the state government funding the bulk of student places until 1988 out of savings from its hospital budget (Martins 1990:212-18). Where most states set up committees or working parties composed of representatives of the various interested groups to oversee the transfer, New South Wales, true to form, went about the task differently:

> We were determined that we were not going to have representatives on the State Planning Group, because if you do that, you slow it down. Senior public servants can work very quickly and very well within the bureaucracy. You can't do that if you're constantly having to wait while representatives go back and get views...We used these other [representative] working parties as advisory to the interdepartmental committee. But the group that was responsible for implementing the transfer was that interdeparmental committee, the State Planning Group. [MMcG/89]

Given that New South Wales had a short 14 month deadline, a small central group with wide powers of delegation was the most practical mechanism. Policy implementation could go ahead in planned stages. In the other states, with groups such as employers and government represented on committees as well as nurses, the method was more pluralist. It was inevitable therefore that other agendas would come to the surface, so that implementation committees had to deal with their own conflicting interests in addition to the mechanics of the actual transfer (McManamny 1991).

Other kinds of nursing

Education within nursing itself was still not uniform. The question of education for psychiatric nurses began to worry at least some nurses as the first flush of victory for general nurse education faded. The Senior Nurse Adviser in the Commonwealth Department of Health urged these nurses to lift their education out of its neglected state by supporting the change of psychiatric nursing to a postgraduate diploma taken after the basic comprehensive course (*ANJ* 1985 May:33-4). Some psychiatric nurses felt strongly however that their training and practice were neither understood nor appreciated by general nurses and wished to maintain their separate identity in the face of the comprehensive or integrated curriculum, as one of them explains:

> Nurses believe too much in the myth of holism, and they have taken that to the *nth* degree with the integrated curriculum. I don't think that a lot of them appreciate the difference between a mental health problem and a mental illness, and they've confused the two in their curriculum. [TH/90]

They were also angry that they had not been consulted about the transfer and doubted as they had 10 years before that the new college 'comprehensive' courses could prepare even beginning practitioners in their specialty (Arthur et al 1983).

At the next 'goals' conference—the Nursing Targets of 1989—it was evident that the differences between general and psychiatric nursing had become acute. In Victoria the government, with persuasion from the union to which most psychiatric nurses belonged, the Hospital Employees' Federation (HEF), had agreed to a separate program in a CAE; and in Western Australia psychiatric nurses were determined to have a separate course. As well as doubting the adequacy of mental health content in comprehensive courses, many feared that few graduates of comprehensive courses would choose to do postgraduate mental health, so that the workforce in psychiatric institutions would have to be augmented with unqualified staff. The tensions between psychiatric nursing and general nursing remain, linked as they are with difficult issues of status:

> General nurses are not prepared to give any ground when it comes to comprehensive nursing…the status of nursing knowledge compared with that of other professions is low, but the status of mental health nursing within nursing itself seems to be lower…that's my real concern. [TH/90]

In New South Wales, where mental health became a postgraduate qualification, some psychiatric nurses feel more confident about the status of mental health in the preregistration comprehensive course:

> We have a fairly high incidence of our students who go to work in the mental health area—that's probably because I'm a high profile *pushy* person who talks about mental health nursing…the dynamic things about it, so that they get

> exposed to it constantly. And agencies...have come round in a full circle: from at first being very resistant now they are trying to attract our graduates. [LS/90]

Education for the second level, the state enrolled nurse (SEN), was also changing during the transfer period. In 1989 the WA SENs achieved a two year associate diploma course (UG3) in TAFE which would enable them to get credits in the college nursing courses. The decision to set up this program (within a tight five week schedule) was largely the result of successful political action by the WA Enrolled Nurses' Association (part of the Federated Miscellaneous Workers' Union, the 'Missos'), using recommendations from a 1984 state report:

> They're a very vibrant group...[and] I think it's reasonable to say that the government was more open for convincing in that pre-election year [1988]. Politicians don't necessarily agree with that but—the decision was made, it would be implemented by February next year, which was really on the eve of the election...[BB/90]

Like the general nurses, the WA enrolled nurses had to convert their existing practitioners to the idea of the new course, though in their case there was little time since the decision to implement it was so clearly political. The persuasion turned out to be a last-minute exercise precipitated by an embarrassing association meeting when the state Minister for Health was in the audience:

> The Minister was sitting there, and speaker after speaker [said]: 'What's in it for us? What are you doing for us? Why are we going to TAFE? The old system's the best!'...the Enrolled Nurses' Association, they were all going redder and redder. In fact they'd been lobbying the Minister, how wonderful this was, and the members were behind it...[But] really the leaders of the association were ahead of their members. [BB/90]

States with larger numbers of SENs have proceeded more cautiously. In New South Wales a Ministerial Review has recommended that the course in TAFE be upgraded to a comprehensive advanced certificate with a 420-hour theory curriculum, replacing the present 360-hour certificate course (*The Lamp* 1991 October:11-14). The advanced certificate will make it easier for SENs to be given credits in the proposed degree courses in general nursing, but it will remain a 12-month program. Not all SEN educators favour a two-year course:

> I would personally fight against that...Our registered nurse has a diploma—how close do you want? If you look at England that's where they went wrong. They allowed their enrolled nurse...to impinge [on the registered nurse's job] so much that in fact the enrolled nurse could be in charge of registered staff...that's why they're getting rid of them. [MS/90]

A 600 hour pilot program began in 1990 at the major Victorian SEN school, but the course remained a 12 month one. The report on this course has recommended upgrading to TAFE. The local ANF branch supports this and wants a new program to articulate with existing registered nurse courses so that SENs can improve their career opportunities (*ANJ* 1991 October:35). The head of the (now closed) Melbourne school explains why upgrading is vital, whether in TAFE or not:

> Patients now, most of them have IV drips and tubes and drains, so that there are very few patients who need basic care...some of the SENs had been doing these procedures [insertion of nasogastric tubes, bladder washouts, female catheterisations, components of IV therapy] without any education whatsoever, but unofficially. Most people acknowledged it. [IK/91]

In both these sectors of nurse education the federal system has enabled diversity to be maintained, probably in the absence of nationally powerful unions like the ANF to represent either group of nurses with one voice. In midwifery the professional body, the Australian College of Midwives, supports a significant degree of separation of midwifery from general nursing and is pursuing 'direct entry' courses on the grounds, first, that general nursing is 'illness oriented', an ironic criticism given nurses' efforts over the last 20 years to demonstrate their rejection of such a bias; and second, that direct entry would attract those who wished to devote themselves wholly to women giving birth without having to train as general nurses beforehand (HDV 1990:14). Unlike psychiatric nurses, midwives seem to be influenced not by perceived status differences but by an understandable rejection of the tendency of some nurses to subsume midwifery under general nursing. General nurses might agree however with a former RVCN secretary:

> [Direct entry]...that's a bit dangerous isn't it? I mean, there's a lot attached to a pregnant woman apart from her pregnancy. [MC/90]

Nursing in the universities

Many researchers will assess the impact of the transfer, especially its implications for nursing practice. So far, two major issues have emerged during the process, both related to professional autonomy and control. First, can the profession maintain control over its curriculum when in many cases academics from other longer established disciplines also contribute to the nursing programs? Nursing is also in competition with other departments for resources so that it has to assert its claims against opposition just as it did in the hospital. Second, the clinical education of the student takes place away from the nursing department in surroundings not necessarily sympathetic to the nurse academics' beliefs and teachings.

By late 1988 Neal Blewett was able to report the steady progress of the transfer with only Queensland lagging behind. The Commonwealth had by that time contributed $13.83 million under the States Grants (Nurse Education Transfer Assistance) Act, amounting to $5700 for each student's three-year course, and excluding the costs of student living allowances (*CPD* 29 September 1988:1314). By this time too the higher education sector that nursing had fought so hard to join was itself about to undergo major change, and in a direction likely to be congenial. The new unified national system which would replace the Martin Committee's 1965 binary creation would emphasise access for a wide variety of students, fields of study with special relevance to economic goals, and applied research. So, just a few years after achieving its ambition of college education, nursing found itself in the universities—though in many cases not initially part of the actual campus—all in the cause of 'educational effectiveness and financial efficiency' (Dawkins 1988:18, 27). From there the heads of nursing departments have been fighting the final battle in the degree or diploma controversy.

Nursing students now

This chapter began with Australia's student nurses in 1960. How different are the nursing students of the 1990s? As women they are different in being reportedly less docile and submissive and in having many other careers open to them. As students they tend to be recruited from school leavers with relatively low level results in their final year: a study of the secondary school results of half the tertiary entrants in 1989 showed that, with education, nursing had the lowest proportion of high scoring and the highest proportion of low scoring students (DEET 1990). South Australian research has found that an increasing proportion of nursing students are slightly older and slightly more likely to be male than previously and that they are also probably from less privileged socio-economic social groups than are the majority of students (Neill 1987). Some of these characteristics will reinforce the view that nursing has lesser claims to academic status, though the growing numbers of male entrants suggests that its status in general may have risen now that nursing education has entered the tertiary sector.

The entry into higher education has been confidently assumed to bring 'acceptance as an equal partner in the health care delivery team' (Duffield 1986). This is expecting too much of the educational advance, that it should translate into an instant and equivalent rise in status in the workplace where medicine is accustomed to pre-eminence. But whatever their future experiences in the workplace, for today's nursing students there is the openness, the relative freedom of university life—a contrast with the enclosed, narrow existence endured by their 1960s aunts and mothers, as a Victorian nurse remembers:

> I hated the subjugation of the pecking order. I hated the subjugation of nurses by other nurses...I hated the subjugation of the intellectual too, as a thinking person. There was no space and no place to ask a question...why we did things a certain way...why things were the way they were—and how come we kept on being like this as nurses? [SMcM/91]

The vision of the leaders, the support of so many other nurses, the years of political effort, have at least brought the possibility of changing that picture of student life.

REFERENCES

Arthur D, Ogilvie S 1983 Comments made at a seminar 'Implications for nurses of the moves towards college-based education'. Lincoln Institute, Melbourne, 17 November

Boxall S 1981 Nurse education correspondence: a report. Australian Nurses' Journal, September:7-12

Cochrane J 1989 Influencing the politics of health reform. In: Gray G, Pratt R (eds) 1989 Issues in Australian Nursing 2. Churchill Livingstone, Melbourne

Cockburn S 1966 Call for higher nursing skills. UNA Nursing Journal, September:239-240

Cohen J 1948 Minority Report. Working Party on the Recruitment and Training of Nurses (the Wood Report). Great Britain. Ministry of Health, Department of Health for Scotland, Ministry of Labour and National Service. HMSO, London

College of Nursing, Australia 1969 Education policies. Melbourne, May

CTEC (Commonwealth Tertiary Education Commission) 1984 Report for the 1985-1987 Triennium. AGPS, Canberra

Congalton A A (ed) 1962 Young people look at nursing. New South Wales College of Nursing, Sydney

Creighton H, Lopez F 1982 A history of nursing education in New South Wales. Lopez, Sydney

Curry G 1977 Educating for nursing professionalism—status or competence? The Lamp, October:5-7

Dawkins J S 1988 Higher education: a policy statement. AGPS, Canberra

DEET (Department of Employment, Education and Training) 1990 Tertiary Education Scores, Higher Education Series, Report no. 9, October, AGPS, Canberra

Duffield C M 1986 Nursing in Australia comes of age! International Journal of Nursing Studies, 23(4):281-284

Duke C (ed) 1975 Nurse education—what future? Goals in Nursing Education: report on a conference in the ACT. Centre for Continuing Education. ANU, Canberra

Durdin J 1991 They became nurses. A history of nursing in South Australia 1836-1980. Allen & Unwin, Sydney

Fellows M P 1971 Education—process of evolution. Australian Nurses' Journal, September:30-31

Fox C 1989 Industrial relations in nursing—Victoria 1982-1985. Australian Studies in Health Administration no. 68. University of New South Wales School of Health Administration, Sydney

Godfrey J 1978 Diversification of higher education in Australia. Australian Nurses' Journal, October:41-43

Guy M F 1964 The practice of nursing. Annual Orations 1953-1976. New South Wales College of Nursing, Sydney

Hamilton J 1986 Australian nursing: a political and social perspective. In: Dubree M A, Culpepper R C, McLean B M (eds) The destiny of nursing: interaction of the discipline with society. Vanderbilt University Medical Center

HDV (Health Department Victoria) 1990 Ministerial review of birthing services in Victoria. Final report. Having a baby in Victoria. HDV, Melbourne

Henderson A R 1990 The politicisation of nurse education in Australia. Paper given at the 16th Convention of the Australian Congress of Mental Health Nurses, Perth, September

Jago A H 1972 Nurse education in NSW. Letter to the editor. Medical Journal of Australia, 17 July

Jayawardena Y 1961 Whither nursing? Australian Nurses' Journal, November:264-269, December:290-296

Jayawardena Y 1962 The ICN and educational criteria for membership. International Nursing Review, 9(5):55-58

Jayawardena Y 1983 The integration of basic nursing education into tertiary education: possible repercussions on the nursing workforce. School of Health Administration, University of New South Wales, Sydney
Keane B 1987 Study of mental health nursing in Australia. Commonwealth Department of Health (Nursing and Health Services Workforce Branch) Canberra.
Lambert P 1975 New horizons in nursing. Australian Nurses' Journal, November:31-34, 44
Larkins N 1972 Nurse education in NSW. Letter to the editor from the AMA New South Wales Branch. Medical Journal of Australia, 22 July:222
Lawson J S 1969 Who will nurse the sick in the seventies? A study of the nursing service in Victorian hospitals. Medical Journal of Australia, 26 July:195-200
Lublin J R 1985 Basic nurse education in CAEs—the educational evidence for transfer. Australian Journal of Advanced Nursing 2(2):18-28
Lyons B 1978 Regional schools of nursing. The Lamp, August:18-21
McGrath M A 1973 Letter to Elizabeth Reid (Prime Minister's Adviser). The Lamp, November:27
McGrath M A 1984 Nurse education in New South Wales. Nurses Education Board of NSW, Sydney
McGrath M A 1987 Transformation through transfer—the re-organisation of nursing education in New South Wales. Paper given at a seminar conducted by King Edward's Hospital Fund for London, London, 19 June
MacGuire J 1969 Threshold to nursing. Occasional Papers on Social Administration, no. 30. Bell, London
McManamny S 1991 Personal communication
McMillan M A, Dwyer J 1989 Changing times, changing paradigm (1): from hospital training to college education in Australia. Nurse Education Today 9:13-18
Martin C 1978 Major confrontation over bans on degree in nursing course. Australian Nurses' Journal, December-January:11-12
Martin L 1964-65 Report of the Committee on the Future of Tertiary Education in Australia to the Australian Universities Commission (Chairman Sir Leslie Martin). AGPS, Canberra
Martins A C 1990 The transfer of nurse education from hospital schools of nursing to higher education institutions: a study of the implementation of educational policy in a federal system. Unpublished PhD thesis, University of Western Australia
Neill J 1987 Tertiary nursing students: a changing demographic profile? Australian Journal of Advanced Nursing, 4(4):52-60
Olesen V L, Whittaker E W 1968 The silent dialogue. Jossey-Bass, San Francisco
Parkes M E 1971 Goals in nursing. (Paper read at the 22nd Annual General Meeting of the College of Nursing, Australia, June). Australian Nurses' Journal 1972 April:35-37
Parkes M E 1986 Through politics to professionalism. In: White R (ed) Political issues in nursing: past, present and future, Vol. 2. Wiley, Chichester
Parkin F 1979 Marxism and class theory: a bourgeois critique. Tavistock, London
Parsons R 1971 The nursing reformation. The Lamp, January:26-35
Parsons R 1973a The transfer of the formal teaching functions of the New South Wales College of Nursing to the School of Nursing in the New South Wales College of Paramedical Studies. The Lamp, May:37-39
Parsons R 1973b Trends in nursing education in colleges of advanced education. The Lamp, June:26-32
Parsons R 1978 Nursing education reform—ten years on. The Lamp, October:9-13
Patten M E 1979 Key letter to Senator Carrick (letter from National Steering Committee to the Minister for Education). Australian Nurses' Journal, October:10-12
Patten M E 1980 Nursing education and patient care. Australian Nurses' Journal, September:41-43
Pilkington M P 1972 A study of basic nurse education in NSW. Australian Nurses' Journal, November:17-18
Pilkington M P 1977 Nursing education—what can we afford? Florence Nightingale Oration, National Florence Nightingale Committee, Brisbane, 27 October
Powell M 1963 The art of nursing. In: Annual Orations 1953-76. New South Wales College of Nursing, Sydney
Russell R L 1990 From Nightingale to now: nurse education in Australia. Harcourt Brace Jovanovich, Marrickville

Saint E 1971 Nursing in Queensland. Report of the Committee of Inquiry into Nursing (Chairman Professor E G Saint). RANF Queensland Branch, Brisbane
Sax S 1978 Nurse education and training. Report of the committee of inquiry into nurse education and training to the Tertiary Education Commission (Chairman Dr S Sax). AGPS, Canberra
Slater P V 1963 Comprehensive training. UNA Nursing Journal, June:202-210
Slater P V 1969 The preparation of the nurse today and in the future. National Florence Nightingale Committee of Australia, Melbourne
Slater P V 1970 Address to the College of Nursing, Australia, Victorian State Committee Annual Meeting 1970. UNA Nursing Journal, July-August:10-16
Slater P V 1971 Comments on the Report of the Committee of Enquiry into Nursing in Victoria. National Hospital 15(5):15-17
Slater P V 1979 Implications for nursing services of proposed changes in nursing education. Seminar on nurse education and training—the Sax Report. Woden Valley Hospital, Canberra, 5 April
Slater P V 1982 The role of nursing organisations in professional education—challenges for the future. 16th Patricia Chomley Oration. College of Nursing, Australia, Melbourne
Summers P 1985 Nurse education under the microscope. Journal of Advanced Education, July:13
Treyvaud E R, McLaren J 1976 Equal but cheaper. Melbourne University Press, Melbourne
Turner K 1985 Back to a contest:1981-1984. In: Chaples E, Nelson H, Turner K (eds) The Wran model: electoral politics in New South Wales 1981 and 1984. Oxford University Press, Melbourne
Willis E 1983 Medical dominance. Allen & Unwin, Sydney
Wood P 1990 Progress through partnership. Commonwealth Government, Department of Community Services and Health, Canberra

4. Nursing work: a few more degrees of freedom

Nurses had been exploited 'financially and physically' according to a member of the federal parliament speaking in 1970 (Hayden CPD 20 May 1970:2391). 'Exploited dedication' (Hayden CPD 20 May 1970:2391) referred to the long hours of hard work rewarded by very low salaries compared to those of other health professionals, and to the vocational nature of nursing work which was seen to justify the poor pay and conditions. The political and industrial activities of nurses, through their unions and professional organisations, have led to substantial gains in pay and conditions of work, and in levels of education, and it is probably because of these gains that nurses are concerned now with different issues in the workplace. Nursing work has changed and this has introduced its own difficulties and opportunities; not least from the mix of attitudes, experience and levels of expertise present in any but the smallest of health care agencies. Change, and reactions to change, are dominant concerns in those trying to bring it about and those who are, sometimes without apparent recognition, struggling with feelings about the value of those changes.

But change *is* occurring and the pressures for change are coming from inside and outside nursing:

> It's from management, from the health system as a whole, from patient demands, from different sets of requirements, from a less paternalistic structure generally. Within this, nurses are beginning to discover a few more degrees of freedom. [JP/90]

Nurses (registered and enrolled) are the largest single occupational group in the health industry. In 1989, they represented approximately 60% of the health workforce (Grant & Lapsley 1992:141). The next largest group was medical practitioners who represented approximately 11%. The Appendix (pp. 319–26) gives health employment statistics from the 1986 and 1991 censuses.

Nurses, as a group, are with their patients over a 24 hour period on every day of the week. They are present in every aspect of health and health care, either in hospitals and nursing homes or in the community. But:

> nurses have become increasingly frustrated with their lack of autonomy within the traditional institutional structure where accountability is seen to be to the

institution rather than to the patient/client, and where they have unequal opportunity to participate in decision making about matters which affect their practice. (Jenkins 1989:203)

Decision making is inevitably a political process, whether it is viewed as a reconciliation of conflicting interests, or as the exercise of power by the stronger over the weaker participants so that the resultant policies or decisions reflect those powerful interests (Gardner & Barraclough 1992:7–9). Power is viewed as the ability of an individual or group to make others do something that they would not otherwise have done, or as the ability to prevent change occurring with or without intervention.

In some ways, the issue of nursing and power is enigmatic. Nurses have always had power—power over each other and power over their patients, more covert power over medical staff, and legitimate power from position—and yet have been described, and have described themselves, as powerless. The nursing hierarchy had provided nurses with the opportunity to hold powerful positions but nurses' right to participate in decisions about their work had not been acknowledged. Part of the explanation lies in definitions of what is perceived to be worthwhile work. Such definitions have tended to be gender related and to include as worthwhile only work carried out by men (Chs 5 & 6). If an occupation is, or becomes, predominantly staffed by women then its perceived status is lowered and opportunities for appropriate remuneration and influence are concomitantly reduced (see, for example, Williams 1988; Rimmer 1991). Nursing, banking and teaching are examples of this process of occupational segmentation. Within the health care agency, particularly in hospitals, the issue of power is closely linked to changes in nursing education and to changes in thinking about nursing practice. It is about nurses being recognised for what they do and participating by right in making decisions about health and how care is delivered, on the basis of their expertise:

> It's no good changing education if you don't change the hospital. Changing the hospital side of nursing practice, and the whole ethos of care, and relationships, and getting nurses to take on appropriate power not inappropriate power, is very difficult...It is about the patient as of primary importance rather than the nurse; empowering the patient, rather than being the controller. [MP/91]

A collaborative approach to defining and clarifying nursing and the role of the nurse was undertaken by the Royal Australian Nursing Federation, the College of Nursing Australia, the New South Wales College of Nursing and the Florence Nightingale Committee Australia to produce a new national document to 'be used by nurses, and nursing and health care organisations, to explain and promote nursing and the role of the nurse within the wider community' (*Nursing in Australia: a national statement* (ANF 1989)). The emphasis in the statement is on the nurse as a clinical practitioner within the social context, experiencing a range of settings from institutions of acute and extended care through to the community, and with broad and complex roles in promoting health as well as caring for the 'physically and mentally ill'. To facilitate this practice an 'essential requirement' is a career structure which 'offers nurses the opportunity to achieve...with recognition in terms of status and remuneration for demonstrated competence, educational qualifications, and experience in all areas of nursing'.

There is now some recognition from outside (from government, from commentators on the health system) of the changes that are taking place in nursing which stem

> from the changed education system, with the changed demands from the new career structure, with women remaining in the workforce, with professional rates of pay, with demands for higher education...[JP/90]

The 'few more degrees of freedom' combined with higher expectations have provided opportunities but there is a great deal of confusion with some nurses feeling inadequate or incompetent. This confusion has been exacerbated by the pressures upon nurses to accept a number of different paradigms of nursing practice and knowledge as 'the truth' (Ch. 2). Nursing is still, not unexpectedly, in a transitional stage. It is in the process of change, but the advantages of improved pay and conditions, a new career structure, and a larger role in decision making do not come without costs.

Reclaiming the caring role

Until recently, decision making for nurses, in parallel with career paths, had been assumed to lie mainly with those in administrative positions. That is, increased participation in decision making was a concomitant of an upward movement through the organisational hierarchy whereby there was an inverse relationship with direct patient care. As decision making increased, patient care diminished for the individual nurse. There have been a number of changes to nursing structures and practice which have attempted to alter this relationship on the assumption that if direct patient care is taken to be the primary role of the nurse then nurses should be making decisions about that care. Decision making should be delegated to the level where direct patient care is carried out rather than being mediated through supervisors who were in the main carrying out administrative functions, while the bedside nurse carried out a number of clinical functions or tasks.

Nurses have to accept some responsibility for the difficulties involved in a changed thinking about nursing practice. This is because of the hierarchy of nursing care created by the hospital based system of training which produced a hierarchy of nursing tasks:

> That euphemism called basic nursing care, which is the core of nursing, was at the bottom of the hierarchy. [MP/91]

Student nurses, after a short preliminary training, entered the hospital and were immediately involved in direct patient care:

> So what did you do? You gave them the relatively well child to sponge and to feed. You gave them those nursing functions, basic nursing care, anyone can do that, because after all a student coming out of PTS can do that, can't she? (or he). So we said that that really was the lowest care. Then we said things like 'As you get a bit more time on the wards, and a bit more experience, you can do things like simple dressings.' Then you might be allowed to give some tablets and some medications. Then in your second year you might be allowed to manage 'intravenouses' and injections. By your third year, you're really good, you can manage technology? Dear God! We created the hierarchy of nursing tasks! No wonder people see technology as being the pinnacle of a nursing career. [MP/91]

So nursing care became devalued in favour of technical competence, whereas it is really the linkage of these which should be important in nursing practice:

> People who provide excellent direct care, very good support for the families, wonderful support for the patients, have still found it enormously difficult to change to working from principles, to work on individual planning, to be the point of articulation between technology and the person...To be able to use the knowledge they have in making connections from the cross-application of that knowledge. You really do need nurses who can make complex judgements in complex situations. That to me is what nursing is all about. It is about linking complex technology and human beings together and making it bearable for patients. It is about getting the patients involved in their own care. [MP/91]

The emphasis on task allocation had begun to break down in the 1970s, to be replaced by either team or primary nursing (see Sellick & Russell 1983, Thomas & Bond 1990):

> The biggest change I noticed when returning in 1976 after a two year break was that task allocation was gradually changing to individual patient allocation. So that on night duty it had been the most junior person who did the pans, observations and sponges, the next up did the more responsible or technical work, and the person in charge co-ordinated and gave out the drugs etc. In 1976, there were still three people on duty but each person had his or her own group of patients and was totally responsible for those patients. One person was in charge and directed the actual allocation of patients. [MS/91]

But change from within is difficult when established structures reinforce hierarchical relationships and attitudes:

> Many nurses are still very traditional in hospital practice because it has more or less been a closed system. Medical training has been such that it rein-

forces particular sets of attitudes; it's very narrow,...it's very much based on the need for people to get the approval of seniors. So it's very conformist, and it's very much based on reciprocity, with a very clear separation or division of labour between doctors and nurses...What has happened is that nurses who could tolerate the clearly structured sets of role relationships stayed there and reinforced them...So it was difficult to get change from within. [JP/90]

The recognition of the need for change in nursing practice so that nurses can make independent decisions about individual patient care is similarly hampered by these traditional role relationships, but as one nurse with over 20 years experience said in response to being asked what she saw as the biggest change in nursing:

The nurse who asks questions, who is not just going to be told 'This is the way you do it'. I think it is valuable for all nurses to be questioning. It wouldn't have occurred to us to ask questions. It is positive because it keeps us 'on the ball'. The negative side is that sometimes the questioning is inappropriate and it might not be backed up by information, which is a problem when it concerns senior nursing or medical staff. [EH/90]

Questioning is a way to learn and to assert one's knowledge, and the comment suggests that nurses have in the past been discouraged from questioning because others believe, or have believed, that they ought not to question and do not need knowledge other than the ability to carry out certain tasks.

A registered nurse who had returned to the hospital after some years and worked in the relieving pool across a number of areas put it this way:

I like people who are open and honest and able to discuss things. If you have fear like I did when I was training you didn't learn, you couldn't ask questions. You were virtually told what to do and you didn't really think a lot either. In that respect it has changed for the better. [RG/90]

Her view is supported by the ANRAC competencies (see below) where the nurse is expected to question (1990:13.1-13.4).

However willing nurses might be to question and to have an input into decision making, they are sometimes thwarted by existing hospital and medical practices. For example, with admission and discharge policies:

If a visiting medical officer in the public system has two sessions a week and has to see the patient before they are discharged, the patient can wait three extra days before discharge...Where nurses are having an effect on admission and discharge planning [it is] in individual work places where there are people able to work together, through medical superintendent, chief executive officer, director of nursing and clinical nurses in the various wards and units, who are working together to facilitate flow through and proper discharge planning. [MB/92]

If the primary concern of nursing is nursing practice, and administration is its support and not its core (Silver 1986:44), then the need for extensive reform in the organisation of clinical nursing becomes obvious. People who choose nursing generally gain their job satisfaction from caring for patients (Rowe & Manning 1987, Walsh & Bruni 1983) not from administration. A number of job satisfaction surveys in the 1970s and 1980s had shown that nurses were experiencing a decrease in satisfaction (Silver 1989:225–6). This lack of satisfaction involved salary, working conditions, status and opportunities to make use of their training. For career advancement, it was necessary to move out of clinical work and into administration or education. The expansion of community health in the early 1970s and of rehabilitation in the 1980s provided further sources of escape for some nurses from the rigidly bureaucratic hospital nursing structures with their diminished access to decision making for all but those at the top of the hierarchy.

Dissatisfaction with pay and conditions of work together with the lack of a career ladder for clinical nurses increased during the 1970s and 1980s until there was such widespread unrest throughout Australia that unprecedented political and industrial action by nurses became a feature of the states and territories (Ch. 6). The intensity varied according to the personalities of the leaders of the state branches of the nursing unions and the intransigence or otherwise of state health ministers, but there was a strong undercurrent of unity of problems and purpose which often transcended state boundaries. However, federalism, or the division of power in the Australian political system between the states and territories, and the federal or national level, unfortunately resulted in different salary and career structures being implemented at different times in the different states. (The career structures in the states and territories can be seen in Figs 4.1-3). More has been written about the South Australian experience of its new career structure than about the other states. In South Australia there had been a six month trial involving 11 health units before implementation throughout the state ('A program for Career Structure' Parts 1-6 *ANJ* August 1986, September 1986, October 1986, November 1986, January 1987, February 1987, Silver 1989, Koch 1990). There are, however, similarities as well as differences, with one of the similarities being changes not only to clinical nursing but to nursing management as well. As Silver (*ANJ* August 1986:44) says, 'The development of a structure which included advanced clinical roles necessitated restructure of management and education roles'.

As early as 1972, the amount of time which nurses spent on administration and other tasks rather than on clinical care was documented. White (1972) argued that:

> since 90% of available personnel are to be found in employment in hospitals and nursing homes, it can be assumed that the majority of nurses are available for the role of direct care...It is appropriate, therefore, to examine the extent to which that role is being fulfilled at the present time.

Level	Management	Clinical	Education
5		Director of Nursing	
4	Assistant Director of nursing: Management	Assistant Director of Nursing: Clinical	Assistant Director of Nursing: Education
3	Nurse manager	Clinical Nurse Consultant	Nurse Educator
2		Clinical Nurse	
1		Registered Nurse	

Fig. 4.1 Career structure model (South Australia).

Level	Education	Clinical	Management	Research
5		Director of Nursing		
4	Coordinator Nursing Staff Development	Coordinator Clinical Nursing	Coordinator Nursing Management	Coordinator Nursing Research
3	Staff Development Educator	Clinical Nurse Specialist	Nurse Manager	Nursing Researcher
2	Staff Development Nurse	Clinical Nurse	Area Manager	Research Nurse
1		Registered Nurse		

Fig. 4.2 Career structure model (Western Australia).

Level	Management	Clinical	Education
7		Director of Nursing	
6	Deputy Director of Nursing	Clinical Nurse Consultant D	Principal Teacher
5	Assistant Director of Nursing	Clinical Nurse Consultant C Supervisor	Deputy Principal Teacher
4	Charge Nurse	Clinical Nurse Consultant B	Teacher
3	Associate Charge Nurse	Clinical Nurse Consultant A	
2		Clinical Nurse Specialist* Registered Nurse	
1		Registered Nurse (1st Year)	

* Personal classification not from position

Fig. 4.3 Career structure model (Victoria).

She described nursing practices as 'the provision of nursing services directly to patients and members of their families' and identified three areas which this involved: clinical practice, administration and teaching. She argued that 'many elements of clinical practice [such as maintenance or restoration of basic functions, changes in a patient's condition and providing support] are common to primary, acute and long-term care and form the fundamentals upon which specialist expertise is later built'. Administration involved the 'co-ordination of services for patients and ancillary personnel, integration and supervising of the activities of personnel and some services' and that the 'supervision of clinical practice and patient welfare generally, involves a teaching function also, particularly with student nurses and junior trained staff' (White 1972:2.2.1).

White (1972:2.2.3) found that while the proportion of time spent on each varied from ward to ward, 'there is a noticeable pattern which shows that less time is spent in clinical practice than in administration, and that minimal time is available for teaching'. Further, that of the total nursing time available per patient only 50% was available during the day shift, 31.7% during the evening shift and only 18.3% at night (1972:2.2.4). Of the non-nursing activities, which represented 39% of ward activities and did not require nursing skills, 68% utilised nursing resources (White 1972:2.2.5).

Following implementation of the new nursing career structures in the late 1980s, changes to the organisational structure and processes have been described by Silver (1986) as a change from the classic bureaucracy identified by Weber (Parsons 1964:329-36) with a rigid, hierarchical structure incorporating legal-rational principles of organisation, to a professional bureaucracy where the structure is a flattened pyramid. In the professional bureaucracy responsibility does not flow downwards and accountability upwards but rather responsibility and accountability are found together. In other words, in the classic Weberian bureaucracy supervisors are responsible for those below them on the bureaucratic level and accountable to those immediately above, and so on up the line. In the professional bureaucracy, as most of the work of the organisation, defined as those procedures most closely linked to the goals of the organisation, is carried out in the 'operating core' (Mintzberg 1979), those doing the actual work were responsible for that work but only *indirectly* accountable to their employing organisation, and not accountable to the patient or client. The new structures thus attempt to 'provide for devolution of power, authority and decision making down the line, resulting in decentralised rather than centralised approaches to management' (Silver 1989:228).

Those trying to bring about change, whether in increased involvement in decision making for nurses, or in implementing different ways of delivering patient care, give the impression of an almost mammoth struggle to carry nursing kicking and screaming into a future where nurses are responsible and accountable, informed and credible, competent and caring. These are seen as necessary if nurses are to be recognised as professionals.

Accountability for care

> If you have people who will not become accountable, you will not become professional. Nurses had developed the dreadful habit of not wanting to accept accountability. To be professional you have to become accountable. [JK/90]

Acceptance of accountability is perhaps made more difficult for nurses by the longstanding attitude of medical practitioners that it is they who make the orders for nurses to carry out and it is they who are accountable, so that 'nurses can hide behind vicarious accountability'. [GL/88] This is in spite of legal requirements which make the nurse accountable for her/or his actions:

> We had an incident a few weeks ago where a doctor ordered 10 times the recommended dosage for a particular drug and the nurse refused to give it and the doctor reported her. He would not understand that because she knew that that was the wrong dosage, had she given it she would have been accountable. [MS/91]

Why isn't the accountability of nursing staff accepted by the medical profession?

> It's a threatening concept and doctors aren't taught about it in their courses. I was arguing at an ethics committee over informed consent and professional accountability and the medical members not only didn't, but refused to acknowledge that nurses had any degree of accountability at all...They find it surprising that not only do other disciplines learn these things in their courses but that they understand them...Doctors have been disadvantaged by their education. [MS/91]

Accountability for nursing care has been enhanced by the stress placed on the clinical role in the new nursing career structures. Increased accountability at each level of practice was included in the objectives for the development of the new career structures in South Australia (Silver 1989:228), and Western Australia (Steering Committee for the Implementation of the Nursing Career Structure 1987), and has been incorporated into the national competencies for the registration and enrolment of nurses. The registered nurse 'demonstrates accountability for nursing practice by accepting responsibility for actions, clarifying unclear instructions, questioning interventions which appear inappropriate, and making sound, independent clinical judgements, (ANRAC May 1990:13.1–13.4). As Cameron (1989:214) argues, the development of national competencies:

> represents a significant milestone for the nursing profession in Australia as, together with the standards for nursing practice already developed (1983) by the Royal Australian Nursing Federation, it typifies the nursing profession's continuing acceptance of accountability for practice.

Concern by governments about the standard of services, and increased costs and declining resources for health care, have led to a need to demonstrate accountability. The increased emphasis on accountability has provided nurses with an important forum for decision making. Quality Assurance (QA) committees have been established in hospitals at senior management level with representation from a wide range of areas, including nursing, in order to prepare detailed quality assurance programs. In addition, the nursing department, or division, is likely to have its own QA committee chaired by an assistant director of nursing (ADON) to prepare a quality assurance program which is consistent with, and complementary to, the hospital program:

> Quality assurance...is mandatory. Nurses had to become aware of quality assurance because it's in their new job descriptions...We started quality assurance programs which have now been reviewed and modified...We asked questions of staff and patients...and have brought in clinical reviews. [MA/90]

In addition to quality assurance (which is now beginning to be overtaken by Total Quality Management), the nursing division is likely to have a large number of committees relating to nursing practice. These can include committees on nursing policy, practice and procedures, or on education, ethics, and equipment. They are usually chaired by a nurse at assistant director of nursing (ADON) level or by a clinical nurse consultant, who selects the membership from different levels and with representation from different areas.

The nursing practice and procedures committee (however styled) reviews every practice and procedure to ensure that they conform to regulations and to accepted standards of practice. The nursing division establishes a policy, which must conform to and be adopted as hospital policy, and then the procedures that actually go with the policy are worked out in detail, taking into account ethical and legal constraints. This is not always easy because nursing policy guidelines established by outside boards responsible for registration and standards are often vague, open ended and difficult to interpret at a practical level. The committee decides on the education and competencies that are required by nurses to undertake certain procedures and to understand the possible side effects of, for example, carrying out glycerin trinitrate (GTN) infusions for pain relief. This has become particularly necessary with the extension of specialist procedures to general wards, where the expertise may not always be available.

Clinicians or managers or both

In spite of variation between states, the emphasis in all the new career structures is on the expert clinical role of the nurse in patient care rather than on the nurse as manager. They thus provide a clinical career ladder as the central feature of the organisation of nursing with nurse managers, educators, staff developers, and clinical researchers as the support staff.

Silver's (1986, 1989) discussion of the South Australian career structure, its development and implementation suggests quite clearly that the decision in that state to divide the charge nurse role into two was based upon the difficulty charge nurses faced in effectively carrying out the management of care and the management of resources. So that in general only one aspect of their role was effectively fulfilled (Silver 1986).

The charge nurse position had been a pivotal role. She or he was the key link between the nurses at the bedside and senior management. Charge nurses were in a position to assert the importance and credibility of nursing in many areas, for example in quality assurance, in staffing, in budget management, and in staff development. Their role was however not clearcut: 'They were administrators, who were not really administrators. They were in a no-man's land' [JK/90]. They were in the position to receive an enormous amount of information but have been described collectively as 'the sponge level', where information is absorbed and only small drops might be squeezed out by those at ward or unit level. In delegating now, there is the need for them to be confident and assertive enough to say 'you must make decisions but make them with me' [JK/90]. Charge nurses had always had a great deal of control and while the changes in the career structures, where the charge nurse position has been maintained as in Victoria and New South Wales, have in some sense given them a larger role in decision making, it has changed their role from one with the potential for the autocratic use of power by direction and supervision to one where the emphasis is on delegation of authority and facilitation through support.

The separation of clinical from management roles at the former charge nurse level in the new career structures in the other states and territories, has however introduced an element of ambiguity. The division of the role does indeed mean that the clinical nurse consultant's (CNC's) role is in clinical practice, but that this also involves clinical management in planning nursing care, and in teaching, guiding and evaluating personnel (Silver 1986:45). By placing the management of the unit itself with the nurse manager, the CNC should have more time for clinical care, planning, education and research. The division between management and clinical work is however not always clear. As a South Australian nurse said:

> I just can't get away from the fact that whether you are in charge of the management of a ward, or whether you are in charge of the clinical aspects of the ward, you are a manager. The clinical nurse consultant has to co-ordinate patient allocation, and organise clinical care and education which involves management in function if not in title. The nurse manager doesn't have a clinical input but does stores and the inventory, rosters and so on. Both are involved in staff selection with the nurse manager carrying out the procedural side. [EC/88]

For the nurse manager the change was often perceived as a loss of status and power, which required sensitive support from those implementing the new structure:

> So we had to improve the communications system, because the one 'linchpin' had gone. What followed from there was of course this division between management, clinical, and staff development, and 'I belong here, and you belong there'. That's started to roll back again, it needed that team spirit: 'We're all here for the one thing, and this is what the clinical nurses are here for and you're here to support them, and they can't do without you'. That's one of the things they say to the management staff development people all the time: 'Yes the clinical nurses are there to deliver the care, but they can't do without you, you've got to provide them with people, with the resources, and you've got to support them in relation to that, so you are part of a team, and a very significant part.'
>
> I think that's one of the things that got lost. 'I'm here doing my bit, but I used to be in charge.' As I said, it's going to take five years; I think my prediction is right. [DMcC/90]

It was perhaps the change in the role of the charge nurse which created the most concern from doctors, particularly in Western Australia where a number of clinical nurses are responsible for patients and no one person is 'in charge':

> I think the teaching hospitals have the biggest trouble because of the key role that the charge nurse had played. The consultants, who had never spoken to the 'plebs' in their lives, had to look at a board to see [who had been allocated to their patients]. So instead of someone giving them third-hand information about their patient, they were expected to be directed to the caregiver. Well, the number of times they wrote long, involved complaints about it! I believe they have quietened now, but I think they expected that the evaluation of the career structure would say 'Put back the charge nurse!' And of course it hasn't done that...
>
> So we had to establish different lines of communication, clearly identify who was the resource person for the day. There would be a co-ordinator—when you have a busy situation you need a co-ordinator—and they rotated it through; it didn't have to be a clinical nurse, it could be a good registered nurse. We saw it as developing management skills...Yes, doctor, sure, sister so-and-so is caring for your patient, I'll get her for you. Yes, theatre, I'll get them to pre-med her, right'. That sort of thing took control. They [doctors etc.] had to name them, because they'd never ever asked for anyone but the charge nurse. Suddenly they found they had 30 sisters and charge nurses, and they'd never bothered to find out their names. So we had to identify who the carers were, so that they would look up and see: Mrs Grant—Nurse Jones, etc. [DMcC/90]

The medical response, however, was not uniform. For medical residents, the change could be seen as an improvement as they are on the ward working with the nurses all day and appreciated not having to consult first with the charge nurse, but preferred to work with the nurse directly responsible for the patient's care:

> 'I don't talk to the charge nurses, because I go to the one who's responsible for the patient's care. They're the ones I'm interested in, I have to work with—I virtually work there all day in the ward.' [Residents] were just like the nurses in those busy wards, they rarely got away except to go into theatre. One resident said 'The person I need is the one who's there—when I've got to put up a drip, I want to start IV antibiotics, or I want to do this, or that, I don't run down and ask the charge nurse.' Five years down the track the new interns are not even going to know that a charge nurse exists. [DMcC/90]

While recognising that each state is naturally committed to its own career structure, the secretary of the ANF (Victorian branch) argued that the structure largely developed in South Australia has:

> ...one huge fundamental flaw and that is splitting up the roles of the charge nurse. I think the whole core of nursing, and the quality of care delivered to clients depends on the charge nurse. And the charge nurse must have that tripartite role: education, clinical and management...To me the strength of nursing is its very broad base...and the moment you start carving bits off, you're reducing the power...and the good effect of nurses and nursing. [BM/93]

In Victoria and New South Wales, while the charge nurse position was maintained and not split as in the other states, it was altered in function. Authority was devolved to the charge nurse as a unit manager and the position of assistant charge nurse was introduced.

The charge nurse in an intensive care unit (ICU) in a medium sized hospital in Victoria described the unit and her understanding of her new role and opportunities. When interviewed in 1990, she had been there for four years and had been appointed as the charge nurse after ten years' experience in intensive care in other hospitals. The interview is reproduced extensively not only because it provides insights into one charge nurse's experience but also because it highlights many of the themes which are relevant to nursing today: change; leadership; communication; structure and processes; education; decision making; relationships with other staff—nursing and non-nursing; and above all commitment to clients, their families and to a health promoting role.

In charge of intensive care in Victoria

> I think I am very fortunate in being a charge nurse in intensive care because (I may be wrong) but I don't think that the charge nurse in the wards has as

much autonomy as I have. Decision making in the unit depends on my style of leadership…If you want respect from the people you work with you have to earn it, and make them feel good about themselves. To do this you have to listen to what they say, communicate appropriately, and provide a good environment. A good environment is one which has equipment, and resources for education, for problem solving, for conflict resolution, and for helping them to grow personally and professionally.

When I first came here we didn't even have a pan room. The procedures had been superseded. For example, they didn't monitor cuff pressure, they didn't take core temperatures. These are standard procedures in intensive care. Even charting, and documentation had to be revised. A lot of change had to occur and people don't take change lightly.

However, if people are involved in change and contribute ideas they are more likely to accept and to follow the changes. Communication is very, very important. I recognise the need to be able to communicate well. I have learnt this over the years and study for my degrees, particularly at Masters level, has emphasised this.

The associate charge nurses, the clinical teacher and I meet every Thursday and discuss the general running of the area and we also discuss how people are progressing in the unit, if we are meeting their educational needs and other issues. Every Friday, we have a ward meeting which is minuted and the night staff have recently started to do the same.

We have an education program and staff decide on the content. On Mondays, we have an article or sometimes a video. Staff members choose the article and make it available to the others. We've changed handover so that we allow a complete hour for discussing the particular topic. On Tuesdays and Thursdays representatives come and talk about their products, and on Wednesdays we have a structured lecture by another nurse, or doctor or clinical teacher…We now have a clinical teacher who is a wonderful resource.

Staff in intensive care understand that equipment assists them in providing care and we were very fortunate in obtaining resources for staffing and to buy the equipment we needed…We have been able to get good monitoring equipment, some good ventilators and other technology which makes life easier, and safer for patients…Before this, we needed more staff and better equipment and I wrote a submission to nursing administration, which they presented to medical administration, and then to the state Health Department. The Health Department was looking at critical care services at the same time so it was very fortunate…Together, the consultant and I have struggled to get what we want. We had closed down beds because we didn't have the money for appropriate staffing numbers. It was very, very stressful for the staff, for myself and for the patients …

In this hospital, if there is something you don't agree with there are people who are sufficiently interested and motivated…to do something about it…When I came I was unhappy about the way central lines were looked after. So I went to the clinical teacher. Within a short time, we had set up an IV subcommittee with nurses from other wards and decided to look at intravenous care and treatment across the hospital. We put together a policy which was subsequently adopted for the whole hospital. It's an educational tool, it's a resource for people to refer to and it maintains consistency and a high standard in nursing care…Nursing is about maintaining a high standard of patient care…I have found people to be consistently motivated and caring here and there are appropriate channels for communication, for example through the practice and procedure committee, or the policy committee…

Here I can deal directly with whoever I need to…If I have a personnel problem, I go to the assistant director of nursing in personnel, if I have an allocation problem, to the ADON in allocations, or if I have a problem that I think only the director of nursing [DON] can solve then I go directly to her…Nursing admin. encourages us to be unit managers as part of a more decentralised (and less hierarchical) structure. I don't have to go through nursing to go to medical administration or physiotherapy…

You have to implement change very carefully, because you need to respect staff and not lower their self-esteem, particularly with people who have worked [here] for years and who might be a lot older, and who might not have a degree. So it has been very interesting trying to implement what I thought was right for the unit.

I like to think we provide a high standard of care and extend that care to the family, because the family is very much part of that critically ill patient. Expectations about visitors were different when I arrived. They were expected to stay a short time and then leave. Now our visiting times are 24 hours a day but only two visitors at a time…We try to involve them in patient care. It is very soothing for critical patients to, for example, have a family member give them a foot or hand massage—to extend the care to the family.

We have a non-detailed handover each shift so that we know what is happening to all our patients and then the shift co-ordinator allocates staff to the patients. I might be a shift co-ordinator. The method of allocation depends on leadership style. Some associate charge nurses [ACNs] might be more autocratic and simply make the allocation for the staff member, or they might say 'Who would you like to look after?' Or you can combine the two methods depending on staff competence and preference and the types of patients…I think people should have the ability to say 'I've looked after this patient for three days and I'm really drained, can I have someone else?' I believe that people provide better care when they have input into it. We allocate one staff member to one patient and the shift co-ordinator is usually supernumerary, so she supervises, and co-ordinates and oversees the general physical environment.

All staff who want to work in the unit are interviewed by myself and the personnel officer and we jointly make the decision on whether to accept them or not…I have also developed a bank of people with critical care certificates and I can use my bank to fill numbers in my rosters. I don't have the authority to go to an agency directly but I can go to my bank.

> I don't have any real say on admissions or discharge but our opinion is sought on whether we believe a patient should go to the High Dependency Nursing Unit [HDNU] or to the ward after intensive care because that has to do with nursing management of the patient rather than with medical management. HDNU then rates the patient which in turn gives them a decision making role.
>
> Intensive care does make you a little bit insular...because we don't have as much exposure in terms of patient progress when they go to the wards or home. Especially being in ICU, which is sometimes considered an elitist area, you have to work very hard on public relations...We are here to help one another personally and professionally because gone are the days when you work for yourself and stab everyone else in the back.
>
> We have a lot of contact with the Health Promotion Unit. We refer patients to the Drug and Alcohol unit if they have come to us because of an alcohol related incident or to the Health Promotion Unit, for example, if smoking is involved. A lot of our patients are in ICU because of their own actions. The decision is theirs, whether they accept assistance or not, but I think we should make it available to them once they are out of the unit and in the ward...
>
> I think a tertiary education is very important for nurses, not because we have to prove anything to one another but to prove to people in other disciplines that we have expertise. It increases not my credibility but my self-esteem. It's good for nursing. We, I refer to nurses, are responsible for total patient care...If we are not happy about, say, a patient's medical care or fluid status, it is up to us to go to the doctor and say 'Will you come over and assess this patient's fluid intake?'
>
> I have now been given the opportunity to be a charge nurse proper. When I first started here I didn't have a secretary or receptionist, I was everything. I was charge nurse, I was shift co-ordinator, I took a patient, I was equipment nurse and I was clinical teacher as well. Now I have days when I can think what I want to do for the unit. I am developing a policy and procedures manual, a quality assurance tool and a nursing care plan. I have to develop those for my area but for the rest of the hospital the projects officer does that. [MA/90]

There are, of course, differences between charge nurse positions in different areas, and in different hospitals, but the extract shows how one charge nurse, who happened to be in ICU, responded actively to changed opportunities and worked to create the sort of environment that she believed was appropriate. The new structure and processes of the organisation allowed her to do this but she took advantage of the opportunities provided, and indeed created opportunities for others in the unit. As a senior nurse academic said:

> The introduction of the assistant charge nurse has actually strengthened the ability of the charge nurse to control what is happening in the area because before it was ad hoc...On the other hand, the charge nurse still has decision making power according to personal attributes. It is not so much coming from the structure but from the charge nurse, who is best able to interpret what powers are available to her and uses them. [AW/90]

The scope of decision making in the clinical area has been enlarged by the introduction in all states of a clinical assistant director of nursing who liaises with the clinical nurses and discusses needs or policies for a particular area. These can then be pursued through the appropriate department or committee in the hospital. To some extent this has served to reverse the traditional authority and decision making flows from vertical to horizontal and to enhance the authority of nurses in decisions about clinical care.

The problems arising from the new structure for the clinical ADON stem in large part from the need to adjust to different roles and to clarify in practice what the role demands. Like the splitting of the charge nurse position, it is a question of deciding what is management and what is clinical:

> Organising the clinical work is partly administrative, yes, and we can't get away from that. I guess if there is a weakness in the career structure it is this idealistic splitting up into clear clinical, management, and education, because there are inevitably areas of overlap and that is becoming a real problem at ADON level...
>
> My job is now clinical. I do not have a patient load. I do not do what most people could consider to be 'clinical' work—clinical is looking after patients. I manage clinical services, I guess. That means things like quality assurance, which is a clinically associated program. Now I don't personally believe that's clinical work. It's administrative. It's just my opinion but I think the next thing the ADON level has to sort out is...that we are administrators. We cannot pretend we are clinicians.
>
> We've got clinical nurse consultants, the experts. So if you've already appointed an expert, and put them in charge of a clinical unit, you cannot have another person coming in above the expert...I believe [at this level] we can no longer clearly define management and clinical; they're administrative roles. [SS/88]

The federal secretary of the Australian Nursing Federation argues that the separation of clinical and management roles is problematic in all states and territories, with a tendency to the recombining of the roles, particularly in Victoria and New South Wales where the career structure changes involved adding clinical positions to the existing management positions: 'They were not about completely changing the focus of nursing activities to clinical from management'. [MB/92] She believes that after reviews have been carried out there will need to be another attempt at role delineation, at the proper integration of changes in nursing organisation with changes in the organisation of the hospital generally, and in improvements in dispute resolution about positions, combined with more effective information systems on financial and human resources, to enable the proper devolution of power and decision making downwards. The report on hospital services in Australia in the National Health Strategy review (1991:102) argued that:

> the potential benefits of the career structure, including multiskilling and capacity for more devolved decision-making, are likely to emerge over a long

period [but] corresponding changes to the hospital culture and organisation may be necessary before its full potential is realised.

Nurses and nursing have made gains in their involvement in decision making within the hospital, although this is still dependent on the particular organisation and indeed often on the nursing leadership within that organisation. It is a tentative acceptance which has been a 'long, hard battle' won by the establishment of credibility. That credibility has been assisted in particular decision making areas, such as over admissions and discharges, by gains made in the 1980s through overtly political actions over non-nursing duties and new pay and career structures. Credibility, however, has not only to be gained but maintained. It means having the facts to support arguments in the clinical area, achieving budget or staffing targets, and being prepared to be tough as well:

> Nurses have had a much more visible role in decision making in hospitals in the last few years. I still think that unfortunately one of our strengths is the power of veto, because the bottom line is that it requires nurses to produce the service. [MS/91]

Changes have occurred at senior administrative levels in order to make more effective the involvement of nurses in decision making which affects nurses and nursing care, and which recognises the value of nursing knowledge in health and health care in general. While nurses have achieved the right to be on hospital policy and decision making committees concerned with health and hospital planning, this is not a guarantee of effective participation:

> It depends very much on the leader of the organisation whether the director of nursing is actually a part of senior management or not, even though the DON may be recognised as such on the organisation chart. Nurses tend to be represented on more top level committees now, mainly because of accreditation and sometimes because it is necessary to have a 'token' nurse. It is then often up to that nurse to use his or her knowledge and skill in order to be heard, because it's not just enough to have representation on committees, one also has to have the corresponding behaviour and support network. [MS/91]

This has been assisted by the positions created by the new career structures which have allowed directors of nursing in the larger hospitals to become part of the hospital executive:

> With this structure the DON can now delegate much more to those in the co-ordination positions (to the ADONs) so that she can attend to senior management and committees. [DMcC/90]

The ADONs provide also a pool as acting DONs, allowing continuity and flexibility. In smaller and country hospitals that support is also evident:

> A lot of directors of nursing have said to me, 'It's the first time that I have really felt that I've got support, that I'm not standing there by myself. I'm not imposing on them, it's not a favour but part of their responsibilities'. [DMcC/90]

The support network can be very useful in winning arguments in committees. Nursing can use to its advantage something which has usually been described in the literature as a disadvantage. The management structure of nursing in contrast to the looser collegial relationships in medicine means that nursing can back its arguments with strength of numbers and cohesion even if there is only a single representative of the nursing division on a hospital committee compared to four or five doctors representing medical divisions:

> It's actually worked in our favour because if we put up one opinion everybody recognizes that that is the opinion of some 2000 people. A line management structure is very useful because it is backed up by authority and implementation can be ensured. If the nursing division puts up a researched and agreed opinion, on say ethics, and the medical divisions put up four different views, the nursing proposal may well be adopted as hospital policy. [MS/91]

Gender differences are still a problem on senior management committees with often one woman, usually the nurse, among 15 or 16 men:

> It does make a difference. What nurses have to learn is to be prepared to get in and fight like a man. I know that sounds sexist...We have to realise that ridicule and similar tactics will be used at meetings...We can't just retire into the background and say 'don't speak to me like that' or 'I don't understand'. [MS/91]

Sometimes, negotiating the power and gender relationship can be highlighted by apparently trivial experiences:

> I was on an infection control committee, which was an interesting experience for me to deal with the chief medical officer in the hospital, the microbiologist, the head of pharmacy, the head of maintenance...I actually chaired the committee but it was a conscious effort not to make the tea, because although a small issue it was quite political for me at the time. [ST/88]

The acceptance of an increased role in decision making and the confidence to participate in hospital policy committees is being assisted by the number of committees established within nursing divisions themselves, with only nurses as members. Depending on the particular committee, the membership may be drawn from different areas and from different levels. These committees prepare nurses for a decision making role by providing them with the necessary skills and strategies to participate. They learn the importance, for effective implementation of policies and decisions, of organisational processes, such as communication, delegation, conflict resolution, leadership and managing change. They learn how to develop, implement and evaluate programs. They learn how the whole organisation works rather than viewing it solely from their own or their unit's perspective (see Cuthbert 1992 for useful insights into management in nursing). They can build on their educational experience instead of leaving it behind and perhaps becoming disaffected from nursing. The experience in committees should help to develop a collegial and affiliation oriented climate for nurses, where their arguments are accepted as stemming from knowledge (Donovan & Jackson 1991:58-9).

Structures alone do not provide an increased role in decision making but they can facilitate participation. Effective participation is however dependent on less direct influences. As the Victorian branch secretary of ANF says:

> I don't think you get a larger role in decision making out of structures...You get a larger role in decision making by education, by feeling more confident and being more assertive...One thing the career structure has done is certainly [to create] more positions for nurses to apply for...There's a greater recognition of their responsibilities through the career structure...Given that this society recognises you by your salary there has been greater recognition and with that one would hope there would be greater confidence, and through [this] there's greater say in decision making. [BM/93]

Should microeconomic reform dictate that hospital management is reorganised on the Johns Hopkins model with a number of decentralised clinical directorates managed by a medical clinician and supported by a senior nurse, nursing as a distinct division under a line management structure would disappear and the autonomy of nursing would be undermined. The ANF and the NSWNA evaluated the model as it operates in the Johns Hopkins Hospital in the United States and Guy's Hospital in the United Kingdom and its effects on nursing. Their findings indicated that the functional unit structure for managing clinical and supportive patient services had some positive features for nursing but that the negative ones outweighed these. For example, day-to-day management devolved to clinical teams improved the quality of operational decision making, medical and nursing staff were more accountable for decisions, and there was improved collaboration between them. On the negative side, most management responsibilities were undertaken by senior nurses without formal recognition, nursing career structures had been eroded, and the position of nursing within the organisation was not commensurate with its role and function (Report to the ANF Federal Executive 1991).

Holism and fragmentation

The increased responsibility for total patient care by the registered clinical nurse where primary nursing has been introduced has created both opportunities and fears. A nurse in her graduate nursing program described it like this:

> At the moment I'm in a medical ward but I've done orthopaedics and general surgery and paediatrics...We are allocated between four and six patients depending on their dependency...We have primary nursing; we are just totally responsible for everything that happens to a patient...I make what you could call 'bedside decisions', and occasionally I am in charge of the ward for a shift, which is pretty frightening. [SJ/90]

A registered nurse at the same hospital preferred this method of patient allocation to her previous experience:

> I prefer it because I know what I am doing and I'm not doubling back to check if the patients have had their drugs or if their catheter bag has been changed. [RG/90]

In managing patient care, too, the amount of information processing has increased with nursing care plans, reports on admissions and discharges, patient transfers and so on. Computerised information systems have been introduced into many wards but training in their use appears often to be only at the basic level of input and retrieval required rather than in the use of computers in general.

Earlier discharges have also changed the responsibilities of the nurse so that there is an increased need to know more about the patients and their circumstances at home:

> We are trying now to start discharge planning at admission, no matter how sick the patient is, so that when it is time to discharge we are part way there. We try to work out their background and what the patient's needs have been and will be...It's a big responsibility and the family needs to be provided with information...Some people are in hospital because the extended family has declined...Some people, particularly migrants, have no family. [SJ/90]

There is however help from the 'team'. If the patient is elderly:

> We have a team where each of us, the geriatrician, physios, OTs [occupational therapists] and the social worker are all aimed at placing the elderly person into the environment which suits them best, whether it be at home and getting them everything they need to live at home, or into the nursing home. That is a cohesive team which works together. [SJ/90]

In working with other health professionals in general there is recognition that while the role of the nurse might have been eroded as others encroached on previously nursing territory, it means also that there are other resources available. It was indicative of the mixed feelings about this that both views could be expressed by the same person:

> It's very frustrating having [parts of your role] taken away from you...The doctor can say the physio can do this and the physio can do that...They are all things that nurses are capable of doing, like getting patients with total hip replacements out of bed. We are taught how to do it...

But earlier in the interview:

> You can ask any physio about any patient, even if she/he is not their patient, they will always give you advice...They get to know all the nurses and are only too happy to advise you on how to handle a patient, and it is the same with the speech pathologists and the OTs, everybody...Everybody is homed in on the patient and heading in that direction. [SJ/90]

Parallel with the development of a range of allied health professions, nursing specialties have evolved. The increasing specialisation of medical care combined with changes in the organisation of services, and in technology and in pharmacology, provided the initial impetus for the specialisation of nurses as they were attached to specialised units and areas such as nuclear medicine, cardiology or gastroenterology. Increasingly, however, nurses have developed their own specialist areas, such as stomal therapy or infection control, and the career structures have encouraged their recognition and further development in the role of the clinical nurse specialist (CNS).

For small hospitals, the implementation of the career structure has been difficult, particularly at the clinical nurse specialist level:

> Within teaching hospitals (I think the career structure was developed for teaching hospitals) it works...You've got to make it work for the smaller ones...If you have one CNS for 120 beds and there are 120 beds [in a small hospital] but you have obstetrics, you have gerontology and you have theatre, or psychogeriatrics, all specialties in their own right, do you have one generalist CNS...? This hospital is predominantly surgical but we didn't have a surgical CNS. We do 4000 operations...and the theatre CNS is expected to [be surgical as well] but in caring for patients her skills are different. [BA/90]

There appears, also, to be a tension developing between the establishment of nursing specialties and the stress on holistic patient care:

> The holistic model of care is good, but unfortunately what has happened in many places across Australia is that there is actually a splitting of care, and a splitting of responsibility with the introduction of, for example, breast nurses, weight reduction nurses, the diabetic educator, or the stomal therapist. [RB//91]

The specialist role can work well if it is linked to the total patient care provided by the responsible nurse at the bedside, rather than fragmenting that care by a number of different nurses performing a particular procedure in isolation which destroys the continuity of care, and reduces accountability. Specialist nurses are needed and the tension can be relieved by the adoption of an educative role:

> You need a stomal therapist in a hospital but what that person mustn't do is all the stomal therapy. She must advise the nurse caring for the patient on patient needs, on how she should care for that patient, what are the range of technical aids available, what she should do if the wound breaks down...It must be an educative role where the stomal therapist teaches the nurse how to care for a patient with a stoma and the stomal therapist carries out only the more complex procedures where necessary. Continuity of care must be maintained. [RB/91]

The development of nursing specialties whether in clinical care or in management will continue, and while there is a need to maintain a certain flexibility, patient care can only be improved by the accessibility of expert knowledge and skills. As Jane Salvage, then Director of Nursing Developments (King's Fund Centre), said:

> I think you need to develop expertise in particular areas. Sometimes that may be in a medical specialty, but it may also be in a particular aspect of nursing. What *is* exciting...is that more and more people *are* taking up specialist posts of that sort. So you get people who maybe are expert in staff deployment issues, and can give support to clinical teams...Or they may be expert in care planning...Of course you need people who can really get very skilled and expert. [JSa/90]

Managing technological change

Rapid technological change combined with the introduction of new drugs has had a huge impact on nursing practice:

> In the old days you only saw IVAC machines in intensive care but they have become less expensive and at the same time new drugs are being developed so the IVAC machine doesn't stay in intensive care. They are in all the wards in all large hospitals. [RB/91]

Called as an expert witness in nursing on behalf of the New South Wales Nurses' Association in the professional rates case, a senior NSW nurse was cross-examined about what is nursing:

> I can remember one counsel who was being very difficult. He went through one procedure (I think it was catheterisation) and I could see what he was working up to so I said 'Yes, you could teach a chimpanzee to do it'. They didn't understand that there is a lot more to nursing than doing a particular procedure. We talk to the patients, help them understand what is going to happen, and why, and what we hope will be the result. Then you have to monitor, know what a drug does and the possible side effects. It's no good simply giving someone who can't sleep the proper drug, you have to try and find out why they can't sleep. [PP/89]

Nurses are now having to cope with more sophisticated procedures and equipment; nursing practice and procedures committees provide guidelines on who is permitted to undertake a particular procedure and what level of competence is required by law. For example, the state body responsible for nursing registration and standards might put out a policy on the use of epidural drugs so that a registered nurse classified as competent can 'top-up' the epidural but the nursing committee at the local level must first create a policy on epidural drugs and then formulate the procedures that go with it. Patient safety is still the primary concern, but it is achieved by provision of policies and practical guidelines which nurses themselves develop and work within, rather than from rigid adherence to rules and regulations through training and close supervision. Again, it is the importance of understanding the principle behind the practice which is critical and this is related to the level of qualification and competence.

Because there are detailed policies and procedures for implementation in place, it does not necessarily follow that adherence will always occur, nor that adherence will be achieved without difficulty by those nurses who are at the bedside. There are political and practical difficulties involved. The role boundaries between enrolled nurses (ENs) and registered nurses (RNs) is a particularly fraught area where practices have developed in an ad hoc way over a long period of time. The legal guidelines suggest that ENs can do certain procedures under the direct supervision of a registered nurse, but in practice it is a very, very grey area. It then becomes very difficult on an individual level to withdraw something from people that they have been doing for a long time, and in which they have become competent. For example, ENs might have been using machines for monitoring blood glucose levels and become extremely proficient but it is really a registered nurse's responsibility, as he or she administers the insulin and is therefore responsible for monitoring glucose levels. The ANRAC (1990:II) competencies state that 'the enrolled nurse works under the direction and supervision of the registered nurse' and while 'responsible for his/her own actions...remains accountable to the registered nurse for all delegated functions'.

The extensive use of sophisticated equipment has created difficulties for nursing practice but it, not surprisingly, has also had an effect on nursing resources:

> The impact of technology is frightening in terms of the way it eats up nursing resources. For example, for people who are acutely ill in intensive care and are suffering from renal failure we might do continuous arteriovenous haemodialysis, in addition to the patient being on an IVAC machine and ventilator. Instead of having one nurse looking after that patient you need two, so it doubles the nursing resources required. [RB/91]

Similarly, the extension of the use of IVAC machines into general wards, as well as in intensive care units and high dependency nursing units, has put more pressure on nursing resources. Patients requiring this and similar procedures are seriously ill and this has increased patient dependency in the general wards. Lengths of stay have decreased so that at any one time there are more patients who are 'sicker' and require more attention.

The introduction of new equipment had usually occurred without consultation with nursing management, let alone with those who were required to use and maintain the machines. There are, however, increasing opportunities for nurses to have an input into such decision making at all levels. In Victoria, nurses are involved in decision making on the introduction of technology at the highest political level through the Nursing Policy and Planning Unit in the Health Department of Victoria. Senior nurses are on hospital technology and equipment committees which have been formed in Victoria as a result of the *Study of Professional Issues in Nursing* (Marles 1988), which in turn was established as part of the agreement reached between the Victorian Government and the ANF after the 50 day strike on the implementation of the new pay and career structure in 1986. Nursing is represented by the DON or ADON on these hospital committees.

Within the hospital, all proposals for new equipment must go through the equipment committees for approval, and all new pieces of equipment are monitored and evaluated by the nursing staff. Nurses designated as equipment nurses are being introduced so that proper education into choice, purchase, use and maintenance of equipment is carried out. The conjunction of equipment committees and equipment nurses appears to be working well and has reduced the ad hoc process whereby the registrar might give the nurse a quick run down on how a machine worked. It has brought decision making to the most appropriate level; the level where the work is actually carried out (Lansbury & Spillane 1983, Milton et al 1984, Aungles & Parker 1988).

Where decision making structures and processes on the introduction, implementation and evaluation of new technology have been established, informal and ad hoc decision making is not absent. Pressure from company representatives who bypass proper procedures can still occur. Nurses, for example in ICU, often develop a relationship with various company representatives and may purchase equipment without the approval of the various committees established to oversee this process. This situation is however made far more difficult by the actual existence of formal structures and procedures for the introduction of new equipment, and individuals whether medical or nursing who ignore the committees 'do so at their peril'. [JK/90] Without such structures there is no means of introducing accountability. Unfortunately, not all hospitals have introduced structures and procedures for monitoring equipment purchase:

> It should be a team approach...Nurses are not usually involved. There are still a lot of hospitals which don't have a divisional structure where every equipment item is approved by the division of surgery or the division of medicine, but even there it is still direct from the department head to the administrator. While that goes on you will have inappropriate selection and no consultation with the people who use it. [JW/89]

While it was once standard practice for doctors, particularly in intensive care areas where they had power and authority from a high status area in the hospital, to simply order costly new machines, there is now more control and accountability. So from a purely political exercise of power at the institutional level, decisions about the introduction of new technology have entered the broad political arena. In Victoria and New South Wales the state governments have exercised constitutional powers to determine which hospitals will have, for example, a lithotripter (Daly et al 1987). Hospitals are accredited on different bases according to the types of procedure they are allowed to carry out.

While nursing work in the hospital has undoubtedly become more complex and new career structures have placed additional demands on nurses to be involved in decision making and to be accountable for their practice, nurses have also had to reassess their values about what is appropriate care, where it should be provided, and by whom. There is an increasing need to improve the links between institutional and community care, with an increased emphasis on and need for liaison and joint decision making between professional groups, clients and non-professional caregivers. This is particularly apparent in nursing patients with HIV/AIDS.

Sensitive caring: HIV/AIDS

The extent and nature of infection with the human immune deficiency virus (HIV) and its manifestation as acquired immune deficiency syndrome (AIDS) has had ramifications for nurses and nursing work, as it has for the community as a whole (National HIV/AIDS Strategy 1989). These include ethical, legal, medical, safety, religious, education, and social considerations, but also the kinds of care provided and the role of the nurse in illness prevention. HIV/AIDS, in common with, for example, drug and alcohol addictions, road trauma and aged care, involves nurses in clinical management, in community based services, and in education and health promotion programs.

The federal secretary of the ANF (*ANJ* May1991:22) argues that it is the responsibility of nurses to focus on the care of those with AIDS and the many more who are HIV positive:

> It is time to stop and take stock of how we go about nursing work. It is not good enough to assume that sex and drugs make AIDS different. A caring consciousness, about our patients, ourselves and other members of the health team should be inherent in how nurses practise nursing.

In assessing the role of the nurse in caring for people with HIV/AIDS, the federal secretary saw it as an opportunity for nurses to demonstrate to others an understanding of the importance of care and to play an active part in policy development and decision making in the community and in institutions. To do this nurses needed to overcome their own prejudices about, and fear of contamination from, sexually transmitted diseases and to become skilled and objective educators (*ANJ May* 1991:21-2).

The recommendations of the HIV/AIDS National Nurses Conference were far reaching in terms of the expression of the political development of nurses. Among others, the recommendations were: that nurses 'become more politically active to ensure that nurses' needs and the needs of...clients are met'; that the Minister for Community Services and Health be asked to recognise nurse practitioners, particularly in the area of HIV/AIDS, as registered health care providers under the Medical Insurance Scheme; 'that ANF Federal Council take appropriate action to expose policies of government and health agencies which insist on HIV testing of persons for whatever reason and whether consent has or has not been obtained'; and further nurses 'will not assist in carrying out non-consensual HIV testing on people seeking care' (*ANJ* May 1991:26).

For nurses involved in caring directly for patients with AIDS, there are additional ethical issues to those outlined above, particularly those relating to confidentiality. Patients might not want their parents or work colleagues to know of the diagnosis from fear of damaging consequences (Kermode 1992:252). Kermode argues that it is the patient who must make the decision about who should be told, and that the nurse must then respect this decision in talking to friends and family members of the patient. There is however a further ethical issue in that the nurse has a concern for others who might be infected in a sexual relationship with the patient: 'Does the nurse protect the interests of the patient and maintain confidentiality, or does he or she protect the interests of the person who is at significant risk of HIV infection?' (Kermode 1992:252). The ANRAC competencies (1990:10.4-10.5) provide that the nurse 'ensures confidentiality of information', but also should act 'to maintain the rights of individuals/groups'.

AIDS is at present a terminal illness and if the patient does not want treatment to continue when death is near, the nurse in the role of patient advocate has to be careful to be guided by the patient and not by her or his own feelings and beliefs. This is of course not confined to people with AIDS. It may, however, be more personalised in that patients suffering from AIDS, because of repeated admissions with opportunistic infections, often become close to nursing staff, as do their friends and families. Treatment for AIDS is rapidly changing and the drugs administered by nurses often have both serious side effects and a lack of information for reference purposes. For these and other reasons, the support for nursing staff from colleagues becomes particularly important in the AIDS area (Kermode 1992).

It is also particularly important for nurses to be, and to see themselves as, members of a team of caregivers:

> Central to the treatment, care and counselling of people with HIV is the range of professional care-givers which may include medical practitioners, nurses, dietitians, dentists, counsellors, social workers and hospital chaplains. Professional care-givers have responsibility for the initial diagnosis and care of people with HIV, and for continuing treatment, care, education and support. (National HIV/AIDS Strategy 1989:7)

The National HIV/AIDS Strategy (1989:6-11) recognised the 'significant support' provided by partners, family and friends, and the 'vital role' of non-government organisations such as AIDS councils and other community based support services. It is perhaps in the care and support for people with HIV/AIDS that nurses have had to become aware of the need to temper dependence with empowerment, and to overcome prejudice. As a district nurse said of one of her patients who had AIDS:

> He liked to keep control right to the end...And his presence is with me constantly as I care for my AIDS people each day. His attitude is his legacy and inspiration (Claire quoted Knepfer & Johns 1989:224).

Nursing mothers and babies

Midwifery has long been recognised as an occupation, but for most of this century its practice has been as a nursing specialisation carried out in hospitals and nowhere in nursing is change more evident. It is an area which has moved rapidly from the treatment of birth as an illness to the acceptance of birth as natural.

In the maternity department of the hospital, which is still where most births take place, the change is evident in single, double, four or six beds to a room, instead of a large open public ward with as many as 30 beds. Nursing care for the newborn in nurseries is giving way to 'rooming in' with demand breast feeding instead of bottle feeds and milk complements. Birthing suites or centres have been introduced, and the partner or a friend is encouraged to be present to provide support at the actual birth. Labour wards however can still be 'overly clinical' and 'routine shaves and enemas are not things of the past and continue to occur in some hospitals' (Ministerial Review of Birthing Services in Victoria 1990:48). Antenatal classes for the preparation of both parents is encouraged, and ante and postnatal exercise classes demonstrate that muscle tone is not simply a matter of chance. The rapidity of the changes has however meant that not all midwives are as well prepared as their clients:

> When I first came here seven years ago, we had a large open public ward with a charge sister to be feared. Now it's very different. We've got unit management and charge nurses and associate charge nurses—a very different structure. Only four years ago it was still nursery care for all babies, with strict four-hourly feeds and now it's all breast feeding. [LT/90]

In this particular hospital, the changes were introduced by nursing and hospital administration with very little consultation or involvement in decision making at the department level, which caused resentment, but:

> You find in midwifery in a lot of places that the charge nurses and the associate charge nurses have very old fashioned ideas. I can see why administration chose to put it in place with little discussion as it would not have happened otherwise, or it would have taken much longer…In the postnatal area breast feeding is still a big problem. Older midwives, or ones who have been here for a long time, still can't cope with demand breast feeding and no bottle feeds. (LT/90)

Although, in this hospital, there were two lactation consultants it tended to be the recently graduated and the student nurses who sought help:

> There are a few of us who try very hard to establish breast feeding the way it should be done, but often the 'mums' get so confused and have very little confidence in their ability to breast feed. I think what will eventually happen is that the more resistant midwives will leave the system and eventually, very slowly it will change. [LT/90]

In this instance, it could be argued that if there had been more involvement in the change process there might have been more universal commitment to that change (see for example, Milton et al 1984; Donovan & Jackson 1991; Cuthbert et al 1992).

There was concern also about the erosion of the role of the midwife, particularly by the physiotherapist:

> I think the physiotherapist has eroded the role of the midwife. She is responsible for much of the antenatal education now, which we used to do, especially pain management, breathing during labour, all the different postnatal exercises, and even dealing with mastitis and engorged breasts...[LT/90]

It can of course be argued that the multidisciplinary team approach is appropriate in antenatal and postnatal care.

While midwives, along with general nurses, are seeing aspects of their former all inclusive role going to other health professionals, they are challenging their traditional relationship with the medical profession and attempting to achieve their independence. Encouraged to some extent by changing community attitudes about the demedicalization of childbirth and recognition that midwives supervise the whole of labour and frequently the delivery as well, some midwives have moved out of the hospital and into independent practice. There is no doubt that if their application to the Medicare Benefits Review Committee (1986) for benefits for midwifery services had been successful, the exodus would have been much faster. As it is, the cost to the potential consumer with limited ability to claim benefits from private health insurance and the costs to the midwife of insurance for home births, militate against the independent practitioner. On the other hand, shorter stays in hospital have provided the opportunity for independent practitioner midwives in postnatal nursing and support in the home, and for lactation consultancy. They receive referrals from obstetricians and paediatricians and it is a growth area with midwives working independently, or as part of a private consultancy service with an average of four or five midwives on call (see Reports of the National Health and Medical Research Council Working Party on Home Births and Alternative Birth Centres 1987 & 1989).

Maternal and child health nurses (baby health and child nurses in NSW) working from local centres continue to provide the expert continuing support needed for mothers and babies when they leave hospital, and their role in the system would have to be regarded as one of the most successful public health achievements. These nurses are skilled not only in monitoring the child's development and administering immunisation programs against the infectious diseases of childhood but also in recognising potentially serious conditions such as jaundice, abnormalities, and even injuries from difficult births, for example, a baby with a broken collar bone after a forceps delivery. As so often happens in nursing, where the real skills often go unrecognised, maternal and child health nurses have faced replacement by less skilled, or differently skilled, people such as mothercraft nurses.

A more recent problem has arisen from budget cuts where mothers and their babies can be discharged from hospital after only 24 hours. With too few maternal and child health nurses and inadequate procedures for immediate follow up, the actual and potential problems and distress for mothers and babies is obvious. This is made worse by the fact that it is often not until about the fifth day when problems such as mastitis appear. The frequent readmissions make nonsense of such practices as a cost cutting exercise.

The involvement of midwives (and paediatric nurses in neonatal care) in ethical decisions about babies with, for example gross abnormalities, is becoming usual practice, as indeed is the involvement of parents. The process of deciding to treat or not to treat can include full information being provided to parents by the registrar and consultant paediatrician with nurses being present at every interview so that everyone involved has and provides consistent information. Should the decision be that the baby or child is not to be treated then counselling is provided for the nursing staff (Cuddihy 1989). The ANRAC National Competencies for registration provide that the nurse 'engages effectively in ethical decision making' (1990:14.3). It would be fair to say, however, that there still is often enormous conflict between nurses and medical staff over decisions about whether to treat or not to treat, and that joint decision making between patient, family, nurse and doctor is not as developed in other areas of the hospital, or in all hospitals (Marles 1988).

It is perhaps in midwifery that the tension between nursing in the hospital setting, and in the community as an independent practitioner is most apparent but there are other difficulties, often related to perceptions about nursing, for nurses working in community settings.

The community spirit

The majority of nurses (registered and enrolled) work in hospitals and nursing homes. The number working in what could be described loosely as 'the community' is much smaller (see Appendix). The costs of institutional care combined with changes in the characteristics of the populations requiring care, such as the aged, and a gradual shift in values towards health promotion and illness prevention have resulted in changes in government policy at federal, state and local government levels in relation to, for example, occupational health and safety, mental health, occupational rehabilitation, community health, and domiciliary and palliative care. The Commonwealth Community Health Program (1973), for example, encouraged the development of community health centres in most states. Stemming from the World Health Organization's (WHO) target of Health for All by the Year 2000 (1977) and the Alma Ata declaration on primary health care in 1978, which were endorsed by Australia in 1979, the federal report *Health for All Australians,* was launched in 1988. This was followed by the strategic framework for achieving Health for All outlined in the National Better Health Program in 1989 (McPherson 1992).

The goals of primary health care, with their emphasis on health rather than illness, the inclusion of sectors not traditionally linked to the promotion of health, such as transport and the environment, and the changed role of health professionals as primary care workers working with individuals, families and the community to promote health, were supported by the International Council of Nurses, the Australian Nursing Federation and the Australian Council of Community Nurses (Schulz 1992). Schulz (1992:238) argues that support for the principles of primary health care and commitment to their implementation 'implicitly broadens nurses' responsibilities to include involvement in health planning and decision making'.

In a survey of the job satisfaction of nurses in different settings, Rowe and Manning (1987) found that sources of satisfaction varied according to nursing area of work and specialisation. For all nurses, (except educators and supervisors) the most frequently mentioned source of satisfaction was patients, but for community health nurses interpersonal relations and communication as sources of satisfaction were higher than for any other group. Responsibility was also important, with community health nurses rating this variable as a source of satisfaction just below nurses in acute care settings.

The opportunity for decision making for nurses in community health falls into three main categories: decisions about the specific health needs of individuals and particular groups; decisions about programs to develop community awareness of major health issues; and decisions on policies for community development.

The first of these is specific and largely individually based and refers to services requiring nursing expertise, for example, in ante and postnatal care and diabetic support. The second is less specific and more related to health education and prevention of disease in such areas as screening, nutrition, and smoking. It refers to conducting particular programs to provide information through campaigns to promote public awareness of disease inducing factors.

It is only the third category which allows for input into policies which encourage community development rather than the more traditional professional roles of direct care and advice to people about how to improve their health.

Mitchell and Wright (1992:250) argue that the two main categories of services and programs in community health, health promotion and curative health care, 'require different approaches and can create difficulties for workers who are new to community health' (see also Schulz 1992). Even experienced community health workers, if they have been trained in the hospital or private practice, find it difficult to combine 'the dual activities of curative and preventive health' and 'the transfer of control to clients and community members' which is the core of a community development approach (Mitchell & Wright 1992:250-5). Some nurses believe otherwise:

> We believe that we educate nurses so that in their capacity as a nurse they can provide care, rehabilitation, extended care, long term care, in the home or in a community agency. That is, that they are adequately equipped to nurse in either a community setting or in a hospital. At the moment they in the main choose the hospital setting. I think they feel this is where they need to develop further and to be a 'real nurse'. On the other hand, I think they haven't been terribly welcome in the community. [MP/88]

The federal secretary of the Australian Nursing Federation recognised this as a problem for nurses and cited a specific example when this was highlighted:

> When the Commonwealth Department of Health amalgamated with the Commonwealth Department of Community Services in 1987 the community services component began to take a much higher profile, and the people who influenced policies were community services oriented, whose view clearly was that nurses belonged in the medical model, the hospital system, and they would be funding a whole range of services that did not include the employment of nurses. Disability services was one area, HACC [Home and Community Care], nursing homes even. Those policy changes brought into stark relief the issue of nurses' work. 'You don't need qualified nurses to do this work, this is not nursing work, nursing work is about working with doctors and looking after sick people...' It was also a view held by organisations such as the Consumers' Health Forum, the Superannuants and Pensioners Federation, and the Aged Care Coalition. A whole range of people that we have communicated consistently with for five or six years, who are now beginning to understand nursing much better. [MB/92]

The stereotypical view of nurses as working only in acute care, high technology areas often portrayed in the media makes it very difficult to provide the alternative view of nurses working within the community which is more difficult to make 'attention grabbing'.

Health professionals may believe that with a more equal relationship between provider and user they will lose professional status and recognition of their skills, but on the contrary:

> Community development in community health relies on workers utilising living skills in conjunction with professional skills. These skills include an understanding of self; communication skills and the ability to impart knowledge in an accessible and culturally relevant manner; skills in participating in a group setting; and an understanding of the political components of the health system and its local context. (Mitchell & Wright 1992:253)

Because a community development approach encourages strategies which directly address inequalities in health status whether related to class and/or ethnicity, as well as providing individuals and groups with the skills to address issues which impact on health, for example domestic violence, much of the work of the nurse, or other professional, is directed towards understanding the context of the particular problem, the language and metaphors of the group and providing initial support while leaving the group to take over responsibility.

Even in community health where multidisciplinary teamwork has been encouraged from the outset, and where peer support is so necessary when colleagues from the same profession are often absent, fears of encroachment on territory have militated against teamwork (Mitchell & Wright 1992). This problem may only be resolved when the allied health professions and nursing each believe that they have achieved full professional status, and are more confident of their expertise.

Health promotion and illness prevention policies have led to an increase in the opportunities for nurses to specialise outside the system of institutional care where their educative and co-ordinating role is expanded, and direct clinical care is reduced. These positions have provided nurses with further opportunities for policy and decision making both within the agency, for example, a community health centre, and in health promotion in general. Again, the opportunities are there but the response is dependent on many factors including individual preference, facilitation by the particular employing organisation, the role of other health professionals, and the education, expertise and skills of the individual nurse.

> Because of these factors, there is little agreement about the extent to which nurses in the community have taken a leading role in policy and decision making. Views range along a continuum of little control over decision making in relation to their own work practices at one end, through control over decision making over work practices but no input into broader policy issues, to taking the leading role in policy decisions at the other. Again, it is a question of looking at the particular agency in order to establish the extent of participation. There is some agreement that the community nurse can and should make an important contribution because of her or his education and the possession of a broad range of skills rather than working from within a narrow therapeutic application. [GN/92]

The extension of care

Aged care spans the 'institutional' gamut from acute care in hospitals, through nursing home or hostel, to support within the home which has been emphasised by policies on deinstitutionalisation (see Home and Community Care Program (HACC) (Department of Community Services 1985).

In the care of the aged, whether in nursing homes or hospitals, there appears to be a view that advanced nursing skills in technical competence and caring are unnecessary. This view is exacerbated by the view that ENs are cheaper than RNs to employ, and as many nursing homes are privately owned this has been influential in staffing practices. It is not, however, confined to the private sector.

The need for increased skills in nursing is not limited to acute care hospitals, but is very much a part of nursing homes:

> Because changes in medical science are keeping people alive longer, the sort of work and the skills required in nursing homes are vastly different from what they used to be. There is an increased dependency in nursing homes and hostels and consequently an increase in skill requirements. [EP/88]

The need for the skills of the registered nurse in monitoring and evaluating side effects of drugs and the effects of multiple prescriptions on the elderly person who often has a range of diseases and disability cannot be overestimated, as it is often the care provided rather than the administration of drugs which can improve the quality and extension of life. For example, fluid retention is often a result of inactivity and can be addressed by increasing exercise rather than by the administration of diuretics, which have adverse side effects. The effects of sleeping pills on the overall health of the elderly resulting in confusion and disorientation is similarly something which has only recently received attention. Nurses have a responsibility to be involved in decision making about the care of the elderly. It is their expertise which is crucial because the focus is care not cure.

The question of traditional nursing hierarchies acting as a brake on an expanded decision making role for nurses is not absent in community nursing. For example, for historical reasons, domiciliary nursing services tended to mirror the institutional pattern in their authority structures, if not in direct supervision of performed tasks. The focus was still task oriented and authority was decentralised only to the extent of carrying out the actual task and did not allow for a larger planning, liaison or co-ordinating role, which was firmly controlled by the DON. This is changing with the implementation of the career structure in domiciliary nursing services.

The changing needs in the aged care sector would appear to provide an opportunity for nurses to be involved in policy and decision making at government level but a nursing officer on a state Nurses Board believes that their input is minimal:

> It's just such a battle to be represented on committees where decisions are made. You have to fight to get there and then when you do get there you're not listened to...They (the registered nurses) really feel that they can't influence decisions at all. [EP/88]

To be really effective in influencing policy decisions in aged care, the same nursing officer believes that nurses have to become more politically active and to be educated to think more broadly about their role so that it extends beyond being able to think only in a clinical situation. In this way more nurses would move into policy positions in the public service and would be capable of influencing change. For example, an area of concern to nurses, and one over which they believe nurses should have control, is in the type of person employed to provide care.

In spite of the need for increased skills in the area of aged and extended care a perceived problem is that registered *and* enrolled nurses are being replaced by less qualified or unqualified staff. When the sorts of problems suffered by this sector are analysed it becomes even more incongruous:

> Especially in aged care, or in extended care, or in the area of the intellectually handicapped there are all these unqualified people being employed. And yet that client population, are our most powerless, are the most vulnerable, often with the most complex medical problems...They'll have a diabetic condition, a CVA, or osteoarthritis. They'll have an overwhelming pathology that the nurse has to work with and that is given, in this particular area, to our most unqualified people. [EP/88]

The reasons for the substitution of registered nurses by others are complex and not necessarily solely related to the belief that employing registered nurses is more expensive, and its converse that other workers because less qualified are less expensive, although this may be the myth upon which such employment policies are based. It is similar to the myth that it was less costly to train nurses in the hospital programs than to educate them in colleges of advanced education. In periods of nursing shortages, there may well have been a shortage of nurses seeking to work in the aged or extended care area because it may have been perceived as less interesting, but this does not fully explain the policy of introducing and educating an array of 'nurses' by another name: paramedical aide, residential care worker, special care worker, health auxiliary...

The argument that registered nurses are more costly to employ is debatable:

> When you employ a whole range of unqualified people, if you take into account the indirect costs, the work output, the need for supervision and the mistakes which are made, they are less cost effective. No one has ever bothered to cost the mistakes, as when people fall out of bed and fracture the neck of the femur, or their incontinence is not properly managed, or they are given insufficient fluids so they get urinary tract infections...[EP/88]

This was supported by the DON at Prince Charles Hospital, Brisbane, who had reorganised the aged care residential section attached to the hospital. In common with most other aged care facilities in Australia, Prince Charles had a few registered nurses, but a majority of enrolled and student nurses. After a pilot program with all registered nurses in the residential care unit, it was decided to maintain half registered and half enrolled nurses, but to employ only registered nurses in the acute cardiothoracic areas of the hospital.

There was also a concerted attempt to change attitudes towards working in aged care so that it was not seen as a depressed and forgotten outpost, and nurses were selected because they had a commitment to working with elderly people. Being part of an acute care hospital had meant that aged care was subject to the same sorts of hospital procedures, like ward rounds, as the rest of the hospital. This was discontinued:

> ...but it took an age to get people into thinking that this really is a residential setting, this is a home, and what we really want is an attitude which sees that people come here to live the rest of their lives and that they should be involved with the community as much as possible. [VC-W/91]

There are two main, but linked, arguments to explain why registered nurses are under threat from below, from vertical encroachment on their territory (Gardner & McCoppin 1989:12). First, there is a general lack of understanding and knowledge about nursing, about what it is and about the skills which are needed. This lack is shared by medical practitioners, health planners and policy makers, and employers, and reflects community values. Quite simply, it is the view that all it takes to be a good nurse is to be a caring person. Nurses themselves have of course been aware of this attitude for a long time and have published numerous articles and books refuting it (for example, Mackay 1989, Marles 1988, Salvage 1985, Wood 1990).

Politicians too have persistently expressed the notion of caring and vocation, while simultaneously downgrading nursing as an occupation not requiring a constant increase in knowledge and skills from education. Because nursing is devalued, it follows that others can be substituted for the registered nurse. With the addition of limited education programs, which nonetheless teach aspects of nursing, the role of the nurse is eroded:

> These courses are being set up all over the country. What is worrying is that the curriculums have been broadened to encompass a whole range of traditional areas of nursing, like drug administration, and the side effects of drugs. The government is devaluing the role of the nurse by allowing this to happen. [EP/88]

Second, nursing has traditionally been seen as caring for the sick; as working within the medical model of the treatment of disease. While the reduction in the length of hospital stays has meant that people going back into the community still require a high degree of intervention for acute needs in hospice care, for palliative care and postoperatively, nurses are not necessarily viewed as the appropriate professionals in primary health care, in a social model of health, in health education and promotion, and in prevention:

> I think nurses have an important role here...but their attitudes need to be turned to a focus on prevention. If they don't others will step in. They will train generic health workers to pick up issues in the community...[EP/88]

The decision makers in the health departments tend also to come from a broad background in the arts or humanities and are not always sympathetic to nurses:

> They just will not listen to nurses. They believe we're inflexible. They believe we come from a disease orientation, a medical model. They believe we make people dependent. We've got to turn all that around. [EP/88]

The implementation of the nursing career structure in aged and extended care might be another factor reducing its attractiveness to registered nurses. For example, in South Australia where the new career structure is generally regarded as a pace setter, its implementation in aged care 'was an absolute abortion of the SA career structure' in general but better than under the previous system:

> The positions, the funding weren't available. I had six separate units, one a day therapy centre, with 45 people coming in every day, with a whole range of services provided. Clearly the person who ran that should have been at CNC level instead of CN level. I had a hospice unit, a rehabilitation unit, two extended care units and a secure unit for people with dementia, needing very different types of skills. I could only get one CNC for the hospice unit, after much negotiating and two for the rest...It was impossible for them to act in their role because the span of control was so enormous...So I had one CNC covering 50 extended beds. [EP/88]

In spite of a professed commitment to aged care by federal and state governments, levels of funding do not appear to match that commitment and it is nursing, family caregivers and the aged who ultimately are the losers (see Minichiello 1989, Minichiello et al 1992). Deinstitutionalisation has occurred at a faster rate than the injection of resources for support services and one is left with the feeling that a certain cynicism related more to cost cutting by reducing institutional care than to improving the welfare of the aged by maintaining them in the community through appropriate nursing and other support has dictated policies. This is apparent also in mental health.

Nursing for mental health

Deinstitutionalisation for those people with psychiatric disorders or who are developmentally disabled has been proceeding in most states after a large number of state inquiries and reports into psychiatric services in the 1980s made recommendations for the expansion of community based services and the reduction of psychiatric hospitals. In 1984, the federal government had endorsed the *Standards for Psychiatric Facilities in Australia* developed by the National Health and Medical Research Council, which had as its first principle that 'the primary functions of any psychiatric facility are to diagnose, to treat, and to restore mentally ill persons to an optimal level of functioning within the community' (Grant & Lapsley 1992). The trend towards deinstitutionalisation has been occurring in practice since the 1970s with utilisation of beds in public psychiatric hospitals declining by two-thirds between 1970 and 1985. Grant and Lapsley (1992:210) argue that the decline can be attributed to a number of factors including changes in community attitudes and the role of community services, in the use of medication, and from policy changes.

Psychiatric hospitals are gradually being integrated into acute general hospitals with hospital closures and mergers, and are linked to community based services which provide treatment, supported accommodation and rehabilitation. For psychiatric nurses, as for other health professionals, these changes have far reaching consequences relating to education, registration, careers, industrial relations, and patient-client care. Even the designation of type of nurse is unclear:

> We call it psychiatric nursing...How accurate that is, is not clear because we call our community nurses 'community mental health nurses' rather than 'community psychiatric nurses'. [EC/91]

One senior nurse academic in New South Wales had no hesitation in designating 'psychiatric' nursing as 'mental health' nursing, which she believed was more appropriate and inclusive of a preventive role. She recognised, however, that for many it was difficult to lose the designation of psychiatric nurse, and that they felt betrayed by the loss of a separate undergraduate program for psychiatric nurses in all states except Victoria, and were resistant to joining the mainstream of nursing:

> Therefore I tend to talk about mental health nurses in a sense of not being just psychiatric nurses. I think many of them can have some difficulty coming to terms with that. I am a head of a Department of Mental Health Nursing, so I feel that there is no loss of identity, and I think probably that I have never felt that there was a loss of identity individually, in the sense that I was a general nurse long before I became a mental health nurse, and so therefore I felt very comfortable in the mainstream of nursing and I have never really got out of the mainstream of nursing except to probably be seen nationally as being accepted as a mental health nurse, and I don't have a difficulty, I don't believe, in being accepted by my colleagues in the mainstream of nursing. But that is because I have been there, and I think that for many psych nurses the transition is too difficult for them. They feel betrayed in a sense, that they no longer have an existing program and because their programs were organised by medics anyway, and there seemed to be no real nursing component in those programs. It was very difficult for them to conceptualise what was different, even though they talk about the differences between the tradition of the general nurse and the psychiatric nurse. Most differences in fact are behavioural science differences, biological science differences, psychiatry differences, and so on—they're not nursing differences. [LS/90]

Another senior psychiatric nurse argued that there is a lot of confusion about the sorts of skills and body of knowledge which psychiatric nurses have and which are different from general nursing skills and knowledge, although those are used as well. Even articulating the role is difficult:

> We often feel threatened because we're unable to articulate it well and begin to make platitudinous comments...So there is a poor self-image...We have in

> the past even tried to call ourselves non-nurses, have tried to call ourselves therapists, as a way of defining ourselves...Because it's really difficult to describe a therapeutic relationship, to be able to describe the strategies that are successful in [one case as opposed to another]...
>
> Our particular speciality is about being able to assess where people are psychologically or mentally, being able to predict what is almost unpredictable in other settings, being able to pick up tiny mood changes...Being able to know intuitively and as an expert...not to precipitate a negative response both for you and the patient. And moving people—as far as is possible from a state of disability, to coping with that in a way which can assist them to live outside [the hospital]. [EC/91]

A Western Australian mental health nurse recognised that nobody had yet been able to define the role successfully but described it as spanning the:

> ...mental health problems of the 'worried well', as well as looking after the mentally ill...So we're dealing with people who are well, and we want to keep well; we have people who have mental health problems, and we want to help them overcome those; and we have people who are mentally ill...Mental health nurses should be able to assess the person's affective, cognitive, behavioural status, identify the significance of their findings and apply them to nursing care. [TH/90]

There is a problem too for nurses who work in the psychiatric area in that, particularly for chronic patients, the sense of achievement is much less apparent. As a mental health nurse from South Australia said:

> Any changes you may see are over months and sometimes you get into a daily routine and don't have expectations at all. [RA/88]

She believed that for conditions to improve for the chronically ill, the consumers themselves needed to have more political power to demand appropriate services but that this was difficult because sometimes the people themselves were powerless and their relatives were 'usually far too drained and too busy to organise'. She went on:

> The other way of course is for nurses to act as the patient's advocate and to have more input into the health system. There are signs that nursing may in fact develop in that general direction, but there are still problems and conflicts...Nurses are in a dual role—they're in a very powerful role as far as the patient is concerned and their needs and the patient's needs are not always going to coincide...So there is a conflict between [being an advocate and their own needs]. [RA/88]

Psychiatric nurses have always had a large degree of autonomy and a role in decision making, probably as a result of the treatment setting. Depending on the stage of the process different aspects of care are emphasised so that the medical psychiatric component is predominant at the acute stage and nurses, occupational therapists, and social workers are involved at the appropriate stage. There is too a role for ENs (mental health aides), particularly in psychogeriatrics.

The planned merger of psychiatric and general hospitals, and the integration of mental health services with community services, has created problems for psychiatric nurses. How, for example, will the psychiatric nursing career structures where they differ from general nursing structures be integrated. To whom, for example, would the director of psychiatric nursing services report and to whom would the psychiatric nurses ultimately be responsible?

> The transition from hospital to the community, and the ability to maintain the crucial emergency intervention and liaison between hospital and community, will take time and resources. It will be difficult both for nurses and for those with intellectual disability or illness, but a report from the New South Wales Department of Health which compared the comparative effectiveness of standard hospital care with comprehensive community care for psychiatric patients consistently favoured comprehensive community treatment according to a number of different criteria. (Grant & Lapsley 1992:211)

Nurses and occupational rehabilitation

During the 1980s, workers' compensation systems in Australia underwent widespread reforms through legislation (Remenyi et al 1987, Swerissen et al 1989). These reforms concerned three main areas: occupational health and safety, workers' compensation for illness or injury, and rehabilitation of the injured workers. The first and third of these provided increased opportunities for nurses.

The occupational health nurse role was transformed from a rather isolated one of treating minor injuries on site to one with a decision making function on occupational health and safety practices and safe working conditions.

As rehabilitation consultants/advisers in worker rehabilitation, the 'nurse' is employed not as a nurse as such but as a health professional with an appropriate background to assist vocational and avocational rehabilitation. As with other allied health professionals, such as physiotherapists and occupational therapists, the original qualification is usually reinforced with a postgraduate diploma in occupational rehabilitation, ergonomics or rehabilitation counselling, although courses and employment practices vary between states.

While nurses would appear to be equally as employable as occupational therapists or physiotherapists as rehabilitation advisers, occupational therapists have gone further than nurses in shedding their background of sole commitment to the client as patient. With return to work particularly, nurses in general have not had the education and training to equip them sufficiently for negotiation/liaison with employers, supervisors, or unions, which is required as much as direct patient care in achieving a successful return to work, in relation to, for example, site assessment or alternative duties. The crucial liaison work appears to be less preferred by nurses than rehabilitation counselling of the client.

Whether it is nurses themselves or rather the perception of nursing as disease oriented which handicaps them in worker rehabilitation as it does in community health is a question which requires detailed research. The changes in nurses' education (Ch. 3) will make a difference where nurses themselves are concerned but no doubt the change in community attitudes will lag behind.

Barefoot nurses Australian style

While it has been argued that there has been an expansion of the role of the nurse in the community and of increased opportunities for participation in decision making, this has long been the case in remote area nursing in sparsely populated rural areas. Remote area nurses have had almost complete control over their work practices and over total patient care. Responsibility and accountability were built in to the nature of their work, particularly in Aboriginal settlements and Bush Nursing Centres where supervision and colleague support were often absent. Accountability was however informal rather than formal and it was not clear to whom accountability was due: to the client, to the employer or to the local community (see for example, Report of the Ministerial Review of Community Health Services in Victoria (1985:162-3)).

Federal and state governments have been forced to respond to the appalling general health of Aborigines, sometimes as a result of alcohol and petrol abuse but more often from unemployment, low incomes and inadequate diet and housing stemming largely from a lack of control over their own lives (Osborne 1982, Winch 1989, Reid & Trompf 1991). Neither the social violence engendered nor the physical degeneration incurred, has responded to western medical approaches. Aborigines and governments have now responded by attempting to place the responsibility for Aboriginal health within their own communities (Nathan et al 1983). This has led to a changing role for remote area nurses. In the Northern Territory, the model which has been adopted is one where Aboriginal health workers, who are registered by law, have the key decision making role and refer clients to the remote area nurse. They belong to separate hierarchies but work together. It is the decision of the community as to who will be an Aboriginal health worker and they are responsible for the health of the community, not the nurse. The nurse is there as an adviser, as a resource, but the actual day-to-day running of the health centres in the Northern Territory is the responsibility of the Aborigines. In Western Australia, this is reversed and the nurse has the primary responsibility. Some remote area nurses are still employed by religious organisations in Aboriginal communities, and Aboriginal control of their own health and welfare has not been pursued to the same extent in these settlements.

In the Northern Territory, the Department of Health and Community Services has established a central policy area which is responsible for overall policies and guidelines in relation to Aboriginal health. Program co-ordinators formulate program goals and objectives and evaluate procedures within the guidelines to ensure equity in the four regions. The regions are autonomous in putting these programs into practice which can result in inconsistencies between regions. There are also differences between the Aboriginal communities which makes it difficult to compare and to evaluate programs.

The aim is a community development approach as part of primary health care which involves and empowers as many people as possible in their own care, and in any programs which affect them. The co-ordinator of the AIDS program for Aborigines has adopted a cultural approach with story telling and symbols from the particular local cultural group to explain how AIDS is contracted. Sex groups are separated for this according to cultural mores.

If nursing staff are not prepared properly they cannot cope within a community development approach. Nurses who have been prepared in the hospital training system tend to want 'to do it all themselves' as the system did not foster a developmental approach. [HB/90] Rather it fostered an approach of 'acting upon' people as 'captive clients'. [GB/90] For the nurse, the ability to analyse the culture and to understand the way people act as they do is required. For example, time is required for the Aborigine to test the outsider and to accept him or her (Winch 1989). The culture shock is such that many remote area nurses stay for a very short time. Those who stay are divided between those who are effective in empowering other people and those who take power to themselves and, for example, run an outlying clinic as if it was in a hospital.

A significant number of Aborigines, particularly in Victoria and New South Wales, live in urban centres where a relatively non-traditional way of life is prevalent, but for these Aborigines too cultural beliefs impact on health and health care. Birth practices are an excellent example. Birth for Aboriginal women is 'women's business' and 'routine antenatal care practices which include vaginal examination and pap smear...are repugnant to most Aboriginal women and discourage attendance [at clinics] (Ministerial Review of Birthing Services in Victoria 1990:77). Not all Koori women are able to attend Aboriginal Health Services and the Ministerial Review of Birthing Services in Victoria (1990:76-7) found that 'the attitudes of both doctors and midwives were...barriers to antenatal care [and suggested] that Aboriginal cultural awareness programs be available for all health professionals and be an integral component of basic and continuing education'. Further, it recommended that 'specific training in the birthing area for health workers, state enrolled nurses and mothercraft nurses of Aboriginal background' be developed.

In hospitals, Aborigines have a much higher admission rate than non-Aborigines (Australian Institute of Health and Welfare 1992:216). They are admitted later, they are more seriously ill and they are more likely to die. They have multiple illnesses requiring multiple treatments and longer stays than the non-Aboriginal population, but they are also more likely to leave before treatment is complete, so that nurses working in the hospitals also need to be sensitive to cultural issues. There is however a high staff turnover which reduces the opportunity for acquisition of local cultural knowledge. The design of the hospital even can be totally inappropriate, as in Darwin where the new hospital was built without verandahs:

> In the old Darwin Hospital you had one Aboriginal tribe behind one of the verandahs and another under the trees...It was all ground level with big verandahs which were cluttered with patients and beds...It was all very 'messy' but it was very comfortable for patients, but whether you are white or black, this hospital has nowhere for you to go. It's not very friendly. [JM/90]

Distance between hospitals, which can be 200-300 kilometres apart, and the inability to provide sophisticated treatment is a major concern for nurses and patients. In Western Australia, the inclusion in the career structure of a staff development nurse has been successful in Roebourne and Whim Creek. These two hospitals are only 10 kilometres apart and share a staff development nurse which it is hoped will reduce the high staff turnover. Roebourne has a large Aboriginal population and previously patients requiring certain procedures would have had to go to Perth:

> Two Aborigines, a mother and daughter need renal dialysis...They would have had to go to Perth and they would have just faded away, away from home, but because of the staff development nurse they can have their dialysis in Roebourne...The nurse is local and every staff member who comes is educated...It would have been unthinkable five years ago because of isolation. [DMcC/90]

The National Aboriginal Health Strategy (1989) recommended mandatory cross-cultural orientation for all non-indigenous staff employed in health and this was confirmed in the *Affirmative Action for Queensland Aborigines and Torres Strait Islanders: A Public Health Strategy* (January 1991). The Council of Remote Area Nurses of Australia (CRANA) in collaboration with the Department of Aboriginal and Multicultural Studies (University of New England) and Aboriginal community organisations has developed an orientation package for non-Aboriginal health professionals. While its focus is on the needs of Aborigines in rural areas it could be adapted for use with other communities because it includes specific cultural rules, attitudes and beliefs provided by local communities. It aims to show the diversity of communities, their attitudes to health, the impact of colonisation on Aboriginal life chances and the experience of cross-cultural communication. For example, case studies present parallels between the culture shock experienced by non-indigenous health professionals entering Aboriginal communities and the experiences Aborigines encounter in white institutions such as hospitals (*ANJ* December-January 1992). The package is used as in service training, distance education and in tertiary courses for health professionals (Anderson 1988). The secretary of the Australian Nursing Federation in the Northern Territory argued that coping with culture shock and conditions in remote areas was difficult for nurses because they were not prepared:

> You might have a nurse one day on a busy ward in Sydney or Melbourne and next week she's 700 kilometres into the desert in a very isolated community... They do not have all the resources available that there would be in a hospital. They're certainly the decision makers. There may be a doctor on the end of a phone but you're the one who is actually there...Accommodation is awful... there is no privacy and as a nurse said 'my wooden floor in my unit caved in and I've got a plank of wood with my freezer balancing on it'. [JW/90]

At the time of the interview, she was trying to gain a commitment from the minister for health (Northern Territory) to provide better accommodation for nurses in rural areas. In Queensland, the ANF/QNU has established a remote area nurses' branch and a remote and rural directors of nursing branch in an attempt to overcome the problems stemming from isolation and a lack of support. Members can communicate through 'teleconferencing' from Cape York to the northern NSW border.

Bush Nursing Services, including Bush Nursing Hospitals and Centres, vary considerably in the functions performed and have been subject to reviews by state governments, particularly in relation to uneconomic services from under utilisation of resources such as hospital beds, and lack of formal procedures for accountability in, for example, drug administration. In some instances this has resulted in the closure of Bush Nursing Hospitals and the 'incorporation' of Bush Nursing Centres as community health centres with a more broadly based function and formalisation of accountability (Economic and Budget Review Committee April 1987).

Wilson and Najman (1982:34-45) found in their study of nursing work in Queensland that there was a relationship between the type of workplace in which nurses worked and the tasks performed:

> In particular, nurses working in rural/isolated areas perform a range of tasks at higher rates than their metropolitan hospital counterparts. Thus rural nurses have the highest rates [of] providing instruction in sexual anatomy and hygiene (59%), providing contraceptive advice (48%)...taking venous blood (67%), suturing (61%)...A higher percentage of nurses working in rural or isolated areas reported that they had provided most categories of medication without doctor's orders.

As the authors point out, it would be expected that:

> Many of these were provided with the understanding that a doctor would subsequently countersign the request...In the meantime, nurses may not only be untrained in some areas where they have no choice but to provide prescribed care, but they may be unprotected (as may be the patient) in an instance where negligence is argued. (Wilson & Najman 1982:33, 36)

This situation remained unresolved in 1992, with remote area nurses continuing to experience the risks arising from exploited dedication. If they acted in response to normative principles of dedication to providing the best possible care, they risked going beyond legal responsibility. Patricia Staunton, Secretary of the ANF (New South Wales branch) and General Secretary of the New South Wales Nurses Association, argued that remote area nurses often worked in 'legal limbo land' and 'needed formal recognition of their services' (Overs 1992). Limited prescribing rights for nurses were supported by the Rural Doctors' Association whose president said that 'nurses were often forced to diagnose and treat illness because of the shortage of rural GPs', and 'while nurses would often ring the local Flying Doctor Service or the closest GP to confirm their decision, legally they were on uncertain ground' (Overs 1992). In remote area nursing the increased responsibility in practice is not balanced by the protection of legal responsibility and accountability.

Legislative reform is often protracted but the federal government is considering the introduction of nurse practitioners in remote areas so that 'nurses working in rural and remote areas may be given Medicare provider numbers and allowed to perform some tasks normally restricted to doctors' (The Age 7 May 1993). The Minister for Health said that:

> It will not be good enough for the medical profession to simply rail against the idea of nurses performing the functions that have hitherto been those of doctors unless it is prepared to assist us in making sure that there is a better spread of doctors (quoted The Age 7 May 1993).

Degrees of freedom

Increased opportunities for decision making for nurses have been provided through the implementation of new career structures where the emphasis is on clinical practice supported by nursing management. There has thus been an attempt to re-establish the importance of the direct caring role at all levels, which had become devalued in favour of a twin hierarchy of technical and managerial competence. Now nursing's focus is back to the patient or client with the potential for increased autonomy for both. With this comes an increase in accountability. The introduction in many hospitals of an extensive committee structure has provided further opportunities for participation by nurses in policies and decisions which affect their professional practice.

Acceptance of the changes in nursing structures and practice is uneven, and an ambivalence about their value is evident, particularly in relation to the separation of clinical from management positions, which if the initial goals of the new career structures are to be met demand a continued commitment by nurses and nursing organisations. Commitment and persistence are required also in overcoming status and gender differences which militate against effective participation in decision making.

These changes are taking place in an environment where resources for health and health care are increasingly scarce but at the same time nursing practice has become more complex. It has become more complex from specialisation, the introduction and more extensive use of sophisticated technology, changes in pharmaceutical usage and in treatment practices, combined with shorter stays in hospital for patients. These changes have had the dual effect of placing a heightened emphasis on nursing knowledge and skills in care of the patient, and in understanding and using equipment. Thus while the role of the registered nurse is crucial in patient care, it is threatened by economic constraints which encourage, however misguidedly, substitution of registered nurses by less qualified personnel.

The registered nurse is, however, responsible for supervising the practice of enrolled nurses, and the development of national competencies for beginning practice of registered and enrolled nurses goes some way towards assisting role delineation. The problem of the erosion of the nurses' role by other health professionals, such as physiotherapists, continues to be a source of frustration combined with recognition of the value for the patient of working with personnel who have different but complementary knowledge and skills. The development by the Health and Community Services Industry Training Board of competencies for all health personnel at advanced practice levels should assist in clarification of respective roles.

Beginning in 1986 in the midst of industrial turmoil but culminating in 1990 in a brief period of relative peace, the Australian Nurse Registering Authorities Conference (ANRAC) agreed in 1986 to formulate two sets of national competencies for the registration and enrolment of nurses (that is, competencies for beginning practice of RNs and ENs), which were approved in principle in 1988. Building on existing state and territory standards and competencies and research commissioned by ANRAC, nurse representatives of each state and territory registering authority developed and refined the competencies which were finally approved at ANRAC and published in May 1990.

Hailed as a triumph of national co-operation over federalism, the ANRAC competencies document sets out a philosophy of nursing and lists competencies for beginning registered nurses and enrolled nurses. Knowledge and skill requirements from educational programs are outlined and the role of the registered nurse is defined as including the integrated components of: 'clinician; care coordinator; counsellor; health teacher; client advocate; change agent; clinical teacher/supervisor' combined with the responsibility for utilising research findings by nurses or others on nursing practice (ANRAC May 1990).

The national competencies for beginning practice (or entry competencies) were approved after implementation in most states and territories of new career structures, and are consistent with changes in the organisational structure of nursing to reflect a professional emphasis, and to contribute to the confidence of the nurse in clinical practice and in decision making.

In practice, however, the progress of the implementation of competencies, like the new career structures, has reflected federalism and has proceeded differently in the states and territories where 'some have taken it up with zeal while others [believe] that it doesn't really affect us'. [MB/92] In 1992, the National Training Board (NTB) in conjunction with state, territory and federal education ministers began a concerted attempt to bring some sort of coherence and integration into education and training and to develop competencies for practice in industry, including nursing. The Health and Community Services Industry Training Board established in March 1992 is the approved competencies development body for the health and community services industry and will refine the ANRAC competencies:

> So that the competencies for beginning practice as a registered or enrolled nurse will fit with competencies at advanced practice levels, and will fit with the competencies at the beginning of practice for the professional groups that are closely aligned with nursing so that we can come to grips with some of the grey areas between what are nursing competencies and what are competencies for physiotherapists or social workers or psychologists or doctors. [MB/92]

The development of competencies for all those in health occupations will assist in resolving the ongoing problem of encroachment on each others' territory (*ANJ* February 1992:19). The establishment of the national Australian Nursing Council (ANC) and the ANRAC competencies are major achievements, but as long as state registering authorities remain, there will be differences between states in the ways that they approach implementation of competencies for registration or enrolment, which will only be resolved when once qualified a nurse is registered with the ANC on a national database under only one national registration act.

Policy changes in community and mental health have provided further opportunities for nurses, but their complete acceptance in a community development role is handicapped by stereotyped perceptions of the nurse as adjunct to the doctor in a curative model focused on disease, rather than on prevention and health promotion in its broadest sense.

Defining the nursing role has proved to be extremely difficult and has given rise to a considerable national and international literature (Benner 1984, Cameron 1989, Lawler 1991, Moorhouse 1992, Rorden & McLennan 1992, Russell 1990). In Australia, this process has been facilitated by a number of professional and industrial issues which necessitated a clear definition of the nursing role. For accountability in nursing practice, state and territory registering authorities and professional associations needed to define what it is to be competent in the delivery of care and what standards of practice are required. The transfer of nurse education to the tertiary sector meant that educational institutions needed to develop curricula which were acceptable both to registering authorities and to employers. For the development of nursing as a profession and to allow registered nurses time for the exercise of skills in patient care, non-nursing duties had to be relinquished and reallocated (Ch. 6). National and state wage cases for equal pay, and for equal pay for work of equal value and recognition as professionals necessitated definitions of the nurse's role (Chs 5 & 6). A mere listing of the different strands, however, leaves out the turbulent industrial and political environment of the 1970s and 1980s in which organised nursing fought for professional recognition and for more control over its own affairs (Chs 5 & 6). Notwithstanding difficulties experienced by nurses in the context of change, it is not credible to view nursing as reverting to exploited dedication in vocational care of the sick. Changes in education and practice, and the few more degrees of freedom provided by new career structures mean that nursing cannot go backwards but can only go forward in the pursuit of identifiable and recognised roles from which they contribute to decision making on the basis of expertise and knowledge. To this end, individual nurses must ensure that they understand that their actions are political. As the ANF Victorian branch secretary said: 'when nurses and the work they conduct are subjected to any change, then how nurses respond to that change will be a political act' whether it is by 'omission' or by 'commission' (Victorian Branch *Newsletter*, November 1991). 'There is no escaping political activity' if nurses want to influence policy on behalf of their clients and themselves, according to the assistant federal secretary of the ANF (*ANJ* April 1990:2). The political and industrial activities of nurses and their achievements over the three decades from 1960-90 would make it difficult for Australian nurses to agree completely with a leading British nurse when she says that:

> The day to day reality of nursing is that it's still a hard slog, with not a lot of people giving you any thanks or valuing you for what is largely unrewarded work. [JSa/90]

REFERENCES

Anderson I 1988 Koorie health in Koorie hands. Health Department Victoria, Melbourne

ANF (Australian Nursing Federation) 1989 Nursing in Australia: a national statement. ANF, Melbourne

ANRAC (Australian Nurse Registering Authorities Conference) 1990 ANRAC National competencies for the registration and enrolment of nurses in Australia. May 1990. Steering committee ANRAC Competency Project, North Adelaide

Aungles S B, Parker S R 1988 Work, organisations and change. Allen & Unwin, Sydney

Australian Institute of Health and Welfare 1992 Australia's health 1992: the third biennial report of the Australian Institute of Health and Welfare. Australian Government Publishing Service, Canberra

Benner P 1984 From novice to expert: excellence and power in clinical nursing practice. Addison-Wesley, Menlo Park

Brewer A M 1983 Nurses, nursing and new technology: implications of a dynamic technological environment. School of Health Administration, University of New South Wales, Kensington

Cameron S 1989 Competencies for registration of nurses in Australia. In: Gray G, Pratt R (eds) Issues in Australian nursing 2. Churchill Livingstone, Melbourne

Community Health Services, Victoria 1985 Report of Ministerial review. Government Printer, Melbourne

Cuddihy L 1989 Is it life at all costs. In: Gardner H, Aroni R (eds) Dying with dignity: ethical religious and cultural perspectives. La Trobe University, Melbourne

Cuthbert M, Duffield C, Hope J (eds) 1992 Management in nursing. Harcourt Brace Jovanovich, Sydney

Daly J, Green K, Willis E (eds) 1987 Technologies in health care: policies and politics. Australian Government Publishing Service, Canberra

Donovan F, Jackson AC 1991 Managing human service organisations. Prentice-Hall, Sydney

Economic and Budget Review Committee 1987 Review of bush nursing services in Victoria. Nineteenth report to the Parliament April 1987. Government Printer, Melbourne

Gardner H, Barraclough S 1992 The policy process. In: Gardner H (ed) Health policy: development, implementation and evaluation in Australia. Churchill Livingstone, Melbourne

Gardner H, McCoppin B 1989 Emerging militancy? The politicisation of Australian allied health professionals. In: Gardner H (ed) The politics of health: the Australian experience. Churchill Livingstone, Melbourne

Grant C, Lapsley H M 1992 The Australian health care system 1991. School of Health Services Management, University of New South Wales, Kensington

Hayden W G 1970 Australia: Commonwealth Parliamentary Debates. 20 May:2391

Jenkins E 1989 Nurses' control over nursing. In: Gray G, Pratt R (eds) Issues in Australian nursing 2. Churchill Livingstone, Melbourne

Kermode M 1992 Nursing. In: Timewell E, Minichiello V, Plummer D (eds) AIDS in Australia. Prentice-Hall, Sydney

Koch T 1990 A new clinical career structure for nurses: trial and evaluation. Journal of Advanced Nursing 15:869-876

Knepfer G, Johns C 1989 Nursing for life. Pan Books, Woollahra

Lansbury R D, Spillane R 1983 Organisational behaviour: the Australian context. Longman Cheshire, Melbourne

Lawler J 1991 Behind the screens: nursing, somology, and the problem of the body. Churchill Livingstone, Melbourne

Mackay L 1989 Nursing a problem. Open University Press, Milton Keynes

Marles F 1988 Report of the study of professional issues in nursing. February 1988. Government Printer, Melbourne

McPherson P D 1992 Health for all Australians. In: Gardner H (ed) Health policy: development, implementation and evaluation in Australia. Churchill Livingstone, Melbourne

Medicare Benefits Review Committee 1986 Second Report. June 1986. Australian Government Publishing Service, Canberra

Milton C R, Entrekin L, Stening B R 1984 Organizational behaviour in Australia. Prentice-Hall, Sydney

Minichiello V 1989 Community care for the aged: benefits to whom? In: Gardner H (ed) The politics of health: the Australian experience. Churchill Livingstone, Melbourne

Minichiello V, Alexander L, Jones D (eds) 1992 Gerontology: a multidisciplinary approach. Prentice-Hall, New York

Ministerial Review of Birthing Services in Victoria 1990 Having a baby in Victoria. Final Report, Health Department Victoria, Melbourne National Health and Medical Research Council 1987, 1989 Working party on home births and alternative birth centres

Ministerial Review of Community Health Services in Victoria 1985. Report May 1985. Government Printer, Melbourne

Mintzberg H 1979 The structuring of organizations. Prentice-Hall, Englewood Cliffs

Mitchell S, Wright M 1992 Community development: creating some confusion for professionals in the community health selling. In: Baum F, Fry D, Lennie I (eds) Community health policy and practice in Australia. Pluto Press, Sydney

Moorhouse C 1992 Registered nurse: the first year of professional practice. La Trobe University Press, Melbourne

Nathan P, Leichleitneir I, Japanangka DL 1983 Health business. Heinemann Educational Australia, Melbourne

National Aboriginal Health Strategy Working Party 1989 A national Aboriginal health strategy. Australian Government Publishing Service, Canberra

National Health Strategy 1991 Hospital services in Australia: access and financing. Issues paper no. 2 August 1991. National Health Strategy, Canberra

National HIV/AIDS Strategy 1989 A policy information paper. August. Australian Government Publishing Service, Canberra

Osborne P D 1982 The other Australia: the crisis in Aboriginal health. Occasional monograph 2. University of Tasmania, Hobart

Overs M 1992 RDA gives support to nurse prescribing. Australian DR Weekly. 20 March:1
Parsons T (ed) 1964 Max Weber: the theory of social and economic organization. The Free Press, New York
Reid J, Trompf P 1991 The health of Aboriginal Australia. Harcourt Brace Jovanovich, Sydney
Remenyi A, Swerissen H, Thomas S (eds) 1987 New Development in worker rehabilitation: the WorkCare model in Australia. World Rehabilitation Fund, New York
Report to the ANF Federal Executive 1991 Evaluation of the Johns Hopkins and Guy's Hospitals management structures: a nursing analysis of clinical management structures, vols 1 & 2. Australian Nursing Federation, Melbourne
Rimmer S M 1991 Occupational segregation, earnings differentials and status among Australian workers. Economic Record 647(198):205-216
Rorden J W, McLennan J 1992 Community health nursing: theory and practice. Harcourt Brace Jovanovich, Sydney
Rowe R, Manning E 1987 Sources of satisfaction for nurses. Australian Health Review 10(2):165-170
Royal Australian Nursing Federation, College of Nursing Australia, New South Wales College of Nursing, Florence Nightingale Committee Australia 1989 Nursing in Australia: a national statement
Russell R L 1990 From Nightingale to now: nurse education in Australia. Harcourt Brace Jovanovich, Sydney
Salvage J 1985 The politics of nursing. Heinemann Nursing, London
Schultz B 1991 A tapestry of service: the evolution of nursing in Australia, vol. 1 Foundation to federation 1788-1900. Churchill Livingstone, Melbourne
Schulz S 1992 Care in the community. In: Cuthbert M, Duffield C, Hope J (eds) Management in nursing. Harcourt Brace Jovanovich, Sydney
Sellick K J, Russell S 1983 Primary nursing: an evaluation of its effects on patient perception of care and staff satisfaction. International Journal of Nursing Studies 20 (4):265-273
Silver M 1986 A vision becomes reality. Australian Nurses' Journal 16(2) August:44
Silver M 1989 Career structure for nurses: the South Australian experience. In: Gray G, Pratt R (eds) Issues in Australian nursing 2. Churchill Livingstone, Melbourne
Steering Committee for the Implementation of the Nursing Career Structure 1987 Implementation guidelines. Western Australia
Swerissen H, Thyer E, Doran J 1989 Workers' compensation in transition. In: Gardner H (ed) The politics of health: the Australian experience. Churchill Livingstone, Melbourne
Thomas L H, Bond S 1990 Towards defining the organization of nursing care in hospital wards: an empirical study. Journal of Advanced Nursing 15:1106-1112
Walsh A, Bruni N, Jonson K, McArthur J 1993 Satisfaction and dissatisfaction amongst past and present members of the nursing staff at the Royal Children's Hospital, Melbourne. Report state 1. Monash University, Melbourne
White R 1972 The role of the nurse in Australia: report to accompany the annotated bibliography. The tertiary education research centre, University of New South Wales
Williams C 1988 Blue, white and pink collar workers in Australia: technicians, bank employees and flight attendants. Allen & Unwin, Sydney
Wilson D A J, Najman J M 1982 After Nightingale: a preliminary report of work undertaken by nurses in Queensland. Australian Nurses Journal October: 31-36
Winch J 1989 Why is health care for Aboriginies so ineffective? In: Gray G, Pratt R (eds) Issues in Australian nursing 2. Churchill Livingstone, Melbourne
Wood P 1990 Nursing: progress through partnership 1921-1991. Department of Community Services and Health. Australian Government Publishing Service, Canberra
World Health Organization 1981 Global strategy for health for all by the year 2000. Health For All Series 3. WHO, Geneva

5. Organised nursing: states of division

The public image of nursing in 1960 was one of 'a noble and worthwhile profession', an Australian academic reported; nurses were 'practical, efficient, industrious, feminine, patient and friendly, and women of high moral ideals' who chose their noble calling in spite of its disadvantages, chief of which were 'long hours, low pay and generally unsatisfactory working conditions' (Congalton (1962) quoted Encel et al 1974:123). A further disadvantage, but one taken for granted at the time, was the unequal position of nurses in relation to members of other health occupations, especially doctors. The major task facing organised nursing during the last 30 years has been to remedy this imbalance, to bring the material wellbeing and occupational standing of nurses up to the level of their professional ideals and public image, while at the same time preserving both ideals and image.

Organised nursing in Australia has existed in an uneasy tension between professional aspirations and industrial necessities, overlaid by the differences and disagreements which a federal structure affords. In the years since 1960 these reasons for divergence and conflict have always been there, and still are, but they have at times come close to solution while at other times they have led to open hostility.

An ideological divide...

From its foundation in 1932 the New South Wales Nurses' Association (NSWNA) was readier to adopt an openly industrial position than its more genteel equivalent, the Royal Australian Nursing Federation* (RANF). The present NSWNA secretary comments:

> I think that the New South Wales Nurses' Association was always perceived by many people, particularly those in the RANF outside New South Wales, as a more industrially oriented organisation, not concerned with the professional interests of nursing...Even those people in New South Wales who were members of the RANF often felt that *that* was their professional organisation, and we were their industrial organisation. [PS/90]

*The Royal Australian Nursing Federation (RANF) became the Australian Nursing Federation (ANF) in 1988. It will be referred to here by whichever name is appropriate.

The RANF in any case spent most of the 1960s in its continuing quest for national unity though it still attended to what the Royal Victorian College of Nursing (RVCN) liked to call 'economic' matters. In South Australia, Joan Durdin (1991:240) says the RANF became more attuned to industrial affairs during the 1960s, especially after Marjorie Ladkin became the first full time secretary of the SA branch. At the national level, a sign of this was the appointment by the RANF in 1964 of an Industrial Officer, Leo Behm. The Queensland branch had actually appointed a secretary in 1959 with some industrial expertise (Dickenson 1975b). This shift towards industrial affairs seems to have come about as a result of two opposing forces bearing on the federation: first, the determined stand of the RVCN on its professional pedestal above the union affray; and second, intermittent threats from other unions which had nursing members. The first, RVCN aloofness from industrial concerns, was more constant during the 1960s, but the Victorians' tenacious adherence to their own version of professionalism (even at the cost of national unity) perversely pushed the RANF closer to a full acceptance of its industrial obligations.

...and federal fragmentation

The federal structure of the Australian industrial relations system has allowed a sometimes disruptive degree of variation in nursing unions. In 1960 there seemed little hope of creating one national association but the divisions, between the RANF and the NSWNA on the one hand, and between it and the RVCN on the other, were more than ideological. They were intensified by federal diversity. In the federal jurisdiction, any association of employees like the RANF must be registered under the Commonwealth Conciliation and Arbitration Act. In four states (Queensland, New South Wales, South Australia and Western Australia) unions are registered under the relevant state legislation, as were the NSWNA and later the Queensland Nurses' Union. The various state and federal acts in effect give unions corporate status and confer certain privileges on those which become registered (Harte 1978). Registration protects a union against member 'poaching' by rivals. Victoria and Tasmania retained wages boards, called industrial boards in Tasmania from 1975. Industrial representation in those states was through unions having direct representation—in Victoria for example, of nurses and employers on the relevant board, the Registered Nurses' Wages Board, which was chaired by a government appointee (McDonald 1975). By 1980 Victoria had moved closer to the South Australian and New South Wales systems with their combination of both compulsory arbitration and wages boards (conciliation committees in New South Wales) and had set up the Victorian Industrial Relations Commission.

These variations have produced some difficulties for a number of unions, including the RANF. In the four states which have arbitration systems, state registered unions are not by law the same bodies as the branches of the federal union, even though both may have the same name, the same members and the same officials. There are therefore (in theory) two distinct groups of nurses, one being, for example, the WA branch of the federal RANF, the other being the RANF WA Branch Industrial Union of Workers. In the 1969 *Moore v. Doyle* case the Commonwealth Industrial Court held (regarding the Transport Workers' Union) that such branches were two legal entities. Rawson (1986b:84) observes that this distinct legal status of state registered unions causes few difficulties, unless state and federal bodies do not have identical memberships and could thus choose different leaders, or in the case of factional disputes within a union. The consequences of dual registration were to affect the RANF twice in the 1980s, first in Queensland and then in South Australia.

In 1960 the federal RANF was still separate from its industrial wing, the Australian Nursing Federation Employees' Section (ANFES) and existed on small capitation fees from state branches. The NSWNA of course dominated industrial coverage in its own state. In Victoria the ANFES acted as the industrial arm of the RVCN (and was held at arm's length), while in Queensland and South Australia the two bodies operated as one. In WA the branches were separate but the membership was the same (Schultz 1974). Other unions had nurse members, such as the Hospital Employees' Federation (HEF), or the Hospital Employees' Association in New South Wales (later the Health and Research Employees' Association—H&REA). Unions like the HEF are 'industry' unions which cover a range of workers in the health industry, whereas the RANF and the NSWNA, based on a single occupation, are 'craft' unions, like the Royal College of Nursing (RCN) in Britain. The HEF as an industry union can enrol nurses, which explains its ability to threaten the RANF or the NSWNA (Fox 1978). The RANF federal secretary even said of the HEF in 1970 that 'our experience in the past has taught us that they do not play it straight with us' (*Journal of the West Australian Nurses* 1970 June:17).

Both the NSWNA and the RANF, whatever their other differences, have consistently proclaimed their status as associations *of* nurses, *for* nurses—however 'nurse' is defined. When the Council of Health Industry Unions was set up in the 1970s, for example, the RANF took part but stressed that this in no way compromised its separate identity (Patten 1976). In this hostility to 'non-nursing' unions, it was at one with the NSWNA, which regularly had to fend off marauders. A South Australian psychiatric nurse who joined an industry union in the 1970s explains, and suggests a potential advantage of such unions:

> I personally believed in industry unions, and that nursing should be better represented in organisations that encompassed other workers in the health field...that's a minority view among nurses, I can assure you...[And] there are a lot of tensions between occupational groups in [industry] unions...[but] you might as well deal with them in the union—as intra-union rather than inter-union. [RA/88]

In Australia the craft union is more common than the industrial kind, but neither is found as a 'pure type'. By the 1980s many unions which appeared to be exclusive to a particular craft had in fact diluted their entry requirements and were recruiting non-qualified or partly qualified employees in their particular employment sector (Hill et al 1982:61).

Beyond these federal complications and inter-union tensions, the major difficulty the RANF faced in 1960 was overcoming the barrier to unity presented by one state, Victoria. The RVCN was to stall attempts to achieve federal unity for nine years.

The struggle for unity...

In 1961 Jane Muntz of Victoria became federal President of the RANF, and the following year Lorraine Jarrett, originally from Queensland, was appointed federal Secretary. It was Jarrett who finally steered the RANF to unity, a goal which must have seemed almost unattainable when she took office. In 1962 the RANF federal council took the first step by making a 'momentous and thrilling decision' to amalgamate with the ANFES by incorporating its constitution into that of the RANF. The following year the council learned that the RANF would have to be absorbed into ANFES, a registered union, rather than the reverse (Anon. 1965; Schultz 1974). This wrong way round method proved to be a further obstacle in the way of unity.

At an abortive 1964 meeting, Jane Muntz acknowledged unhappily that her own state had set its face against unification. The RVCN did not want to lose its separate identity, and it feared the effect that combining professional and industrial aims in one organisation would have on its professional aims, especially if the Victorian ANFES took over the RVCN. Two Victorian nurses look back:

> The RVCN had the economic wing—to which we all belonged...That wing looked after salaries and conditions. But the education side was dominant and the economic side was at a lower key...[GB/88]

There was resistance to unification then because

> ...the RVCN had a royal charter and it was a *college* of nursing, and they didn't want to become just part of the federation. They saw themselves as a much more *professional* body than RANF, which was quite ridiculous. They didn't want anything to do with the union part...[PO/90]

Such views demonstrate the firm hold that the ideology of professionalism, or nursing's conception of it, still exerted over many senior nurses, to the extent that they thought their professional ideals should not be tainted with baser industrial concerns. The RVCN also wished to perpetuate its own prominence and opposed all states having equal representation on the council of the new body. The separation, indeed segregation, of professional from industrial issues was never questioned in Victoria, and in 1964 only Olive Anstey from West Australia spoke against it (Bessant & Bessant 1991:122-3). The Victorian position thus encapsulated both dimensions of nursing disunity: the ideological industrial-professional disjunction, and the federal divisions in the RANF structure which allowed the RVCN to perpetuate it. The RANF quest for unity was also a fight to establish a more equal status for its industrial and professional aims, as some nurses realised:

> ...on the [Victorian] council, I was president of ANFES, and I was a vice-president of RANF at the same time. Others were in that same sort of situation: trying to get the ANFES to think more professionally, and trying to get the others to recognise that there was a place for improvement in conditions of work, including nursing salaries, which were pretty poor. [BS/90]

Nurses in the past were often reluctant to acknowledge the importance of how much money they earned and its effect on their occupational standing. A New South Wales nurse links the unions to this problem:

> ...certainly nurses *need* to be industrially aware. I always quote the good old book: *The Labourer is Worthy of his Hire.* And for too long nurses were the 'el cheapo' section of the health services. [PP/89]

And a former NSWNA secretary believes:

> Pay is crucial in industrial activity. Some people say it's the only issue. I don't believe that. But pay is certainly crucial, and once people become discontented about their pay, they start becoming discontented in other areas. [JHa/89]

The RVCN however 'consistently downplayed' its trade union responsibility to improve members' pay and conditions (Bessant & Bessant 1991:183). The Victorians maintained their opposition to unification after 1964 in spite of assurances from the new RANF President, Joyce Rodmell (Matron of Sydney Hospital), that the International Council of Nurses (ICN) would not disqualify Australia from membership if the RANF became a registered union. In 1967 the RVCN was even invited to withdraw from the federation, so bitter was the feeling against its stand (Schultz 1974; Bessant & Bessant 1991: 126-9).

Yet the RANF was far from neglecting its professional duties. With the National Florence Nightingale Committee (NFNC) it set up in late 1959 the National Nursing Education Division (NNED) as a nursing research and information centre. This was a courageous step to take when unity was uncertain and when, in spite of appeals to several government departments and some lobbying, there was little outside support. Nurses themselves financed the activities of the NNED to a total of nearly £12 000—enough in 1965 to buy quite a reasonable house, and a remarkable effort for women who were not highly paid. This RANF support for the NNED shows that the leadership was very much alive to professional issues, though attention was often diverted from this by the RVCN's stance as self-appointed keeper of the professional flame.

...and the struggle for pay

Under its Director, Yvonne Jayawardena, a European nurse researcher, the NNED carried out the first national survey of Australian nurses to examine why trained nurses left the workforce, with consequent staff shortages. She reported in 1960 that there were 47 255 nurses in Australia and 4259 licensed aides, but discovered to her surprise what Australian nurses took for granted: there was no federal legislation relating to the nursing profession. Each state had its own laws governing quite varied salaries and conditions of employment (Jayawardena 1965). This degree of disparity in Australian nurses' working conditions left a visiting ICN expert 'bewildered, and even dismayed' (Quinn 1963). The NNED survey showed that most nurses (78%) who left the workforce did so for marriage and family reasons. Of those who said they would never return, the low pay, awkward hours (including broken shifts) and poor working conditions were significant reasons. Bess Deakin, who wrote the final report, warned of 'increasing militancy on industrial matters' among nurses (NNED 1967:21, 34-8, 113). This link between unsatisfactory pay and conditions and shortages of nursing staff was a recurring theme for the next 20 years.

In New South Wales, where the shortage of nurses was also acute, the union was active on matters of pay and conditions of work. On the only occasion during his 23 year term of office when he was challenged for his position the NSWNA Secretary, Les Hart, was able to list a number of achievements in improving the conditions and pay of general and psychiatric nurses. The union was affiliated with a 'peak' body, the Australian Council of Salaried and Professional Associations (ACSPA) and took part in ACSPA campaigns. Professional matters were less prominent but not ignored: the NSWNA lobbied to have the state's four-year nursing course reduced to three years, advocated greater unity among nursing organisations and had discussed amalgamation with the Australasian Trained Nurses' Association (ATNA), the oldest nursing organisation in Australia, and even possible affiliation with the RANF. And Les Hart had travelled abroad, including a visit to Russia from where, anticipating Women's Liberation, he reported: 'From my observations only, approximately 20% of women wear foundation garments...' (*The Lamp* 1962 March:1, July:8; Hart 1965).

It was symbolic of the difference between the two unions that in 1966 when the RANF was confronting the RVCN iron curtain between professionalism and unionism, the NSWNA promoted a burst of industrial fervour. There were mass meetings, including one of 3000 nurses in Sydney, in a campaign for a 'reasonable' salary claim. The authorities, reported association officers, 'have underestimated the intelligence and determination of nurses to stand up and fight for their just rights'. The Sydney meeting was judged a success in spite of worries about the 'high-spirited younger nurses' who cheered noisily and later insisted on gathering in front of Parliament House (*The Lamp* 1966 April:5, 15). These nurses were aware that their Victorian and ACT colleagues had received recent wage awards which left them behind, so the Australian doctrine of comparative wage justice warranted their unrest. And at this time R. J. Hawke, for the Metal Trades Unions, was arguing that a buoyant economy proved the capacity of industry to pay higher wages (Paterson 1964).

The Minister for Health in the Askin (Liberal) state government, Harry Jago, speaking to nurses later, seemed disconcerted by '...the nursing profession, so highly regarded by the public, suddenly organising mass demonstrations with all the familiar techniques of mass agitation', and he tried to link the nurses' actions to the party struggle and even to communist propaganda. Les Hart repudiated the minister's criticism, pointing out that other white collar workers such as teachers and bank officers had received pay rises after *their* 'mass agitation' (*The Lamp* 1966 August:8-9, 14-15). The minister seems to have misjudged the nurses' mood, and his red flag waving was by now much less of a threat than it would have been in the cold war era of the 1950s when Prime Minister R. G. Menzies had brilliantly exploited the communist issue.

The 1950s and 1960s were marked by the growing militancy of white collar unions in general, so the New South Wales nurses were aligning themselves with other workers like teachers, who had just been accused of helping to defeat the 24 year old state Labor government (Wells 1966). Their campaign was ultimately successful, though not without a further mass meeting at which 'strike action was only narrowly defeated'. The Premier would not intervene, and the Minister for Health pointed out that hospitals were 'largely autonomous' and said that although they were mostly dependent on public funds, he favoured 'a minimum of interference' with their affairs (*NSWPD* 10 August 1967:361-4, 370-6). This position of state governments as only indirectly responsible for nurses' working conditions was used frequently by politicians as a reason for inaction.

The NSWNA salary appeal produced a variation to the award which for the first time incorporated penalties and shift allowances into the Public Hospital Nurses' (State) Award, the state benchmark award for nurses (Staniland 1969). This followed a general trend towards a total wage (instead of the basic wage with margins for skill) a trend recognised formally in 1967 by the Commonwealth Conciliation and Arbitration Commission when it abandoned the previous system because it had allowed 'leap frogging' to occur based on either part of the wage. The total wage consolidated both into a single unit which could then be adjusted. The total wage decision marked a decline in the commission's influence over wages and the start of a period of wage rises outside the arbitration system (Hill et al 1982:154-5; Deery & Plowman 1991:360-1). Nurses were to become part of this movement against wage control from 1970 when they agitated nationally for higher pay.

The NSWNA meanwhile was able to show its members that they had a lot in common with US nurses, for whom 1966 was the year they 'stopped talking and began battling'. Nurses in a number of American states won substantial pay rises through industrial action such as mass resignations, mass 'sick leave', and in California a threat to drop the national 'no strike' policy of the American Nurses' Association (ANA). The ANA was also aiming to give all nurses a voice in health policy, reported Eleanor Gattoni of its Economic Security Unit. When challenged on an alleged lack of concern with the effect of higher nurses' pay on hospital costs, Gattoni retorted: 'High costs are all around us...After all, the high cost of bourbon doesn't prevent people drinking, you know' (*The Lamp* 1966 December:9-13). The British RCN did not become a trade union until 1977 after 'considerable debate' among the members, and after the Wilson (Labour) Government had given special rights to registered unions (Salvage 1985:104-5, Clay 1987:127, 393-4).

The shortage of nurses in New South Wales was a matter of political concern in 1970, when state Labor MP Kevin Stewart described the position as 'alarming' and proposed that the government should act immediately to 'provide wage justice to this magnificent body of dedicated workers who are fast becoming an underprivileged section of the community'. The Minister for Health replied, as in 1966, that the government was not the nurses' employer (*NSWPD* 19 February 1970:3418-22). In fact, governments delegate some employer functions to health agency managements, which are in theory the employers, but government representatives 'typically assume responsibility for negotiations relating to major claims and for appearances before industrial tribunals'; and the government is always a third party in the Australian industrial relations system (Fox 1989:2).

Bringing it all together

In 1968, the centenary of Lucy Osburn's arrival in Sydney, Lorraine Jarrett held the twin posts of secretary of the RANF and of ANFES, symbolising the desire for unity, but her hopes were disappointed yet again. The revised ANFES constitution, which would have allowed unification, was put to the vote of the entire membership at simultaneous meetings in the states but failed to get the required two-thirds majority largely because of a big 'no' vote in Victoria (Schultz 1974). A more hopeful outcome of RANF Council deliberations that year was the firm decision to produce a national journal. All the necessary money had not been collected, but the small WA branch committed itself to $5000 a year for eight years, noting later that (in contrast to this generosity) Victoria would not take part in the journal (*Journal of the West Australian Nurses* 1970 February:10). In spite of these preoccupations, the RANF did not neglect industrial issues: Jarrett spent some time examining nursing conditions in the Northern Territory (still under federal jurisdiction) and later the ANFES succeeded in getting a full investigation and 'large increases' in nursing establishments (*ANJ* 1968 March:68; 1969 August:173).

Talking to nurses in Adelaide at the end of 1968, Lorraine Jarrett enumerated the six federal and 47 state organisations which had some connection with nursing, either professional or industrial. As a group, she concluded, Australian nurses had 'managed to completely fragment the organisation of their affairs', and had therefore made sure that neither governments nor industrial arbitrators need bother to listen to them. Perhaps thinking of her Victorian colleagues, Jarrett emphasised the contemporary trend towards professional employees becoming members of unions, and affirmed her own position: 'Reconciling all that is desirable in the dignity of the nursing profession...with a belief in proper rewards for our efforts—creates no conflict in my mind.' She envisaged a strong national organisation, but was clear that this did not entail weak state bodies; and at both levels nurses would work to further educational, research, service *and* economic welfare goals (Jarrett 1968). For Jarrett at least, federal unity of the RANF branches meant also professional-industrial unity of purpose. A future federal secretary agreed:

> At that time in the 1960s, it was absolutely evident that whatever else nursing did, we had to be able to get the professional and the industrial running along together...and while they could be run separately, they had to be in harmony. [MP/91]

It was this view which prevailed the following year rather than the outmoded separatism of the RVCN. In spite of 'gloom and despair' at the March 1969 council, further simultaneous members' meetings in July finally approved the amended ANFES constitution. In March 1970 during the federal RANF/ANFES meeting held in Hobart the integration of the two bodies was finally agreed to and became official on 1 July. A pointer to the future was a series of discussions held between the federal and state industrial officers which, as the WA industrial officer reported, led to 'uniformity of actions and a greater awareness of the future industrial activities...' (Giles 1970). After a period of delay because the ICN had to approve the constitution of the new body, the first meeting of the integrated union was held in March 1971. The inaugural president, Violet Hall of Queensland, was soon succeeded by Olive Anstey, the first WA nurse to become federal President. The new federal secretary, Mary Patten, had been appointed earlier by a combined executive of the two bodies (Schultz 1974).

The RVCN remained separate from its industrial arm for the next five years, wishing to retain its independence and holding to its conviction that a trade union should not manage all nursing affairs (Bessant & Bessant 1991:132). An additional reason may have been the serious industrial conflict of the time. A trend towards punitive action by the Commonwealth Industrial Court against striking unionists culminated in the 1969 gaoling of Victorian union leader Clarrie O'Shea, a member of the militant Maoist sect of the Communist Party (Rawson 1986b: 101). Such an event could well have accentuated RVCN antipathy to unions.

The final victory over RVCN obduracy was the result of efforts in the various states to recruit more ANFES members, and of the help of the NSWNA (Bessant & Bessant 1991:131). The New South Wales vote probably came from nurses who were jointly members of the NSWNA and of the old ATNA (*ANJ* 1968 September:192). The new Secretary of the NSWNA was M. V. ('Ronnie') Henlen, a former matron and an office bearer of the NSW College of Nursing, credentials which must have made her particularly acceptable to the RANF. At this time Henlen herself favoured 'one strong nursing body at Federal level'. Further, the RANF had sided with the NSWNA in opposing an H&REA attempt in 1968 to take over industrial cover of NSW nurses (*ANJ* 1968 June:134, 1977 August:7, *The Lamp* 1968 October:7, 1970 April). And the new federal secretary saw that as well as those in the RVCN who had been overtaken by events, there were some Victorian nurses who favoured unity:

> In the end, I think they just had to acknowledge the way the world was going, and the reality, whether they were going to stay isolated or get in with it. Also there had been some changes in the organisation...[through] people like Moira McNair, who believed firmly in the two organisations coming together... You had people like that actually *pushing* the amalgamation very strongly. [MP/91]

The rewards of unity

If unity seemed to become at times a holy crusade for the RANF leadership, a joining of the national sisterhood, there were practical as well as emotional reasons for seeking it. A united voice would gain more attention from policy makers, and a united union could more easily withstand challenges from rivals. As Lorraine Jarrett had argued, nurses' reticence in wage negotiations encouraged these 'non-professional groups' (like the HEF) to meddle in their affairs. 'If we do not negotiate nursing awards', she warned, 'others will...' (Jarrett 1968). Further, governments (state and federal) together constitute the largest employer of nurses. Violet Hall (President of ANFES) reminded members that the government had to be able to deal with registered organisations, a point that 'a lot of nurses don't seem to grasp' (Hall 1968). Nursing leaders also realised in the late 1960s that the Australian Labor Party (ALP) might win federal office and might favour what they saw as threats to organised nursing: a national health service and the HEF, which was affiliated with the ALP (Bessant & Bessant 1991:125-6). At the time the conservative parties in fact dominated national politics, but the new federal secretary considered:

> ...the period we were moving into was going to be one where numbers counted. And in nursing if we didn't have the numbers to support issues...well then, we wouldn't ever get a hearing. We were starting from the bottom of the pile, so to speak, politically, and people didn't really pay much attention to nurses in those days. And I couldn't see how without the numbers we could

> achieve anything. Also...we were all very aware of the different way that [a Labor government] would look at some of these issues. [MP/91]

In the event, Labor was relatively benevolent to nursing. By 1970 the ALP had put behind it the destructive period of the Split and had reconstructed the 'hard left' Victorian branch. Under Gough Whitlam, the leadership had shed its old Catholic and working class image and the party had become more attractive to voters in the middle class Protestant suburbs (Jupp 1982:115).

The passions and practicalities of unity were vindicated in the following decades, especially during the education campaign. They were less obvious in the industrial sphere, since for most unions the day-to-day operational level is typically the state branch and this continued in the RANF, especially since most nurses were working under state awards in state hospital systems. The RANF recognised at the start that it had to establish a desirable balance between a national view and the view of the individual states and territories (*ANJ* 1971 September:13). In 1973 the constitution was changed to allow for proportional representation of branches on council, though only on matters of finance and the constitution itself. This change was made 'to stimulate recruitment and to meet the wishes of the Branches' (*ANJ* 1974 December-January:45). The federation had to perform a continual balancing act between the national body and its sometimes restive branches, a task the NSWNA was spared. A former president saw the difficulties of this balance:

> The weaknesses of the RANF are really its strengths. Federalism is a weakness, but it is a strength in speaking for nurses across Australia. But people have a vested interest in the states. [DW/89]

The publication of the national *Australian Nurses' Journal* (ANJ) from mid 1971 prompted a national view, though there were regrets in the state branches when the cessation of their own journals over the next few years ended an era of close acquaintance with local events:

> If you wanted to find out if anybody died, got married or some other thing, you usually found it in that journal [UNA]. But now...we found ourselves with a few pages in a national journal...[MC/88]

From cloth caps to the white shirt brigade

Australia has had a high level of union membership relative to that of comparable countries such as the US and Britain, initially because the system of industrial arbitration encouraged it early in the 20th century. Women workers, however, while forming a growing proportion of all union members (from 19% in 1920 to 33% by 1982) have always been and are still less likely than male employees to belong to a union: 48% of female employees were unionised in 1981 compared to 60% of male, though the gap had narrowed (Rawson 1986b:25). Nurses have been part of a remarkable trend in white collar or non-manual union membership growth, in contrast to the decline in blue collar unionism as the composition of the workforce has changed. During the 1970s many white collar unions expanded, but the RANF grew most rapidly of all (Rawson 1986b:23).

The newly unified RANF became part of a large and diverse sector of the trade union movement in Australia, the public sector unions. Some nurses work in the private sector (about 20% of RNs and SENs in 1978), but industrial relations in the two sectors have become increasingly integrated since the mid 1970s. Further, public sector employees are almost twice as likely to belong to unions as are private sector workers. The character of the nursing unions as white collar and public sector bodies seems to have offset the initial handicap of their female composition.

One difference between these unions and others is that public sector managers commonly belong to the same union as their workers. Directors of nursing and their staff, for example, may all belong to the ANF. This can bring difficulties for such unions when taking industrial action, but it has the advantage of tilting membership in the direction of those who are better paid and more powerful (Rawson 1986a). In the earlier part of the period under review, nursing organisations were studded with presidents and other (honorary or paid) office-bearers who were or had been matrons (later called directors of nursing). The combination of experience and respectability embodied in these women probably gave the nursing unions more weight and credibility with politicians than they might otherwise have had. The federal secretary of the time believes that:

> Without the matrons...we would have no organisation. I think that nurses need to acknowledge that historically. It was the matrons who got the nursing organisations going, and led them, and got nursing into a reasonable position in this country. [MP/91]

As industrial activities gained momentum, the matrons were probably less of an asset in the daily push and shove of union affairs, and the distance between them and the working nurse may have deterred some juniors from joining. A Western Australian nurse saw an additional problem when she joined the RANF branch council in 1970:

> The council tended to be largely directors of nursing and heads of schools of nursing—I think that would have been true with most branches of RANF. And there was a conflict of interest: quite clearly, you can't be 'director' of the union and do things that are going to give you pain as a director of nursing. [MV/88]

The RANF later acknowledged this problem: 'Recognition must be given...to expertise in various nursing specialties...possessed by members of the Federation as something quite separate from the formal position which a nurse holds within the hierarchy of the organization...'. Members were equal in their status as employees, the RANF said, and urged them to deal with interlevel conflict inside nursing (*ANJ* 1980 July:10). The growing professional specialisation and expertise of nurses was eroding the bureaucratic line authority of the matrons.

Federal unity, but turmoil in the states

By 1970 Australia was no longer a forgotten imperial outpost but becoming part of the world economy. Its prosperity now depended less on the proverbial sheep's back and more on manufacturing (behind tariff protection) and on mining. But the long boom period of the postwar years was drawing to a close. Over the next few years the annual rate of increase in the Consumer Price Index (CPI) went from the 2.5% it had been during the 1960s up to 8.2% by 1973. In parallel, the rate of increase in average weekly earnings rose from 5% in the 1960s to 8.5% by 1970, and continued to rise. The federal Arbitration Commission was forced to grant a 6% increase in the minimum wage less than a year after awarding a 3% rise, which speeded up price inflation (Crowley 1986:15-16). Nurses were inevitably affected by this sharp rise of both wage and price levels, the more so because their pay and conditions were already behind those of comparable workers. The final triumph of RANF unification was greeted by an upsurge of industrial unrest.

A visiting US nurse told her Australian colleagues in 1969 that there were three major problems which affected nurses everywhere: deficiencies in their education, shortages of staff, and poor pay and working conditions (Elliott 1969). In late 1969 the HEF had served a log of claims for salary increases for nurses at the Canberra Community Hospital. The hearings for this claim continued until April 1970 and generated a high level of interest among nurses around Australia with bus loads of sympathisers arriving in Canberra. Canberra nurses were necessarily members of the HEF, since the local RANF branch was 'a professional body' only. A few weeks later they set up an ANFES branch (*Canberra Times* 26 June 1970).

This case constituted the first Arbitration Commission Full Bench review of nurses' work: that is, it required at least three senior members of the commission to decide a matter of economic significance. The local press reported that nurses wanted recognition as a profession, and regarded the case as 'a national test case' (*Canberra News* 10 & 11 February 1970). The HEF asked the commission to 'consider only the work and responsibilities of nurses, without regard to rates in other states', and to reassess nursing 'as a profession' across Australia: 'We have to break this circle of each of the states simply following each other for pay rises', said the HEF industrial advocate, Raymond O'Dea; but the commission said it could not overlook other rates (*Canberra Times* 5 June 1970). The circle of comparative wage justice kept nurses' pay low partly because it was related only to that of other nurses, not to the pay of those doing what might be judged similar work.

In the states nurses were also dissatisfied. Members of the RANF (SA branch) agitated so effectively during a state election campaign that the

(Coalition) state government announced a new system of training and recruitment; and the Leader of the (Labor) Opposition, Don Dunstan, promised to improve conditions if elected—which he was. One of the reported complaints of the Adelaide nurses was of the 'hopelessly conservative' members of the RANF (SA branch) Executive (*Canberra Times* 23 June 1970). The RANF failed to placate the 'stirrers', but it was 'preparing for action' (Durdin 1991:241; *SA Nurses Journal* May/June 1970). Lorraine Jarrett reported 'high feeling' among nurses across the country, and said that the RANF had been pursuing an 'increasingly active' industrial program at both state and federal levels to avert 'unprecedented action' by nurses. 'Let nobody underestimate the capacity of nurses to be militant and to fight aggressively for their demands' Jarrett warned, but added 'even though we will never contemplate doing anything that could in any way harm our patients'. Queensland nurses had made a significant advance in 1969 by getting a 'living out' wage which gave them for the first time wage rates comparable to those in other states, but in 1970 many were still dissatisfied and 2800 attended a public meeting at which they proposed a ban on non-nursing duties (*The Tasmanian Nurse* 1970 March:7-8; *Hobart Mercury* 19 March 1970; *Journal of the West Australian Nurses* 1970 June:17; *RANF Review* 1970 February-May).

The Canberra judgement handed down on 14 May 1970 (two days after the 150th anniversary of the birth of Florence Nightingale) granted much less than nurses wanted. The Matron of Canberra Hospital, Margaret Guy, was reported to have called the situation 'crass and idiotic', since tribunals in some states had already granted higher salaries (The *Australian* 15 May 1970). A particular outrage was the Arbitration Commission's opinion that 'a Grade 1 sister at the Canberra Hospital was exercising a skill and responsibility no less than that of the average "tradeswoman"'. This had left most nurses 'in a stunned state', said the hospital's assistant matron. The commission had compared nurses with fitters, as members of an apprentice trade, rather than with other professions (Kennedy 1970)—fitters are the traditional 'benchmark' for determining margins for skill.

In Canberra '400 angry nurses' (including Margaret Guy) stood on the steps of Parliament House until the Prime Minister, John Gorton, appeared, accompanied by visiting Canadian Premier Pierre Trudeau (*Canberra News* 20 May 1970). The case had now become an issue in a current ACT by-election, and the federal (Coalition) government, 'to its great discomfiture', found it 'rapidly becoming a national issue'. Also an unwelcome one, when the government was having a 'running fight' on doctors' fees and its health policy was under 'concentrated fire' (*Canberra News* 21 May 1970)—this last over deficiencies in the voluntary insurance scheme. Under pressure, Gorton and the Minister for Health met an HEF-led delegation of senior nurses including the NSWNA secretary, who said afterwards that the meeting had brought no results for pay, but that the Prime Minister had said he would 'give nursing education a push' (*Canberra Times* 27 May 1970).

The HEF went on to lead a walk-out of nurses from the Canberra Hospital—they were officially on 'special leave' for two weeks. At the time measures such as work bans or special leave were considered daring, but since the RANF outlawed strikes there were only limited actions which dissatisfied nurses could take. Finally, after three weeks of leave, intervention by two federal government ministers and ACTU support, the nurses returned to work hoping that the 'spirit of Canberra' would promote responsible unionism. New pay rises were awarded a few days later: a modest $3.20 to $5.80 which was met with an understandably 'mixed reception' (*Canberra Times* 9 & 10 July 1970). Both the RVCN and the Queensland Branch sympathised with the Canberra nurses but did not support their 'special leave' action. The Queensland branch Secretary, Bartz Schultz, made a careful distinction between RANF methods and those of the HEF: the way in which nurses tackle their problems, she thought, 'will determine whether or not they will be recognised as "professionals" or "tradespeople"' (*RANF Review* 1970 August). This statement suggests that nursing leaders wished nursing to maintain a professional and implicitly middle class image. This forced them to reject any connection with more proletarian occupations and with the industrial methods of most unions. Even rank and file nurses, although they were ready to adopt at least some of the industrial methods of working class unionists, disliked the obvious implication that they too were 'tradespeople'.

Nurses in a number of states also achieved pay improvements in 1970 through the various state industrial tribunals. Victorian nurses held a rally of 4000 in May and instituted a ban on non-nursing duties. They also attacked the Minister for Health, who was replaced by the Bolte (Liberal) state government after the next election, and they began a work value case accompanied by 'several hundred' meetings (*ANJ* 1971 August:16). Queensland nurses were awarded pay increases in July, but as the RANF branch realised, they would never get salaries which recognised the full complexity of their work and responsibilities without expert assessment and comparison with salaries paid to other occupations. Without this, Queensland nurses, like others, would be left with the interstate comparisons and 'leap frogging' pay rises which left them 'somewhere between the best and the worst' (*RANF Review* 1970 December). The RVCN Industrial Officer (and acting federal industrial officer), Geoff McDonald, a man with left wing connections, reminded members of the celebrated *Engineers' Case* of ten years earlier (McDonald 1971). The Arbitration Commission then had 'tacitly acknowledged' relativity between engineers and other professionals like doctors and had awarded them 40% salary increases. The case demonstrated 'a form of comparative wage justice directed at desired, rather than established, relativities' (Deery & Plowman 1991:397). Nurses in 1970 realised that the established relativities put them at a disadvantage because, partly on the grounds of their apprenticeship training, it compared their skills with those of tradespeople such as fitters. Like the engineers, they had to aim at a more favourable baseline for comparative wage justice.

The 'spirit of Canberra' briefly infused nurses, and an additional stimulus may have been the widespread agitation of the time against the Vietnam War. The WA branch industrial officer reported that the previous industrial apathy had gone and members were taking more interest in industrial activities, 'especially students and junior sisters' (Giles 1970). RANF branch officers began to realise that conducting industrial relations was not only an important part of their work, it was an onerous job. The WA branch industrial officer, 'highly gratified' that members recognised his growing workload, pointed out, for example, that there were 12 separate awards for nurses in the state, with that for public hospitals the 'parent' or primary award. Changes in that award usually meant 'flow ons' to other awards. Other states faced similar complexity but the RANF was not yet fully equipped for its industrial responsibilities. The Queensland branch industrial officer pointed out that it had none of the usual industrial back up of similar organisations, such as job representatives 'or as they are more commonly known, Shop Stewards' (Catterall 1971). This was a deficiency the RANF had to make good in the future, said WA Councillor Hilda Jury, if nurses were to leave behind their 'rather amateurish' way of conducting their industrial affairs, and show that they were 'a force to be reckoned with' (*Journal of the West Australian Nurses* 1971 February:12-13). The RANF industrial officers (at the time nearly all men) clearly recognised that the RANF had to be better organised. They had to look no further than the HEF, whose astute secretary, Keith Mitchell, reorganised the No. 1 branch in the early 1970s by setting up a network of shop stewards, and then used the union's organised power to achieve substantial wage gains (The *Age* 24 May 1975; Hill et al 1982: 82-83).

Right, left—or fancy free

The ANJ from the start proclaimed the non-political, especially non-*party* political position of the RANF, which it shared with the NSWNA in the 1960s and 1970s. At least that was the public position of both unions in the sense of not being openly partisan. In practice, many nurses seemed to equate 'political' with 'left wing', as a former RANF president found:

> I think nurses were naive in the main. Their political minds were that the Liberal Party was OK and the ALP was all wrong. So if you invited people to come and speak...if you had a Liberal Party member that would be great, but if you had a Labor Party member...it would be seen as communistic, 'red-ragging' and all those other sorts of things...It was only with the advent of the 'goals in nursing education...' that nurses started to approach both parties. [DW/89]

In fact, public sector unions are inevitably political since it is impossible for them to maintain a clear line between industrial and political questions: the size, composition and decisions about pay and working conditions in the public sector are decided by the government of the day, so that a public sector union like the RANF 'may therefore have wholly industrial reasons for adopting a political policy—even a "party political" policy of seeking the return of one party and the defeat of another' (Rawson 1986a). This reality would eventually affect the nursing unions.

Most nurses at this time probably did not expect their associations to be politically active or to be a recognised part of the policy making process. Many seem to have accepted medical domination in health policy as well as in the workplace, though Mary Dickenson has shown how the Queensland branch of the RANF learned in the 1960s to act with at least some of the methods of an effective political pressure group. As she makes clear, however, several handicaps had to be overcome, including RANF disapproval of 'any activity which could be construed as having a party political bias' (Dickenson 1976a).

In 1969 the RANF published details of the federal (Labor) Opposition's proposed health insurance scheme, Medibank, as seen by the Australian Medical Association and in 1972 the NSWNA published a Labor account of this innovative policy (*ANJ* 1969 April: 86-7; *The Lamp* 1972 October:27). The scheme was a major federal election issue in both years, but in neither case was there any nursing comment except as implied by the contrasting sources of comment and information. A few years later RANF President Olive Anstey was more outspoken, referring to the federal Whitlam (Labor) Government's policy of providing 'a health service which is a national responsibility and a service to which the whole population is entitled' (*ANJ* 1974 November:7). From 1971 the pages of the ANJ show that senior members of the RANF, though they avoided partisan comment, were aware of the changes taking place in health policy during the decade and recognised the potential for the RANF to contribute to policy making—for example, there were articles on Aboriginal health and on community health. The federation also made regular submissions to the many government bodies and committees connected with health services which the Whitlam (Labor) Government established. Senior NSWNA officers were similarly aware of political issues but similarly restrained in airing political views until the mid 1970s.

Both the RANF and the NSWNA lobbied consistently to have nurses appointed to statutory bodies, with some success. The Whitlam Government appointed Mary Patten and Sister Paulina Pilkington to its new Hospitals and Health Services Commission, and Sister Paulina in 1975 became the first Director of Nursing in the Commonwealth Department of Health (*ANJ* 1974 October:7; 1976 September:7-8). This central position brought advantages to nursing, especially when it was upgraded:

> That was my object: to set up a forum whereby we all got together...the nurse advisers from the states and territories, who'd meet in Canberra...I was committed to the fact that you needed a strong voice in Canberra if you were going to bring about any change...[and] there was a need to have a [2nd division] position, because unless you are a senior officer within the bureaucracy no one really takes much notice of you. [PP/89]

As it became fashionable for state governments, led by New South Wales, to set up Health Commissions during the 1970s (following various reports), nursing organisations had the chance to seek representation. In 1975 the small ACT branch admitted failure, despite 'strenuous lobbying', to gain a full time commissioner on the new ACT Health Commission, but it was able to report a significant achievement when, in line with federal Labor Government policy, Jennifer James became the first Australian nurse to chair a registration board. Queensland's 1977 Act followed this precedent, and Joan Foley, Adviser in Nursing at the Health Department, was the first nurse to chair the Queensland board (*ANJ* 1975 August:42; 1977 May:63; 1980 June:73). Other significant appointments included Joyce Rodmell's in 1976 as Director of Nursing in the NSW Health Commission, and later Janette Noble's as a Commissioner (*ANJ* 1976 March:8; 1979 October:17). The RANF, said Olive Anstey, had established itself as 'the authoritative resource' for advising governments and health agencies, and was poised to 'rocket nursing into the 1980s' (*ANJ* 1974 November:8).

The non-partisan position remained: the RANF was non-political in a partisan sense, an editorial proclaimed, but it was 'intensely political' when it came to fighting for the progress of nursing (*ANJ* 1974 December:5) as the 'goals' campaign demonstrated. By the end of the decade, the federal secretary thought that nurses had been recognised as a significant group who could influence policy (Patten 1979). Nursing was achieving more recognition from politicians during the 1970s, but even an 'authoritative resource' has to force the government to listen to its advice. The RANF leadership apparently failed to query whether their industrial reticence did not deprive them of a vital source of political power.

The missing foot-soldiers

An initial weakness of the RANF was its relatively low membership. In 1970 and for some years after, its total membership was lower than that of the NSWNA, which included psychiatric nurses and SENs. It grew rapidly in the 1970s, but from a low base. A further problem was that the national journal, the essential mouthpiece for any unified policy statements, produced a deficit in the early years partly because federalism reduced possible classified advertising revenue since most job recruiting was in the states. Nurses themselves lent a total of $15 250 to keep it going but the number of subscriptions remained small—about 14 000 in 1975. In 1976 it was saved by the decision of the Queensland, Victorian and SA branches to include a subscription in their membership fees, bringing the circulation up to over 27 000 (*ANJ* 1977 April:10, 1981 February:5). The ANJ was at last on the way to becoming an asset and justifying the faith of the dedicated few who had started it.

Neither the RANF nor the NSWNA openly advocated compulsory unionism, though both regularly inveighed against 'free loaders' who accepted hard-won pay rises without contributing membership fees. The Queensland branch's industrial advocate thought RANF members should encourage non-members to join, since they shared 'a clear moral duty to contribute' (Steinitz 1979). In some states with Labor governments (South Australia under Don Dunstan, or the Tasmanian régime of Eric Reece, for example) there was a system of job preference to union members, though a Tasmanian nurse claimed that the RANF was not a professional body if it condoned this 'compulsory unionism'. In Queensland the branch was disturbed by threats from the Bjelke-Petersen (Coalition) state government to remove preference clauses (*ANJ* 1977 November:6, 1978 October:71). While industrial gains depend on a reasonable level of union membership (Hill et al 1982:85), most nurses would probably have objected, for example, to the South African Nursing Association's policy of compulsory membership.

The RANF did want political influence, so the various branches were naturally concerned about member apathy. If the policy makers overlooked nurses, warned WA branch president Beryl Grant, this was the fault of their 'passive attitude and lack of interest in the broad social and political issues of health'. The Victorian and Queensland branches lamented members' low level of interest in union affairs, as did the NSWNA. A Tasmanian sub-branch president thought the lack of interest was an abrogation of professional responsibility, and regretted that 'a lot of nurses...would not be unduly concerned should the Southern Sub-Branch cease to exist' (*ANJ* 1974 October: 37-8, 1979 December-January:71, March:55; September:63; *The Lamp* 1970 July:10). That working nurses were apathetic about their unions and about politics in general is not surprising—it would be more surprising (even alarming) if they were incessantly active. Unions which are apparently well run, which have open elections and which satisfy the needs of their rank and file members are unlikely to have a very active membership (Hill et al 1982:83-4). Large and lively meetings and high voting rates in elections may signal member dissatisfaction, as events in 1970 showed. And the working conditions of students and of junior RNs also made active participation difficult, a South Australian nurse observed:

> The rank and file was too difficult to organise because of the shift work....[And] you don't have a stable student body because there is this constant turnover...it was very difficult to organise a large student body. Your beginning workers—well, they'd survived three years of training and they weren't about to put that on the line...[SMcC/88]

For many nurses there was also the daily absorption in their clinical work which deflected interest from events beyond the workplace, as a New South Wales nurse sees in retrospect:

> It's frightful when I think about it. I was *immersed* in spinal injuries as my clinical specialty—and that was fine, a good thing. But for broader issues...! [RP/89]

US nurses were told in the 1970s that they left themselves open to charges of political naivety (Kalisch & Kalisch 1976). 'The time has come', one nurse considered, for them 'to poke their apolitical heads out from under their caps' and recognise that they had to take the political route if they wanted respect from other professions and attention from legislators (Powell 1976). Political apathy becomes unprofitable when, for example, it hinders nurses from protecting their own job territory or stops them challenging other staff on ethical issues. A South Australian nurse regrets these consequences:

> ...they don't like the physios and social workers moving in...especially when nurses do everything at the weekend. It's ironic that it seems they're apathetic and don't want to do anything about it...From my experience too, when we start to talk about ethical situations...The fear that 'I'll lose my job if I don't do as I'm told or if I make a fuss, or I'm labelled as a trouble maker—so I'll put up with these things'. [JW/88]

Joining a man's world...

Mary Dickenson, then Assistant Secretary of the RANF Queensland branch, observed in 1975 that 'Australian nurses generally do not think very seriously about their unions and have little conscious awareness of being part of a trade union movement' (Dickenson 1975a). It was probably also true for most that they did not feel part of the labour movement in the sense of having even vaguely socialist sympathies. In this they were like their unionist comrades, since the aims of Australian unions 'are largely restricted to the negotiation of limited improvements within the framework of capitalist work relations', whatever the more radical oratory of leaders may suggest (Deery 1989a)—practical results are preferred to ideological inspiration.

The RANF and the NSWNA differed from unions of manual workers in that in addition to industrial activities, a significant portion of their resources was (and is) devoted to professional matters and there are likely to be members who join primarily because of their professional rather than industrial interests (Fox 1978). This was true at the time also for British nurses joining the RCN (Bellaby & Oribabor 1980). But nurses who did not see themselves as part of the union movement lacked both knowledge of and sympathy for union aims and methods. A US nurse noted ruefully, 'Most nurses welcome higher salaries and better working conditions, but many reject collective bargaining and collective action as means to attain them' (Grand 1971). The nursing unions were like right wing unions, which may recognise a range of goals wider than the strictly industrial, but are less likely than left wing unions to take industrial action in their pursuit (Davis 1987). Nursing union leaders have usually been moderate in that they have not generally espoused radical causes, with a few remarkable exceptions. The long held antipathy to strike action was one sign of this moderation.

The Australian system of conciliation and arbitration gives unions a secure place, but in return it demands some control over how they administer their internal affairs, including democratic procedures for electing officials and conducting ballots. The registration system gives unions some protection from rival organisations but this provides therefore less of a check on the power of officials. Unions are legislatively controlled to an extent unique in Western countries, primarily to prevent abuses of power or financial irregularities and to ensure that leaders are responsive to rank and file members. (Deery & Plowman 1991:282-3). The federal RANF in 1970 was not a wholly democratic body in that branch councils, *not* the general membership, elected the branch secretaries, just as the federal council (made up of two branch councillors from each state) elected the federal secretary (*ANJ* 1969 June:124-32). This indirect election method was to cause tensions in the federation's dealings with the NSWNA, whose members had elected their secretary since 1962.

There were efforts however to improve both the representation of members and communication with the rank and file. The RANF (SA branch) in 1971 installed a system of 'key members' (analogous to shop stewards) and soon most states had done so, though the Queensland branch reported in 1978 that its efforts to set up the system had been 'disappointing' because some members claimed that they would be victimised if they took part (*ANJ* 1971 February:12-13; November:40; 1978 October:70). Yet the RANF retained 'a distinct lack of interest', Mary Dickenson thought, in bringing rank and file members actively into its affairs by encouraging them to take part in the industrial relations process and become fully aware of their entitlements (Dickenson 1976b). Many junior nurses seem to have thought that the RANF did very little to represent them, and, given its continuing domination by senior nurses, they probably felt (as in 1970) that the leadership was too conservative. An ACT nurse who trained in Victoria in the early 1970s found:

> There wasn't very much industrial activity at all. The RANF was not considered to be really worth joining...But in Melbourne we started a [non-union] nurses' industrial group. We campaigned a bit on the wages issue and had a rally in Melbourne...it wasn't a very big rally...The RANF was seen to be a hospital management organisation more than a union. [KK/88]

Junior nurses may have believed also that the RANF was preoccupied with professional matters such as the 'goals in nursing education', a WA branch council member considered:

> ...a lot of members thought so, that we weren't attending sufficiently to their conditions of work and salaries and so on...[MV/88]

...but 'the ladies came to stay'

Australian women have been members of unions for a century, but until recently they have seldom attained elected executive positions. In the nursing unions, by contrast, women have always held most of the senior positions

(Pittman 1985), though their impact on union policy has until quite recently been made from the viewpoint of the single woman rather than from that of her married colleague. In the 1960s the nursing workforce was 95% female and 73% unmarried (NNED 1967). The young single women were expected to toil at the lowlier tasks until they left nursing, summoned by wedding bells, while the older single women (the 'battle-axes' of legend) commanded them from the senior positions. It is not surprising therefore to find little discussion in the journals about matters such as child care and maternity leave. These were not however the concerns of any trade union at the time, and the union movement remained very much a 'man's world', as the NSWNA secretary found:

> [My predecessor]—*his* concern was that I wouldn't be able to go into the pub and have a beer with members of the [hospital] board. Well, that was about the easiest thing that I could think of to overcome! [MH/89]

The impact of the women's movement began a slow process of change. In the 1970s the Trade Union Women's Conferences drew attention to the demands of women workers. Male unionists realised that women were a potential source of membership since they were a growing proportion of the workforce, and in 1977 the Australian Council of Trade Unions (ACTU) adopted the Working Women's Charter (Doran 1989).

The nursing unions' female composition may also explain why other unions did not always take them seriously. During a 1975 pay dispute in Victoria, for example, the HEF acting secretary claimed that the RANF and its Industrial Officer, Geoff McDonald, were 'unfortunately treated as a joke' in industrial affairs (The *Age* 29 March 1975). And even senior RANF members exhibited the supposedly 'feminine' trait of excessive modesty, a former WA councillor thought:

> Nurses undervalue themselves, which from a union point of view is stupid. For a long time [federal] RANF had meetings at weekends. To travel from WA [to Melbourne] by plane you would arrive buggered, so we changed to travel first class. That was much better, but they wanted to take that away to be the same as everyone else. I said 'Look, I'm likely to be sitting next to [WA Senator] Fred Chaney on the way over, and I can beat him up'. [DW/89]

Equal pay—half way

During the 20 years of post war economic boom in Australia unions had gained considerable improvements in pay and working conditions. But economic expansion stimulated widespread expectations of an affluent style of living amid a plethora of consumer goods. This contributed to the rising proportion of married women in the workforce: from 13% in 1954 to 35% in 1970, at least partly brought about by the perceived need for additional family income (Hudson 1974). The changing character of the workforce was reflected also in nursing: in 1978 the Nursing Personnel Survey found that of 62 548 responding RNs who were in the nursing workforce, 95% were female and 63% were married; the proportions for the 14 584 SENs were similar (1979 vol. I: viii, ix). The sex composition of nursing had not changed in ten years but the marital status of working nurses had. The revolution in the workplace coincided with the second wave of the women's movement and encouraged some progress towards equal pay.

The pronounced labour force segregation in Australia handicaps women because they are concentrated in a small range of occupations and industries which are female dominated and characterised by low pay and a higher than usual proportion of part time workers. In the professional and technical segment of the workforce, women are overwhelmingly located in a few occupations: one-third are teachers and over one-third are nurses. The high proportion of women employees who work in predominantly female occupations has changed little over time: from 84% in 1911 to 82% in 1971, and is likely to remain high in the future (Whitfield 1987; Deery & Plowman 1991:479-83). Similarly, in Britain most occupations are dominated by one or other sex, 'feminised' occupations tend to rank lower than male dominated, and gender has implications in all occupations for social status and for income (Murgatroyd 1982).

As in many other cases of improvements to working conditions, state industrial tribunals, particularly in states with Labor Governments, took the lead in deciding on equal pay for women (from 1958) and the federal Arbitration Commission had to follow. In 1969 R. J. Hawke put the unions' case, pointing out that the early discriminatory rates had been based on 'the assumption that working women were mainly young single girls filling in time until Prince Charming arrived' (exactly the assumption made about junior nurses) whereas now many working women were married. The employers opposed the change. The commission, while rejecting the unions' claim for complete equalisation, accepted the principle of equal pay for equal work, but (in principle 9) specifically excluded cases 'where the work in question is essentially or usually performed by females...' (Encel et al 1974:161-2, Deery & Plowman 1991:126, 367). Rosalind Denny of the RANF WA branch explained the decision, quoting a union official: 'What has happened is that the discrimination that fixed wages on sex has been removed. Instead we have a new discrimination based on what is traditionally women's work' (*Journal of the West Australian Nurses* 1969 October:13).

Nearer to equal

The decision was of little help to nurses, or indeed to most female workers, since it preserved the idea of women's work being of lesser value than work performed by men. As long as the notorious '9th principle' remained nurses were unlikely to receive equal pay (*ANJ* 1969 October:211). In 1971 Hawke, now ACTU President, pointed out that with the 9th principle nurses and other female workers such as typists could not receive equal pay. The 1972 Equal Pay Case then led to the adoption of the new principle of equal pay for work of equal value: that is 'the fixation of award rates by consideration of the work performed irrespective of the sex of the worker', and made provision for comparisons of value between work performed mostly by women and male award classifications which had some affinity (Encel et al 1974:163; Deery & Plowman 1991:368-9). This case brought women a 'substantial rise in female relative pay' (Whitfield 1987). The NSWNA welcomed the change, though it had already achieved 95% of the male nurse rate for female nurses.

The setting up of offices for equal opportunity was a further initiative designed for women and other disadvantaged groups. In South Australia, for example, the Commissioner for Equal Opportunity investigated a case where a nurse was dismissed because she was pregnant, and the hospital subsequently reinstated her (*ANJ* 1979 March:62). Discrimination worked both ways, as the Victorian industrial officer found when she inquired in 1979 about accommodation for male nurses in hospitals. At the time the supply of accommodation was exceeding the demand as more nurses 'lived out', yet a significant minority of hospitals offered no accommodation for men, with one commenting that it had done so in the past but this had caused 'too much trouble' (*ANJ* 1979 June:68).

Treading the tightrope

The RANF was always concerned to maintain its professional and educational interests, and to demonstrate to its members that it was dedicated to doing so. New South Wales nurses, an ANJ editorial said approvingly, had just been awarded increases of up to 35%, the 'highest on record in any state', and they had achieved this 'without compromising their professional code' (*ANJ* 1974 July:5). In the same year the WA branch Industrial Officer, Mick Jahn, looked back over the previous few years and assured members that 'we have advanced industrially without any undue harm to the professional image' (*ANJ* 1974 August:42). There were industrial advances, but members had to be reassured that they had kept their professionalism intact.

It had been only in 1969 that federal rules were registered which incorporated both industrial and professional objectives, and when the newly unified RANF began to publish its journal in 1971 the federal secretary commented that the past split between professional and industrial activities embodied in the previous dual RANF/ANFES structure 'was always an artificial one, for so often they are inseparable' (*ANJ* 1971 August:11). Since 1969 the RANF had advanced in both spheres, she considered, thus 'demonstrating the compatibility of the two' (Patten 1979). This integration of the two major functions was also an NSWNA tenet: on her return from the 1973 ICN conference in Mexico, the secretary reported that her travel experiences had confirmed her conviction that 'the professional organisation without industrial involvement is doomed', and later she reiterated this position (*The Lamp* 1973 July:3; 1975 July:3). Not all nurses agreed, as a former RANF federal president found:

> They used to say to me 'You look after the industrial and I'll look after the professional side'. I said 'Don't be stupid...because everything on the industrial side reverberates on the professional side, and vice versa'. [DW/89]

The unions could not satisfy all members at all times, because the demands of professional as against industrial interests are not evenly distributed over time. A WA nurse now in the federal ANF office explains:

> ...there ought to be a balance between them, I agree, but I think it may be that the balance is not necessarily at the same time but at different times. I think that if we analysed it out [over time] we would find that there was a balance...[MV/88]

The RANF's Federal Industrial Officer, Jack Wilson, quoted the view of other unions that nursing was 'riding a tightrope' between its professional and industrial interests (*ANJ* 1977 May:20). In the 1970s the unions were balancing on the tightrope with growing surefootedness.

If industrial issues were becoming more prominent, officers of both unions were far from seeing themselves as leaders of a working class occupation. An ANJ editorial rejected the Commonwealth Public Service Board's classification of nurses in the fourth division of the public service together with ship stewards and forklift drivers (*ANJ* 1973 June:4) and as the Canberra case showed, they did not want to be ranked with fitters. Nurses probably saw themselves as what at the time were called 'reluctant militants': like airline pilots, who also regarded themselves as professionals, they 'were adopting working class means in pursuit of a distinctly middle class objective' (Roberts et al 1977). The growth of unionism among non-manual workers like nurses could signify a decline in the traditional view that trade unionism is characteristic of an underprivileged or working class part of the population. Alternatively, it could be evidence of the emergence of 'a broader and ultimately more powerful "working class"' (Rawson 1986b:4). In Marxist terms, middle class groups like nurses are proletarianised through discovering their true position as workers in capitalist productive relations. If so, then this might partly explain the greater openness of the RANF to state enrolled nurses (SENs).

The RANF moved in 1973 to admit nursing aides/SENs to full membership, with only one branch objecting. At the end of the year the ICN had admitted the second level nurse, but left it up to individual countries to decide their own policy. The following year the federal RANF, over the objections of the HEF, was granted coverage of SENs in repatriation hospitals in four states and in the Northern Territory (*ANJ* 1974 June:16). South Australia gained the 'undisputed right' to admit SENs as members in 1975, something it had been trying to do since the early 1960s (*ANJ* 1975 August: 43-4). The federal Public Service Arbitrator's decision in a work value case for SENs in 1976 (presented by the RANF jointly with the HEF) had the effect of recognising 'an undeniable shift in emphasis' in the use of the aide, making her 'a more integral unit' within the nursing care team (*ANJ* 1977 December-January:18). Even the Victorian branch accepted the aides in 1974 and later set up a Nursing Aide Special Interest Group (*UNA* 1976 July-August:28). There was an element in this of making up for past neglect in addition to the attraction of greater numbers. The NSWNA secretary comments:

> For many years...the RANF consistently, by way of policy and by way of attitudes, more or less distanced themselves from enrolled nurses and enrolled nurse education. They essentially took the view that there was really only one sort of nurse in this country and that was the registered nurse; and that was all they were interested in. So...for all practical purposes [RANF] abandoned the enrolled nurse by way of industrial coverage. And the other unions naturally of course came along and picked them up. [PS/90]

The slide into stagflation

If nurses were not yet politically minded, political events affected them. The Whitlam (Labor) federal government, elected in late 1972, suffered the fate unfortunate for a reform government anxious to enlarge health and welfare spending of having to preside over an economy afflicted with rapidly rising inflation combined with growing unemployment (stagflation) and a chorus of wage claims from the unions. The new instability of the international economy, especially in early 1974 when the price of oil more than doubled, sent the Australian economy quickly into recession. This was immediately followed by a wages explosion as the inflation rate accelerated, stimulated by rising taxes (the notorious bracket creep), so that wage earners' purchasing power actually declined (Sexton 1979:272-7; Crowley 1986:98-104). Over six million working days were lost in 1974 through industrial action, the highest ever recorded, with wages the major issue (Rawson 1986b:98). The Arbitration Commission's loss of control of wage fixation since 1967 had reached the point where unions were operating outside the arbitration system and wages were out of control. Finally in 1975 the commission introduced wage indexation: it would adjust wages in line with movements in the CPI but wage rises from other sources had to be kept to a minimum or the system would not work. Indexation allowed however for exceptions such as 'catch ups', changes in work value, and anomalies. It became the major source of wage movements until 1981 and thus achieved some stability (Hill et al 1982:157-8, Dabscheck 1989:28-30).

Nurses and their organisations were inevitably part of this inflation induced surge of agitation. Mary Patten told members of the SA branch that the RANF considered it a matter of urgency to catch up on wage relativities (*ANJ* 1974 July:44). Staff shortages were still common: Queensland's health system 'tottered' while nurses tried to keep going in understaffed wards (*ANJ* 1974 June:12-13). New South Wales nurses, also facing acute staff shortages, turned out in their thousands at mass meetings in Sydney and Newcastle, and in June 1974 received full equal pay with a new award (*The Lamp* 1974 June:5; July:7, 11, 13). The Victorians began a pay claim in September 1974 but there was still no decision after six months. Enraged by the delay, 4000 nurses stormed up the steps of Parliament House in Melbourne. Once again, the connection was made between low pay and the shortage of staff: a nurse with five years' experience earned less than an air hostess. Finally the Industrial Appeals Court acknowledged relativity between nurses and physiotherapists—much to the dismay of the physios (*The Age* 13 March & 27 June 1975; *ANJ* 1975 July:14-16). Beyond pay dissatisfaction, a New South Wales nurse claimed that staff shortages increased the pressure of work so that it made inroads into off duty time and ultimately exacerbated the shortages: 'Thousands of young single sisters give up work in Public Hospitals, because men are not prepared to sit in their cars outside hospitals, waiting for their beloved to get off...' (*The Lamp* 1974 April:23).

One effect of inflation was a rise in union subscriptions: to $30 a year in the RANF WA branch and in the Northern Territory. By 1976 the NSWNA had to raise its subscription to $40 (in 1969 it had been $6). The secretary tried to calm members' alarm at this 'major jump' by reminding them that during her term of office the association had grown to over 30 000 members (from 14 000 in 1968) while the staff had not even doubled, and that RNs had gained a pay increase of $12 a week during the year (*The Lamp* 1976 September; October; 1977 January). Subscriptions of $40 were similar to those of many unions at the time (Rawson 1978:69), but the nursing unions, particularly in the smaller state RANF branches, faced the difficulties of a relatively low income membership and therefore limited resources. The WA branch (under 6000 members) reported that it had kept its staff costs down to 42% of income, which was at the low end of a comparative cost scale, and Brenda Wilson, secretary of the tiny Northern Territory branch, went 'into orbit' with exasperation when a member wondered if she was getting value for money (*ANJ* 1975 September:39; 1976 December-January:36; May:41).

Wage indexation changed the usual assumption of the RANF that a particular rate of pay would be adjusted in line with wage movements in other states. The Victorian branch Industrial Officer, Carol Fox (always energetic in educating members), pointed out that the only ground for a wage claim outside indexation was a change in 'work value', which was measured by 'changes in the nature of the work, skill and responsibility required, or the conditions under which the work is performed'. The only alternatives for the RANF were to proceed to a full work value case, or accept an unsatisfactory result: after two years of indexation, the 1976-77 wage increase for nurses was 8.4%, less than the CPI rise for the same period (*ANJ* 1978 March:20; 1979 December-January:67). The effects of wage indexation were particularly clear in the case of repatriation nurses in Victoria and WA, who had instituted work bans in 1975 when they realised that their pay (under a federal award) had fallen behind the levels in the states. Having failed to have the existence of an anomaly declared, the RANF had no choice but to mount a full work value case. Significant in this ultimately successful case was the federal Public Service Arbitrator's recognition that the emphasis in the nurse's work had changed from the performance of set tasks to that of independent decision making based on her theoretical knowledge. The federal secretary believed that her industrial officer's expertise and the RANF 'no strike' principle won these cases:

> A lot of the things that happened in the work value cases were from Jack Wilson's skill, [Commission President] Sir John Moore's appreciation of his ability, and of the fact that nurses *wouldn't* go on strike. We actually got mileage out of that...because we got put to the top of the list of work value cases. Mind you...we worked our backsides off! [MP/91]

The results of work value cases are however unpredictable: Tasmanian nurses, for example, did less well than those on a federal award. The state Public Service Board awarded increases which were 'most disappointing', thought RANF branch secretary Enid Gibson, especially since the work value case was the longest ever undertaken in the state (*ANJ* 1976 February:17-18, 43).

The results of wage indexation became still more unsatisfactory: the Fraser (Coalition) Government was anxious to contain wage rises, and in 1976 the Arbitration Commission began a policy of providing only partial indexation, except for the lowest paid (Hill et al 1982:159).

A (technological) man's world

The existence of a highly segregated workforce allows different standards to be applied in evaluating work mostly done by women from those applied to men's work, since work tends to be evaluated in ways which reflect pervasive social and cultural stereotypes (Burton et al 1988:30, 33). Further, technological change in health care has been dominated by organised (male) medicine, which has allowed subordinate workers to perform the more routine production tasks associated with a new technology (Daly & Willis 1988). Nursing unions took a limited interest during the 1960s in the effects of technological change, and it was not until 1975 that the ACTU drew up a formal policy on the subject (Markey 1987).

In nursing the acquisition of skill was seen as part of an educational rather than a labour process. The professional ideology of the leadership was centred on the bedside nurse, but because student nurses (and SENs) did most bedside nursing, the impact of medical technology on their work received attention in the 1960s and 1970s as an argument for improved education, rather than as a case for better pay and conditions. As with other subordinate workers in the health division of labour, medically imposed technological change reinforced nurses' subordination (Daly & Willis 1988), though it also gave them additional skills. Its effects on their work included increased specialisation of nursing functions and the threat of competition from other workers such as technicians (Brewer 1983:18-20, 52-3).

There was also a possible connection between changing technology and nurses' growing industrial militancy. The impact of technology on industrial relations occurs as a result of certain problems encountered by workers, problems familiar to nurses such as: '...faster tempo, lack of control over pace of work, the necessity for constant alertness and close concentration, and the heavy burden of responsibility imposed by awareness of the serious consequences of an error...[and] a considerable increase in shift work and night work...' (Stettner, quoted Deery & Plowman 1991:40). Such elements of working life were clearly affecting nurses by the 1970s. Some, such as a lack of control over the pace of work, and the necessity for shift work, had always been present, but the faster tempo in the hospitals and the greater demands being made on nurses' skills and responsibility were not matched by any increase in their control over their work, or by a commensurate recognition of the authority they needed to fulfil their responsibilities. Forward (1984) thinks that women workers are less well equipped (through their socialisation) than men to adjust to the structural change which accompanies technological innovation. And, she adds, 'women's work' which is mechanised often becomes 'men's work'—operating theatre technicians for example.

One impact of the growing specialisation within nursing which followed these developments in the 1970s was the rise of specialist groups or sections in the RANF. It was clearly in the federation's interest to avoid fragmentation through the creation of outside groups, but the price was a high degree of autonomy for the sections and the right to levy their own subscriptions (*ANJ* 1974 April:45-6). Groups such as occupational health and critical care nurses thus became nationally representative of their specialties and were able to link up with similarly interested bodies outside nursing. Midwives had no national body until 1979 when the federation set up a national association. A number of these groups showed separatist tendencies from time to time, such as the midwives, whose NSW secretary protested against the inclusive use of the RN initials, claiming that most saw themselves as midwives first, not as nurses (*ANJ* 1978 June:16; 1979 June:16; 1981 February:8-9). The SA branch was unique in having a Research Officer, Genevieve Gray, and the first with a nursing research interest group. The NSWNA already had its Crown (psychiatric) and general divisions, and was less affected in the 1970s by the trend to specialist sections.

Where have all the nurses gone?

The World Health Organization and the International Labour Organization reported in 1976 that nurses worldwide were in short supply, overworked and underpaid, blaming this on a persistent but false belief that 'nursing is a matter rather of motherly care than of technical specialisation' (*The Lamp* 1976 May:15-17). In Australia even in the mid 1970s comprehensive and reliable information on the nursing workforce was scarce or non-existent, a casualty of federal devolution to the states (Wood 1990:97-8). By 1978 the Sax Committee had commented on the 'abysmal ignorance' about the total number of nurses in Australia, although a 1975 committee had recommended a survey of nursing personnel as a matter of urgency (Sax 1978:37-8). In 1975 the RANF council endorsed the principle of the 35 hour week, and some branches took steps to facilitate the introduction of shorter working hours but realised that without workforce information the impact could not be forecast. Federal council therefore initiated a detailed analysis of the usage of nursing personnel (*ANJ* 1977 April:14). The federal Hospitals and Health Services Commission set up a Committee on Nursing Personnel Survey chaired by Sister Paulina Pilkington, then Senior Nurse Adviser to the federal Department of Health, who had herself been critical of the 'dearth of studies' investigating nurse staffing needs and projections (*ANJ* 1974 November:10-12). Just at the time when the survey committee was gathering data, the economic recession of the late 1970s caused some unemployment among nurses, the first since the 1930s depression.

A research officer for the Victorian Hospitals' Association examined what was still quaintly called nursing 'manpower' and confirmed a 10% shortfall in the supply of RNs, but commented that a stable workforce was available: nurses with children. Child care was the one significant difference among hospitals in attracting nurses (VHA 1977). This pool of potential labour had been neither recognised nor integrated into the hospitals, and nurse administrators apparently disliked the complicated rostering arrangements required for part time staff (Syme-Townsend 1975:102). There were also proposals to encourage retention of clinical (bedside) nurses, including more automation and labour saving innovations, and, from a Sydney nurse, a recommendation for team nursing (Spencer 1975). In the same year the NSWNA published an account of the US Resource Monitoring System, which had been tried out in three Sydney hospitals with the aim of determining staff requirements for nursing units (Hope 1975). The Nursing Personnel Survey reported relatively high staff turnover in Australian hospitals (1979 vol. 1:201), and both the RANF and the NSWNA showed interest in ideas for promoting job satisfaction and reducing staff turnover.

Not going all the way

The unions were thus aware of staff dissatisfaction but the RANF at least did not connect this with militant action. Talking to student nurses in 1975, Mary Dickenson acknowledged that over the past decade the RANF had become more active in industrial affairs, but it continued nevertheless to be 'ultra-moderate' in its approach, she thought, especially on the question of 'direct action in pursuing industrial objectives' (Dickenson 1976b). An important reason for the RANF's objection to unions like the HEF was its perception that their militancy entailed striking and was therefore inimical to patient care.

Senior RANF members also saw strike action as a threat to nursing partly because they were convinced it would alienate public opinion. The federal secretary made this clear at a time when nurses around the country were agitating for pay rises: RANF members would not leave their patients, she said (in capitals) 'because to do so would be to tear out of the body of nursing its central life-force'. But she warned employers: '...if those responsible choose to ignore us we will not rest until they have paid the price. We have ALL of the people on our side' (*ANJ* 1974 June:8-9). Although striking was an 'inalienable right' of workers, for nurses the withdrawal of their labour 'negates the very thing we say we stand for professionally'. Refusal to use the strike weapon presented 'a formidable challenge to our ingenuity', the secretary added, particularly as the RANF wanted both higher pay and professional recognition for nurses (*ANJ* 1974 September:10). The antipathy to striking rested especially on the belief that it was unprofessional to leave patients. As the then federal secretary sees it:

> I still believe that I couldn't go out on strike in that situation [Victoria 1986]. I simply can't put patients as the meat in the sandwich. That's the be-all and end-all of it. [MP/91]

The NSWNA secretary had more practical reasons in early 1976 for avoiding strike action:

> I said to [members of the state Labor Opposition] that I wouldn't have any trouble organising what you might call a rally—the kids were wanting to put on a show—but...there was no way I could have a successful strike. It would be a fizzer, because half would be for it and half against it, no matter what we were fighting for. But I said we could put on a bit of a show. [MH/89]

The job of a union, says Mary Dickenson (1976b), is to restrict management's 'allowable area of unilateral decision making'. Unions exist so that their ordinary members, who are individually weak, can become stronger through mobilisation. But union power is at least a potential threat to the individually powerful, such as business leaders or politicians (or even directors of nursing). This makes unions controversial and inevitably political because they challenge the existing distribution of power. In Australia unions achieve their aims in the various industrial tribunals and by getting concessions from management through other means, including strikes (Dickenson 1976b; Rawson 1986b:12). These 'other means' the RANF chose to limit. In the US when hospitals became 'big business' managed by skilled administrators, nurses began to find that their usual methods of moral persuasion were inadequate. By not striking they enabled management to use them as strike breakers, and some groups of hospitals even formed cartels to fix their wages. The movement to use collective force which had begun in

1966 culminated in the American Nursing Association removing its 'no strike' pledge. By 1970 US nurses were exhibiting a new militancy, influenced by the gains made by other female workers (Bullough 1971). The British RCN ('for the nicer nurse') has stuck to its 'no strike' rule, though at least one British nurse considers that this restraint has not been rewarded (Salvage 1985:113, 122). Australian nursing in the 1970s seems to have sat somewhere between these two imperial relatives, not as daring as the Americans but less inhibited than the British.

New South Wales for nine dollars

Nursing unions avoided partisan comment on the major political event of late 1975, the dismissal of the Whitlam Labor Government. The RANF federal secretary alluded to the deferral of supply by the Senate which had cut off government advertising in the ANJ, but remained determinedly impartial in hoping that 'political dinosaurs from whatever part of the jungle will go the way of all dinosaurs' (*ANJ* 1975 November:3). The NSWNA published a reminder 'during the present political upheaval' that it was 'NON-POLITICAL' (*The Lamp* 1975 December:9). This disclaimer was difficult to credit the following year when the association's industrial action had unquestionably political effects. New South Wales nurses gained a 'catch up' pay rise of $9 a week at the end of 1975 (*The Lamp* 1976 January:5) but the NSW Health Commission successfully appealed against it. The NSWNA held a mass meeting in Sydney in March 1976 at which nurses decided to impose a number of bans on various duties and to keep a 24-hour vigil outside Parliament House. The then secretary looks back on events:

> [The nurses] marched on Parliament House...the cry was 'What do we want? Nine dollars! When do we want it? NOW!' It rained cats and dogs, and the wharfies 'borrowed' tarpaulins and tied them to the fence at Parliament House, and there [the nurses] stopped...We probably had about 50 there for four days. [MH/89]

Public demonstrations of support for the nurses eventually forced the (Liberal) Premier, Sir Eric Willis, to intervene. Finally a joint Health Commission-NSWNA working party was set up which decided that a work value case could proceed (*The Lamp* 1976 May:3).

Nursing, motherhood or the flag

The case was undertaken by a four person working party (including Heather Johnson and Valda Wiles of the NSWNA) with nine expert witnesses. The 'quote of the year' came from the Health Commission barrister: 'Your Honour, to be against Nurses is to be against Motherhood or the Flag'—gratifying if anachronistic sentiments. These NSWNA activities, combined with those of the Nursing Organisations Representative Committee (NORC) were influential during the state election campaign then under way: the ALP Opposition included a number of undertakings to nurses in the party election platform and the government made an election-eve announcement of education initiatives (*The Lamp* 1976 May:5-9; *ANJ* 1976 May:45; June:48). The final outcome, a flat increase of $12 a week, was disappointing. The secretary was reported to have said that matrons would 'go through the ceiling' since the NSWNA had applied for 25% increases for the senior grades as against 15% for juniors. The RANF WA branch had faced a similar problem in 1975 with a flat increase of 27% which 'drastically affected' the relativities between senior and junior staff (*ANJ* 1976 June:47; 1978 October:62). The salary structure reflected the nursing hierarchy, and the senior ranks were anxious to maintain their relative position.

The agitation on both education and industrial fronts in New South Wales probably contributed to the defeat of the Willis (Liberal) state government and the election of Neville Wran during a dark period in ALP history. The NSWNA secretary was well aware of the political impact of the rally outside Parliament House, but the union's non-partisan principles ruled out public support for the ALP:

> I didn't feel that ethically I could go to nurses and say 'If we put Wran in, we'll get the nine bucks. If we don't, we won't'...I wasn't even able to say that I'd discussed it with Wran...[MH/89]

Like other white collar unions, the RANF and the NSWNA were theoretically non-partisan and neither was affiliated with the ALP. This fitted their desired professional image. Nevertheless, like unions of any shade, they could make life difficult for an incumbent government through industrial action and thus help the opposition. Yet they stopped short of publicly supporting the victory of a particular party, however much they actually contributed to that result. A British nurse thinks the RCN has steered a successful course between the extremes of outright partisanship and a politically neutered quiescence:

> ...affiliating too clearly with either party—that's of course the long term danger: if you say the Labour Party is much more likely to plough money into the health service—they are. You then put all your eggs into that basket, and when the Tories [Conservatives] are in power they're not going to negotiate with you very sympathetically. [JW-B/90]

This is the usual explanation of a non-partisan position, but it is unconvincing: even left wing unions affiliated with Labor have worked with conservative governments. The nursing unions maintained their non-partisan stand at least in part because many nurses were still committed to middle class professional ideals and were therefore reluctant to join fully in what they saw as a working class union movement. In fact the NSWNA leadership was close to the right wing of the state ALP (Neville Wran's faction), while the federal RANF leaned towards some members of the ALP centre left such as Senator Neal Blewett, or Senator John Button of the Victorian independents group which worked in Canberra with the centre left (McManamny 1993).

The nursing organisations did not join the widespread union strike action in July 1976 against the new Fraser (Coalition) Government's changes to the Medibank scheme, changes which in effect began its dismantling in spite of Fraser's election promise to maintain it (Gray 1984). The RANF did however publish a white collar 'peak' council's comments on the Medibank changes and criticised the large reduction in funds for community health (*ANJ* 1976 July: 25-7; August:5, 17). An ANJ editorial was later critical of the 1978 changes to Medibank, the third since its inception, saying that the original scheme despite expected problems had been 'sound and desirable' in offering universal health insurance (*ANJ* 1978 July:5). The NSWNA secretary, outspoken as usual, accused the Fraser Government of having 'mangled' Medibank and also criticised its curtailing of community health programs (*The Lamp* 1978 July:3). The health policy of both unions was clearly closer to the Labor Medibank scheme than to the government's modifications but, as with the 'nine dollar' agitation, this was never translated publicly into partisan support.

'A little yes and a big no'

Nursing unity was further consolidated in 1975 when members of the RVCN voted by a 97% majority to become the RANF (Victorian branch), thus creating 'one professional nursing organisation in Victoria' (*ANJ* 1975 June:40). Then the NSWNA announced that it had 'taken over' the 76-year-old ATNA (which preferred 'amalgamation') after more than ten years of negotiation and legal procedure. This was a major step, said NSWNA Secretary Ronnie Henlen, 'towards the ultimate intention of the New South Wales Nurses Association to amalgamate all nursing bodies in the State' (*The Lamp* 1975 July:3, 7).

The origin of interest in union amalgamation in general has been the belief that there are too many unions in Australia. In 1977 there were 281, but more than half of all unionists belonged to the 16 largest unions. These had over 50 000 members each, like the Australian Teachers' Union which had 125 000 members in 1979. Both the RANF and the NSWNA were two of the 36 largest unions (more than 20 000 members) which together contained 78% of all unionists. The NSWNA was among the minority which operated only in one state.

Relations between the RANF and the NSWNA were cordial in the early 1970s. The small RANF NSW branch, with Patricia Tarlinton from the ATNA as its inaugural secretary, covered only Commonwealth employed nurses so did not encroach on NSWNA territory. An ANJ editorial commended Ronnie Henlen's 'redoubtable battles' for wage justice and described the NSWNA as 'figuratively speaking, a model of virility' (*ANJ*

1974 July:5). In October 1973 there was a 'gruelling two day meeting' of the full RANF council to discuss proposed rule changes to enable the RANF (NSW branch) to amalgamate with the NSWNA. A meeting in October 1975 produced a 'heads of agreement' document. The association in December 1975 sent its own harmonisation document (which had been discussed with the RANF at the October meeting) to RANF branch councils in an effort to enlist their support. Further negotiations were held up by the NSWNA's industrial action in March 1976 but the RANF agreed to a special council meeting in May. After 'intense and long' discussions a revised 'heads of agreement' was drawn up and the RANF was to let the NSWNA know by 20 May the result of its branch votes on the document. Members of the RANF federal council had made a commendable effort, the secretary thought, to look beyond their immediate interests:

> The New South Wales Nurses Association put up a whole lot of conditions that our council had to accept. Olive Anstey [President] and I decided that we would recommend [the document] to our council...[the council] actually agreed to it, with lots of misgivings...They were very courageous in doing that because they didn't like it, but they really tried hard to look into the future for the benefit of nursing...[MP/91]

All RANF branch councils in fact voted in favour of the agreement. Members considered the terms 'fair and reasonable', and thought that the harmonisation would benefit Australian nursing. Then the NSWNA (whose members were not asked to vote) pre-empted this result by informing the RANF on 11 May that the proposals were unacceptable.

It is clear from the accounts of both unions that the major 'heads of disagreement' were in the end much the same as they had been in 1973: voting rights and money. The 16-member RANF Federal Council wanted to keep its Senate style voting method of two votes for each state or territory, with proportional voting limited to matters of finance and the constitution. But this would have deprived the NSWNA of the major say it obviously expected within the federation, based on its large membership. The RANF argued that even the limited proportional vote would give New South Wales financial control. Further, 'it was considered that any attempt at outright domination by any one state had to be resisted *particularly* in New South Wales' (*ANJ* 1977 August:8 emphasis in original). From the RANF point of view, the association appeared to want a power of veto and to be demanding rules of such detail as to rule out any future flexibility. On the NSWNA side, its officers were trying to establish what they saw as a reasonable *quid pro quo* at the start of negotiations and to guarantee that the association would not lose its initial advantages. On finances, the association wanted a ceiling of $100 000 on capitation fees, but the federation preferred a ceiling for each branch of 38% of total capitation, to guarantee enough federal funding (*ANJ* 1976 May:8; June:7-12; 1977 August: 6-10; *The Lamp* 1977 April:20-1). A WA branch councillor of the time sums up one view:

...New South Wales were greedy and they wanted to come in and take over the organisation...[Other states] were certainly aware that New South Wales could take over and they would lose their identity...New South Wales didn't want to lose their identity either and I could understand that...[and] Ronnie Henlen was seen as a strong character. [DW/89]

NSWNA officers obviously concluded that the benefits of harmonisation would not make up for the loss of independence. Trying to get the support of RANF branches can only have been intended to attract Victoria in particular, which stood to gain most from a proportional system of voting—a system which would hardly have appealed to the smaller branches.

Table 5.1 Nursing union membership 1976 and allocation of federal council votes to each branch under the proposed proportional system

	Membership *	PR Branch vote
Vic	11234	7
WA	7283	5
Qld	6634	5
SA	2287	3
Tas	1247	2
ACT	877	2
NT	439	2
NSW	1200	-
RANF Total	**32941**	**26**
NSWNA	**30000** (approx.)	**15**
Total	**63000** (approx.)	**41**

* RANF figures based on RNs and students only—capitation to the federal body not being paid on other categories (*ANJ* 1976 November:40, 1977 November:63)

As Table 5.1 shows, proportional voting would have put the premier state in a dominant position, but one which could have been challenged by Victoria with the help of two or three other states. The then federal secretary thinks that the negotiating process ultimately had an impact:

...it really did change the face of RANF, because it also then got RANF going down the track of proportional voting...And the Victorians said they wanted it that way, because that gave them greater power...[MP/91]

The Victorian branch had voted in 1976 for the limited proportional system, but full proportional voting was less attractive if its ancient rival had a weightier presence at the same council table. The Victorians had not lost their fear of the giant next door: 'They were always getting up in the morning and saying "What's New South Wales doing today?"' (Heath 1993).

The NSWNA later alleged that disagreement about election of the federal secretary by the whole membership had started the breakdown of negotiations. Although the RANF Federal Council would have agreed to this NSWNA demand, the then federal secretary had reservations about direct election for her position. As she argues:

How could you possibly have a sensible, informed electorate to vote for a federal secretary Australia wide? It didn't make sense. The other thing that

> was obvious was that once you went to that, you were really into party politics, not just power politics, because you'd start getting factions and tickets, and outside organisations interested in funding for their own purposes, because of political issues...I just didn't see that as the way to go. [MP/91]

This view marks a major difference between the two unions, with the RANF at this time still clearly in the 'professional' camp and claiming a distaste for party political factions, as against the more pragmatic and 'industrial' NSWNA which the RANF feared might push nursing irrevocably into active unionism. The differing political allegiances of the two unions (above) further widened the gulf between them.

The breakdown of this first attempt at harmonisation was a loss to both unions. The NSWNA would have gained the national platform that its size and political capacity warranted, and its loss of authority in the early 1980s might have been mitigated by the checks and balances of a national forum. The RANF lost not only a numerical and financial resource, but also the support of a nursing leader, the redoubtable NSWNA secretary, who had a sharp appreciation of political power:

> I figured you had to put government into a difficult position, [get them] by the jock-strap, so to speak...You'd find it hard to believe that [at a conference in the early 1970s] one girl stood up—and this was after we'd talked a lot about what was going on. She said 'Oh now, don't let's upset the government, because we seem to have them on our side at the moment'. I said 'Well really, if you *don't* upset the government you won't get anywhere'. [MH/89]

Relations between the two unions deteriorated after the negotiations ended. The RANF (NSW Branch) moved its office to the NSW College of Nursing, as it was 'no longer appropriate' (and probably embarrassing) to share with the NSWNA. The branch Secretary, Katrina Zepps, a local David facing up to the NSWNA Goliath, had to repudiate several accusations of misrepresentation from the association over the next year, including Henlen's warning that NSW nurses should not 'fall for the thimble and pea trick' of the RANF claiming (she alleged) that it could represent them. In August 1977 the NSWNA withdrew from the Nursing Organisations Representative Committee (NORC). Henlen apparently blamed this decision on the absence of harmonisation which she affirmed as the association's long term goal, and in 1979 the NSWNA sought federal registration and tried to set up a rival national organisation. The attractions of a national platform still beckoned, but the provisions of the federal and NSW Arbitration Acts prevent similar attempts at dual registration (*ANJ* 1976 October:43; 1977 April-November; 1979 September:67-68; *The Lamp* 1977 February-September; 1979 July:3; Plowman & Spooner 1989).

A more amicable note was struck in 1978 when the NSW College of Nursing affiliated with the College of Nursing, Australia, nearly 30 years after the initial NSW-Victoria rift (Ch. 1). The two had worked in harmony for some years, including their joint commitment to the 'goals in nursing education'. The NSW College became the NSW state committee of the now national College of Nursing, Australia, with Betty Lyons, former President of the NSW College, chairing the state committee. A New South Wales nurse reflects on the past rivalry:

> They've done different things of equal importance, apart from working together...I think they'd been gradually coming to the idea that it's really absurd for the River Murray to go on dividing us...For all their divisions, when the [nursing] organisations have pulled together, the federal organisations and the NSW College of Nursing, which is often in there, a lot has been achieved...[RP/89]

For the moment anyway, the Murray was in full flood between the nursing unions.

A more accommodating suitor

The RANF could look back at its first years as a unified body with some satisfaction. The federation had expanded rapidly and it had gained recognition 'by nurses, governments, other organisations and statutory authorities', though it was still threatened by other unions 'which often recognise the potential power and influence of nurses acting collectively more readily than many nurses themselves' (*ANJ* 1977 April:16; 1978 May:12).

The rise of white collar unions like the RANF and the NSWNA has transformed the composition of the ACTU: between 1979 and 1985 it absorbed three major public sector union associations, starting with the Australian Council of Salaried and Professional Associations (ACSPA). It did so with surprisingly little fuss, considering that these associations had remained aloof for years. A major reason for this sudden rush into the arms of the ACTU was the trend towards centralised wage fixing, and the position of the ACTU as the mouthpiece of the unions. In spite of this, however, these white collar unions have not taken the next step of affiliating with the ALP, although the ACTU does not hide its preference for a federal Labor Government. The industrial interests of public sector employees, their pay, conditions and possible promotion, have become a party political issue: both major parties now favour a smaller public sector, but the Coalition's preferred reduction in size is usually more stringent than that of the ALP. Public sector unions in fact have 'a prima facie case for preferring Labor governments, however much they may later be disappointed in their actions' (Dickenson & Rawson 1985; Rawson 1986a; 1986b:10, 20-3, 65).

The RANF had to decide in 1977, the 50th birthday of the ACTU, whether it wished to remain with ACSPA which had decided on ACTU affiliation, to stand alone, or to affiliate with the ACTU in its own right. Among the benefits of direct affiliation, the federation cited government recognition of the ACTU irrespective of the party in power, so that the RANF would be recognised as speaking for nursing; the congruence of the broad aims of the RANF with those of the ACTU, especially the aims of establishing equitable standards of living for members and maintaining full employment; and affiliation through the ACTU with the International Labour Organization (ILO). Federal council stipulated that it would proceed only if at least one branch agreed to affiliate with its state Trades and Labour Council (TLC), and if at least five (out of eight) branches were in favour of federal affiliation with the ACTU.

The question of affiliation became contentious in a number of states. In WA members insisted on a referendum and voted 'no' (Hobbs 1980:179). Two Victorian nurses felt 'dismay' at the idea of associating 'with the ACTU, anarchism, power grabbing or any other...forms of people domination' (*ANJ* 1977 October:4-5). Branches which decided against affiliation had three queries: the ACTU attitude to the RANF 'no strike' clause; the question of funds going to a political party (the ALP); and the ability to disaffiliate. Federal council later told the branches that the ACTU President, Bob Hawke, had assured the RANF that affiliates were autonomous 'professionally, industrially or politically' (*ANJ* 1978 June:20). The Victorian Branch Council also noted the 'drift' towards professional organisations affiliating with the Victorian Trades Hall Council (VTHC), which it stressed was not affiliated with any political party (*ANJ* 1978 May:84).

By the 1978 federal council meeting the ACT branch had affiliated with its local TLC and the Victorian branch had decided to do the same with the VTHC, so the RANF moved to leave ACSPA and to seek affiliation with the ACTU. This was achieved on 4 July 1978 for its 37 500 members (Harte 1978). The affiliation expanded the arch between the federation's twin pillars of professionalism and unionism by adding the 'industrial' ILO on one side to counterpoise the 'professional' ICN on the other.

NSWNA members were also asked to vote on joining the ACTU. To persuade them, Ronnie Henlen used her old rival, pointing out that the RANF had already affiliated, and therefore 'it is vital that the Association accept this move, in order to be in a position to influence Federal policy decisions'. The secretary realised that some members would be alarmed, seeing this as a move to the left:

> I felt...that we should have been...involved with the Trades and Labour Council. There was no reason why we couldn't remain a right wing union—that was OK. We were members of ACSPA at that stage...at the same time they were working, somewhat behind the scenes, to become a member of the ACTU. And the ACTU—never, absolutely *never!* The feeling in the organisation, and...I suppose in the whole area of nursing, was 'Oh no, not with those communists!' [MH/89]

As in the RANF, the proposal upset some members but the majority voted in favour. Two years later the NSWNA affiliated with the local TLC (*The Lamp* 1978 October:3; 1980 April:37; 1980 July:42). Nurses could now influence the union movement from inside—for example, in the decision of the ACTU Executive to set up an Occupational Health and Safety Unit (Marsh 1980). In turn they were inevitably likely to be influenced by the factionalism of the state Labour Councils.

In joining the ACTU the leadership of both unions moved ahead of at least a section of their membership. Perhaps if ACSPA had not decided to become affiliated the nursing unions would have hesitated to take the first step, but by 1978 a labour movement link which would have seemed revolutionary in 1950 was now almost commonplace.

The end of an act

In the late 1970s nurses and their unions were affected by the federal Coalition Government's budgetary policy, including a 'razor gang' of senior ministers set up to cut government outlays. State governments consequently had to reduce health service spending. The New South Wales government started a program of hospital 'rationalisation' ('beds to the west') and even closed part of the venerable Sydney Hospital. Both the NSWNA and the RANF were disturbed. The RANF Industrial Officer said it was time to 'apply maximum pressure wherever appropriate at every opportunity' to maintain standards in the health service, standards which he believed were threatened by the cost cutting (*ANJ* 1980 December-January:22). Over 1000 New South Wales nurses held a 24 hour strike, the first general strike by nurses in the state—unlike the RANF, the NSWNA was not constrained by a 'no strike' rule. This action forced the Premier to appoint a new chairman to the rationalisation consultative committee (*Sydney Morning Herald* 18 & 19 January 1980). The RANF Victorian Branch Council reported that many members had complained, in what was to become a refrain of the 1980s, that 'work loads were too heavy, insufficient staff were on duty at any one time and patient care was falling below acceptable levels…' (*ANJ* 1980 May:52-3).

The 'goals' campaign had been for the RANF the 'single most important activity' of the 1970s (Patten 1981) but it was clear that industrial affairs would soon become equally demanding. The RANF 1980 annual report referred to 'the complex interlocking process of apparently disparate activities…the two main strands of RANF work—the professional and the industrial'. 'Each year', the report continued, 'the importance of each strand becomes more apparent as does the need for them to run in harmony within an organization capable of dealing with both' (RANF 1980).

By the 1980s the nursing unions had travelled a long way towards becoming a recognised political force and seeing themselves as part of the policy process. The then federal secretary reflects on the decade:

> What we were learning to do in the '70s to influence policy was to look more analytically and more carefully at what data were available. I think we had started to influence policy. But again, a lot of it's how you do it. It's not always easy, and you get trodden on. [MP/91]

In spite of being 'trodden on', the RANF remained active in making submissions on policy, such as its submission to the federal government's 1980-81 Commission of Inquiry into the Efficiency and Administration of Hospitals. RANF officers were later critical of the commission's report for its failure to recommend an extension of community health services, and they opposed one of the consequences of this inquiry, the (Coalition) government's final unmaking of Medibank, and the return to voluntary health insurance and the 'user pays' principle (*ANJ* 1981 March:7-8, 10-14; *The Age* 2 February & 29 August 1981). It is fair to say however that the RANF was still a submerged voice in policy making, largely because it was not until 1980 that it began to use outright political tactics in pursuing the 'goals', and it was later still that the use of industrial strength came to be seen as a source of political power.

Nursing was however becoming more integrated into the union movement, especially as many unions in the 1980s moved towards 'strategic unionism', putting more emphasis on education and research services and in general broadening their interests (Plowman 1989). The RANF noted that its presence in the ACTU had sharpened other unions' appreciation of its dual professional-industrial character (RANF 1980). And as women, nurses had been a significant element in union growth during the 1970s, which raised the proportion of women who were union members to 43% compared to 36% a decade before (Hill et al 1982:99).

There were significant changes on the way for the nursing unions. In 1980 the long terms of office of both Mary Patten at the RANF and of Ronnie Henlen at the NSWNA were coming to a close. Symbolic of a time of transition for the RANF were Patten's resignation as federal secretary in early 1981, and the death in 1983 of Olive Anstey, not long after the end of her term as ICN President. In Victoria Barbara Carson became branch Secretary in 1980, and was to lead the movement for deletion of the 'no strike' rule. A local union leader told a group of Victorian nurses the following year that 'Anyone who does not have the right to strike is a slave' (Cotton 1981). Nurses who would later achieve prominence were already holding positions in the early 1980s, such as Marea Vidovich at the RANF WA Branch, Marilyn Beaumont at the SA Branch, Pam Wright on the Tasmanian Council, and Patricia Staunton at the NSWNA.

In the NSWNA there were internal disputes and a challenge to the leadership. A serious quarrel broke out between Henlen and one of her assistant secretaries and the council asked her to resign to avoid a split in the union. She refused, characteristically defying council to remove her (*Sydney Telegraph* 6 March 1980). Nurses Reform, led by Jenny Haines, later accused Henlen of being out of touch, of financial mismanagement, and of standing in the way of determined action against the Wran Government's hospital closures. The Haines group offered 'a different style of leadership...younger, more energetic and more determined to pursue our claims...' (Margo 1982). Nurses wanted change, Haines believed:

> ...they wanted a union that...if there was trouble, they could go to the union, have some support. I think we did get that message across. We made that very clear in a number of the disputes we handled. We supported that in our paper, in our leaflets—'this is how we are doing it differently for you'. [JHa/89]

For Henlen, it was a bitter ending to what had been a dynamic if not always tranquil reign, especially since the challenger came from the Labor far left. Those who like her had led a 'quiet revolution' in the 1970s (Margo 1982) now found themselves being replaced by a new generation of leaders, younger women who were less likely to be directors of nursing. A future RANF WA branch secretary describes standing for council in 1980 on a change platform:

> [WA Senator] Pat Giles, who's an ex-nurse of course...said, 'Why don't you get involved in the union?'...I said 'I can't, because I'm not a director of nursing...' I thought I was really stepping out of line. But of course once I understood what it was all about, and understood the rules, I thought 'Right!' and I got elected to council, and I had a wonderfully big vote—I had more votes than Olive Anstey, for example! Because people were ready for a change. [PM/90]

The change was rather an accelerating speed in an established direction: towards more active unionism and more concern for the pay and conditions of the clinical (bedside) nurse.

Organised nursing faced the 1980s with a major professional goal, tertiary education, still to be achieved, but with its industrial position consolidated by the experience and growing expertise of the unions, and through the ACTU affiliation. The ideological, federal and political divisions remained. The NSWNA was still more militant in industrial affairs, while the RANF was relatively restrained industrially and more dedicated to professional aims, especially the 'goals' which had pre-occupied the leadership for seven years. The RANF had to maintain its federal balance between national and state demands, always difficult given the domination of the Victorian branch, while federalism confined the NSWNA to one state and deprived it (or helped it deprive itself) of a national platform. And the two unions were aligned with politically opposed factions of the Labor Party, though these alignments shifted in the 1980s with the emergence of leaders from the far left in the two major states. This political change was to turn the RANF more decisively towards industrial activism and to show both unions that they could no longer sit publicly on the political sidelines. By the early 1980s the foundation for these changes had been laid. A former president of the RANF (NSW branch) reflects:

> We came in [in the early 1970s] and were regarded as young Turks, with an 'old guard' who accepted us. We had now reached a stage where we were being perceived by young industrial activists as 'old guard'. It was time to get out. It was obvious it had gone full circle. [JH/89]

REFERENCES

Anon. 1965 What is the ANFES? Australian Nurses' Journal, November:277-278
Bellaby P, Oribabor P 1980 'The history of the present'—contradiction and struggle in nursing. In: Davies C Rewriting nursing history. Croom Helm, London
Bessant J, Bessant B 1991 The growth of a profession: nursing in Victoria 1930s-1980s. La Trobe University Press, Melbourne
Brewer A M 1983 Nurses, nursing and new technology: implications of a dynamic technological environment. Australian Studies in Health Service Administration No 47. School of Health Administration, University of New South Wales, Sydney
Bullough B 1971 The new militancy in nursing. Nursing Forum X (3):273-288
Burton C, Hag R, Thompson G 1988 Women's worth: pay equity and job evaluation in Australia. Australian Government Publishing Service, Canberra
Catterall O R 1971 Improving welfare of nurses. RANF Review, November
Clay T 1987 Nurses: power and politics. Heinemann, London
Committee on Nursing Personnel Survey 1979 Nursing personnel: a national survey. vols I & II Commonwealth Department of Health, Canberra
Cotton G 1981 Strikes. Talk given at Lincoln Institute School of Nursing, 28 September
Crowley F K 1986 Tough times: Australia in the seventies. Heinemann, Melbourne
Dabscheck B 1989 Australian industrial relations in the 1980s. Oxford University Press, Melbourne
Daly J, Willis E 1988 Technological innovation in health care. In: Willis E (ed) Technology and the labour process. Allen & Unwin, Sydney
Davis E M 1987 Roles of Australian unions in industrial relations. In: Ford G W, Hearn J M, Lansbury R D (eds) Australian labour relations: readings, 4th edn. Macmillan, Melbourne, ch. 12
Deery S 1989a Union aims and methods. In: Ford B, Plowman D (eds) Australian unions: an industrial relations perspective, 2nd edn. Macmillan, Melbourne, ch. 3
Deery S 1989b Unions and technological change. In: Ford B, Plowman D (eds) Australian unions: an industrial relations perspective. 2nd edn, Macmillan, Melbourne, ch. 12
Deery S, Plowman D 1991 Australian industrial relations, 3rd edn. McGraw-Hill, Sydney
Dickenson M 1975a Nurses and their unions. The Lamp, April:11-13
Dickenson M 1975b The anatomy of an attitude. Australian Nurses' Journal, July:23-27
Dickenson M 1976a The nursing profession as a pressure group. Australian Journal of Social Issues 11(2):88-98
Dickenson M 1976b RANF and its branches as union organizations. Australian Nurses' Journal, December-January:17-18
Dickenson M, Rawson D W 1985 Trends in public sector unionism. Australian Journal of Public Administration XLIV(2):118-130
Doran J 1989 Unions and women. In: Ford B, Plowman D (eds) Australian unions: an industrial relations perspective, 2nd edn. Macmillan, Melbourne
Durdin J 1991 They became nurses: a history of nursing in South Australia 1836-1980. Allen & Unwin, Sydney
Elliott J E 1969 I challenge all nurses everywhere (ABC radio armchair chat). Australian Nurses' Journal, January: 2-6
Encel S, MacKenzie N, Tebbutt M 1974 Women and society: an Australian study. Cheshire, Melbourne
Forward A 1984 Technological change and women's employment. In: Lansbury R D, Davis E M (eds) Technology, work and industrial relations. Longman Cheshire, Melbourne
Fox C 1978 Union registration and the freedom to choose. Australian Nurses' Journal, December-January:21-22, 26
Fox C 1989 Industrial relations in nursing—Victoria 1982 to 1985. Australian studies in health administration no. 68. University of New South Wales School of Health Administration, Sydney
Giles D 1970 Industrial officer's annual report. Journal of the West Australian Nurses, August:8-10
Grand N K 1971 Nightingalism, employeeism and professional collectivism. Nursing Forum X (3):289-299
Gray G 1984 The termination of Medibank. Politics 19 (2):1-17

Hall V M 1968 Opening address of the federal ANFES meeting, March 1968, given by the president. Australian Nurses' Journal, May:112, 114
Hart L 1965 The Soviet Union. The Lamp, December: 4-5
Harte C 1978 RANF affiliation with ACTU. Australian Nurses' Journal, October: 24-27
Heath J 1993 Personal communication
Hill J, Howard W A, Lansbury R D 1982 Industrial relations: an Australian introduction. Longman Cheshire, Melbourne
Hobbs V 1980 But westward look: nursing in Western Australia 1829-1979. University of Western Australia Press for the Royal Australian Nursing Federation (WA Branch), Perth
Hope M 1975 Nurse utilisation study. The Lamp, December: 14-17, 28
Hudson W J 1974 '1951-72'. In: Crowley F K (ed) A new history of Australia. Heinemann, Melbourne
Jarrett L 1968 Nursing organization. Australian Nurses' Journal, December: 264-270
Jayawardena Y 1965 National Nursing Education Division. UNA Nursing Journal, January:19-21
Jupp J 1982 Party politics: Australia 1966-1981. Allen & Unwin, Sydney
Kalisch B J, Kalisch P A 1976 A discourse on the politics of nursing. In: Hein E C, Nicholson M J 1982 Contemporary leadership behaviour: selected readings. Little, Brown, Boston
Kennedy P 1970 Is nursing a profession? Letter to the Canberra News, 11 June
McDonald G 1971 Nursing—an organization in the professional mould. Australian Nurses' Journal, August:19-21
McDonald G 1975 Industrial relations officer's report. UNA Nursing Journal, March-April
McManamny S 1993 Personal communication
Margo J 1982 The militant voice of nurses finds strength. Sydney Morning Herald, 22 July
Markey R 1987 Technological change, the unions and industrial relations. In: Ford G W, Hearn J M, Lansbury R D (eds) Australian labour relations: readings, 4th edn. Macmillan, Melbourne
Marsh J 1980 ACTU guest speaker. The Lamp, October:11-14
Murgatroyd L 1982 Gender and occupational stratification. The Sociological Review 30(4):574-602
NNED (National Nursing Education Division, RANF) 1967 Wastage of trained nurses in Australia: survey report. NNED and National Florence Nightingale Committee of Australia
Paterson J 1964 ACSPA basic wage newsletters 1 & 2. The Lamp, March:3-4; April:2-3
Patten M E 1976 The role of RANF. Australian Nurses' Journal, June:37-39
Patten M E 1979 The nurse and corporate action. Australian Nurses' Journal, March:43-45
Patten M E 1981 Federal Secretary's Interim Report May-December 1980. Australian Nurses' Journal, March:14-18
Pittman E 1985 Goodbye Florence. Australian Society, February:8-10
Plowman D 1989 Unions and the industrial relations context: an overview. In: Ford B, Plowman D (eds) Australian unions: an industrial relations perspective, 2nd edn. Macmillan, Melbourne
Plowman D Spooner K 1989 Unions in New South Wales. In: Ford B, Plowman D (eds) Australian unions: an industrial relations perspective, 2nd edn. Macmillan, Melbourne
Powell D J 1976 The struggles outside nursing's body politic. Nursing Forum XV(4):341-362
Quinn S 1963 Australian nursing conditions. UNA Nursing Journal, February:53-60
RANF 1980 Annual report May 1979-April 1980. Australian Nurses' Journal, June:7-24
Rawson D W 1978 Unions and unionists in Australia. Allen & Unwin, Sydney
Rawson D W 1986a Public sector unionism and militancy. In: Rawson D W (ed) New developments in public sector management, no. 8. Industrial relations in the public sector. Conference papers and report. ANU Centre for Continuing Education, Canberra
Rawson D W 1986b Unions and unionists in Australia, 2nd edn. Allen & Unwin, Sydney
Roberts K, Cook F G, Clark S C, Semeonoff E 1977 Trade unionism among the white-collar proletariat. In: Hyman R, Price R (eds) 1983 The new working class? white-collar workers and their organizations: a reader. Macmillan, London
Salvage J 1985 The politics of nursing. Heinemann, London
Sax S 1978 Nurse education and training. Report of the committee of inquiry into nurse education and training to the Tertiary Education Commission (Chairman Dr S Sax). AGPS, Canberra

Schultz B 1974 Along the way. Australian Nurses' Journal, October:10-35
Sexton M 1979 Illusions of power: the fate of a reform government. Allen & Unwin, Sydney
Spencer S R 1975 Planning to maximise staff resources. National Hospital and Health Care 1(7) November:24-27
Staniland M 1969 The anatomy of trade unionism today. The Lamp, May:10-13
Steinitz B 1979 Union support is a clear moral duty. Australian Nurses' Journal, October:47-48
Syme C, Townsend L 1975 Report of the Committee of Inquiry into Health Services in Victoria (the Syme-Townsend Report). Health Department, Melbourne
Wells F 1966 New militancy among the white collar workers. The Lamp, March: 6-8
Whitfield K 1987 Disadvantaged groups in the workforce. In: Ford G W, Hearn J M, Lansbury R D (eds) Australian labour relations: readings, 4th edn. Macmillan, Melbourne
Willis E 1988 Introduction. In: Willis E (ed) Technology and the labour process. Allen & Unwin, Sydney
Wood P 1990 Progress through partnership. Commonwealth Government, Department of Community Services and Health, Canberra

6. Organised nursing: conflict and cohesion

The anger overflows: overt militancy in the 1980s

If the 1970s were akin to the 'build up' to the rainy season in Northern Australia, then the 1980s were the 'wet' and all the drama of electrical storm, with brief lulls in one part of the country and outbreaks in another. It was in the 1980s that the four major professional achievements of nursing in Australia came to fruition through political and industrial means. These were the abandonment of non-nursing duties, the transfer of nurse education from hospital schools of nursing to the tertiary education sector (and later the achievement of an undergraduate degree as the first qualification), new pay and career structures, and professional rates. These were achieved in a political and economic period in Australia when national growth was slowing and increases in wages for most sectors of the workforce were held in line with increases in the Consumer Price Index, softened by concessions from a 'social wage', including Medicare, workers compensation reforms and changes in community care. Nursing stood alone in the industrial arena in the extent of its gains, both in comparison to other sectors and to its previous levels of remuneration, in a period when economic rationalism came to be the accepted wisdom (Considine 1992; Muetzelfeldt 1992). This is even more remarkable when it is considered that nursing was, and is, a predominantly female occupation, and one which had previously largely eschewed industrial activity.

The leadership of nursing organisations laid the groundwork in the 1970s for these achievements but the political and industrial activity of the 1980s was very different from the 1970s in style, intensity and scale. If the aims were to be achieved, nursing could no longer rely on a relatively apathetic membership, on a leadership which was distant from its membership, on a fragmented industrial structure, and on the sporadic resolution of issues on a case by case basis. This is by no means to deny the importance of previous gains nor to relegate to history the achievements of individual members of the leadership, many of whom continued to play a crucial role in the 1980s, particularly in relation to education. The strategies and the extent of participation differed and this often relied on a different leadership style. This brought different leaders to the fore and, as in any period of intense change, there were some in nursing who found this difficult to accept as it appeared to deny previous practice and hard fought gains. It meant above all that there was a coming together of professional and industrial issues. The Australian Nursing Federation (ANF) is both a professional and an industrial organisation and at times it has been perceived as giving more emphasis to professional over industrial issues.[1] In the 1980s, there was some unease that industrial issues had come to dominate. In practice, of course, there is no such simple separation, much of what is achieved in the industrial arena aids professional development. 'Industrial' concerns refer to conditions of employment, conditions of work, and salary and appointment levels. 'Professional' is defined as concerned with status based on specialist expertise and educational qualifications.

As the ANF federal president argued, professional and industrial issues are not mutually exclusive and neither should be concentrated on at the expense of the other:

> They are mutually dependent on each other. There are plenty of examples... The desire for so-called career structures in the various states over the past half-dozen years or more has stemmed from a genuine professional desire to be better recognized and rewarded and to give people career opportunities. How is that achieved? It's achieved through industrial processes, and how then has this moved to professional rates of pay for nurses? This arose quite obviously from the professional desire by nurses to have their education transferred to the tertiary sector. That has an obvious industrial outcome. So to suggest that somehow we can have an organisation looking after things professionally and not industrially, to me is nonsense. I think that it has taken nurses as a group many years, unfortunately, to come to the realisation that their professional aspirations are very much linked to industrial processes... They are much more aware now. [PS/90]

While nurses in Australia have been at the forefront of professionalisation through a combined professional and industrial approach, nurses in a number of countries have shown a growing inclination to try to correct their perceived grievances by taking or threatening industrial action. This trend accelerated in the 1980s, with nurses in the United States and Canada going on strike in 1981 and 1982, in Finland in 1983, in Israel in 1986, on three occasions in Norway between 1986 and 1988, in the United Kingdom and France in 1988, and in New Zealand and West Germany in 1989. Even in England, where the major nursing union outlaws strike action, nurses did resort to it in 1988. Much of this industrial action has succeeded in gaining significant pay rises.

The character of nurses' industrial activity is conditioned not only by changes within nursing itself in the drive for professional status and improved pay and conditions of work, it is affected also by the nature of the particular political and industrial relations systems within which nursing organisations operate. In Australia, industrial relations has been characterised by a system of centralisation and statutory arbitration of wages and conditions (although this is beginning to break down in the 1990s with moves towards labour deregulation and enterprise bargaining). The federal political system meant that most nurses, except Commonwealth employees and nurses in the Northern Territory and the ACT, were under state awards. Thus rates of pay and conditions of work differed and still do, between the different states. It meant, also, that changes had to be negotiated in each state separately, resulting in, for example, new pay and career structures being different, and implemented at different times, in the states and territories.

Nurses in Australia, as in the United States and Britain, had been reluctant to pursue overtly industrial action to achieve their aims, seeing it as inimical to their wish for professional status and concentrating instead on advances in nursing education through lobbying government and opposition. Thus although nurses' associations such as the American Nurses' Association, the Royal College of Nursing in Britain and the ANF act on behalf of nurses in industrial relations, they had in the past abjured overt industrial strategies such as work bans or the strike (Salvage 1985). The RANF removed the 'no strike' clause from its rules in 1984 after a national poll of members, with 65.3% in favour. Within a year, this was to prove a highly significant act. In Australia, there is some evidence that the greater willingness of rank and file nurses to take industrial action is linked to the development of militant attitudes (Arch & Graetz 1989; Gardner & McCoppin 1986, 1989) and to the advent of a more radical leadership. There has also been an increasing tendency since the 1970s for white collar public sector workers, many of whom are women, to engage in industrial activity (Martin 1984; Williams 1988). The more intransigent industrial disputes in Australia since the 1960s have involved teachers, public servants and nurses. The salaries and conditions of occupations largely made up of women have in general been below those of equivalent male occupations (Williams 1988; Rimmer 1991).

The construction of nursing for much of its history this century has appeared to be a social construction from outside nursing (Bonawit 1989). If nursing was involved, it was in acquiescing to, and sharing in, the prevailing attitudes and values inherent in this social construction. It did not appear as a collective either to challenge the image or to attempt to transform it. The construction of nursing was in other words according to rules formulated outside nursing which served interests other than those of nurses.

Indeed, the social construction of nursing can be compared to the social construction of the aged. Townsend (1981) argues that the structured dependency of the elderly is a creation of social policy in the twentieth century. For the elderly, social rules legitimated low incomes (pensions), denied rights to self-determination in institutions, supported the acceptance of early retirement, and assumed that recipients of care were predominantly passive (Townsend 1981:93). It is not too difficult to apply this to nurses and nursing. Nursing has evidenced also a structured dependency, notably that of its well documented subordination to the dominant profession of medicine (Freidson 1970, 1974; Willis 1990). As a predominantly female profession it was required to accept definitions of its worth based on a vocationally oriented dedication to service, where rewards were non-material and linked to assumptions about women's work as an extension of their caring role in the home (Gamarnikow 1978; Game & Pringle 1983; Muff 1982; Speedy 1987). The basis for the legitimacy of nursing work had been its vocational nature and its derived status from medical science. These two factors were thought to require obedience and unquestioning attitudes, which were maintained by socialization into the dominant belief system—that of the medical profession. Nurses should be obedient, dedicated, selfless and above all should accept medical and nursing authority. This had been achieved by 'on the job' training in the hospital but more importantly by the 'total institutional' nature of the nexus between hospital school of nursing, nurses' home, hospital, and the hierarchical organisation of nursing authority itself.

Nowhere was this view more apparent than in the legislatures of the Australian states and the federation. The rule makers, while in the actual process of making or changing the rules which governed nursing, frequently made comments in support of this view. For example:

> Although qualifications are necessary...if ever a profession demanded a love for the job and a desire to carry out the duties involved, it is this one (Manning *WAPD* 1968:1643).

> They go on talking glibly about the great academic standards which are necessary to cope with the advanced techniques in nursing today. It is all so much gobbledygook...They could even wear blue stockings when they have passed the examinations. Perhaps there could be a Bachelor of Science Degree for those who want to be an administrator of a hospital with more than 300 patients. But for heaven's sake, let us keep our feet on the ground (Henn *WAPD* 1968:1645).

> As chairman of a major hospital in New South Wales, I know that the best nurse we have is not the lass with the leaving certificate, but the girl with practical home training (Crabree *NSWPD* 1962:204).

'Early retirement' for the majority of nurses was socially accepted as occurring with child bearing and rearing. The rest, unmarried, remained as the exploited members of health care (Law 1980). Although it was socially acceptable for nurses to return to work when their children were older, especially in rural areas, when 'many of these women, who come back into nursing after having raised families of their own, are better nurses because of that experience' (Borthwick *VPD* 1966:2949). This 'early retirement' with a return to work as part time employment, the assumption that nursing was not a career, contributed to the socially constructed dependency of nursing. It was linked directly to the form of training in hospital schools of nursing, to the requirement that nurses should 'live in' and to inhumane and inflexible rostering. But more important, the system was perceived as supplying an inexhaustible supply of inexpensive labour. The 'cornerstone', 'backbone', of the state health systems (too many references to require citation) were paid less than secretaries (Jenkins *VPD* 1964:2461). By 1975 nurses' salaries were being compared adversely with those of kindergarten teachers and even 'charladies' and one opposition member of the Victorian parliament was moved to advise his colleagues to forbear from recommending nursing as a career for their daughters (Holding *VPD* 1975:4628, 6140).

As early as 1964, however, a shortage of nurses was becoming apparent. In Victoria, for example:

> The situation is not yet grave, but it is developing, and, in view of the fact that no predictions have been made no one seems to be taking active steps to attract girls into the profession...or to improve the conditions under which they work, the Government should consider this urgent problem which affects the health of the community (Jenkins *VPD*1964:2462).

Questions in the parliaments of the states on 'the shortage of nursing staff' became more frequent throughout the 1960s, 1970s and 1980s and debate became focussed directly on improvements in conditions which might be required to attract and retain nurses. The medical profession blamed bed closures on the shortage of nurses. As educational qualifications progressively improved, the debate shifted so that the shortage was perceived to be as a result of the transfer of nursing education to colleges of advanced education. This allowed the states, however, to absolve themselves from blame and to pass the buck to the federal level which is responsible for tertiary funding (Ch. 3). A large degree of hypocrisy was involved here as the states were well aware of the costs to themselves of the state run hospital schools of nursing:

> A cost study undertaken by the Nurses Education Board identifies the greater cost efficiency of tertiary education courses. The Commonwealth has endorsed hospital based training, not because it provides better patient care services or because it is educationally preferable or because it is cost effective, but because in this way a cost burden can be transferred to the state [of NSW] (Landa *NSWPD* 1980:1403).

A patriarchal society thus legitimated low incomes, long hours of work, low status, and increasingly inadequate training for the work nurses were expected to perform. The denial of rights to self-determination in institutions requires only a slight shift in interpretation to be applicable to nursing. While not inmates of institutions in the sense that the elderly were, nurses lacked professional autonomy in that they had little legitimate control over the content of their work practices, and were insufficiently represented in policy and decision making at all levels of the organisations in which they worked. There is a paradox here as Staunton cogently points out:

> The nursing profession has had to wage its battle for professional identity with concomitant educational standards against a background of stringent legislative control and regulation. Nurse Registration Acts have been in existence in all States of Australia since earlier this century making provision for educational and registration requirements and disciplinary provisions on the basis of 'professional misconduct'. The paradox is inescapable—on one hand nurses were encountering significant and sustained obstacles in creating their professional identity while on the other, the legislature on behalf of the wider community seemingly had no such compunction (*ANJ* November 1989:9).

Nurses' legislation in all states has undergone changes since original enactment in the 1920s, for example in relation to entry qualifications, to the inclusion of different categories of nurse, or to the provision for male nurses to practice midwifery, but in the 1980s major changes were enacted in the states, providing amongst other things for a majority representation of nurses on the registration boards, and for a nurse to chair the board.

The reluctant militants change the rules

Federalism, the constitutional division of power between the states and territories and the Commonwealth, complicates the rules which govern nursing just as it does all other areas of Australian life. Nurses are aware of this and have learned, especially in the 1980s, that to empower nursing and to have their own construction of nursing recognised, a strong national organisation is mandatory to achieve both professional and industrial gains through the political, legal and industrial systems in Australia (Beaumont 1989; Gardner & McCoppin 1989). Nurses have shown that they are well able to use the rules and this is reflected in a different construction of nursing and nurses in the legislatures in the 1980s from that of the 1950s and 1960s. Figure 6.1 provides an indication of the remarkable increase in the representation of nursing issues in the parliaments.

Like the recipients of care and the providers of that care, nurses had been assumed to be predominantly passive, and indeed were expected to be passive, hence the somewhat aggrieved responses by parliamentarians to nurses' political activity:

> ...angry nurses...are clamouring outside in the rain waiting to see the Minister ...Normally nurses are humane people and take a lot of upsetting (Boyd *NSWPD* 1983:1897).

> Elements in the Nurses Association are attempting to con the people of New South Wales with these outrageous publicity stunts and claims. They should get back to concentrating on what they are paid to do—namely, providing the highest quality of patient care for the sick and ill in our State (Brereton *NSWPD* 1983:2643).

> I tell you Mr Minister, the nurses may not have been terribly militant at one time but, my goodness me, they are getting militant now and you will have a strike on your hands...if things are not done very quickly (Amos *TPD* 1984:189).

> It is important that all members of this House, especially those who have constituents working as nurses or who might return to the profession be cognisant of [nurses'] increasing politicization (Collins *NSWPD* 1987:12263-4).

With this reluctant recognition of nurses as a political force, came a concern from parliamentarians to show that they were aware of changes in the practice of nursing:

> ...The role of nurses has been continually extended to keep pace with the advances of medical science and technology. Increasingly, and particularly in the past 10 years, nurses have assumed responsibility for more complex patient care. New community activities and expectations, the introduction of highly sophisticated medical technology, changing medical practices and higher educational standards have all created a very different environment... (Keneally *SAPD* 1984:2190).

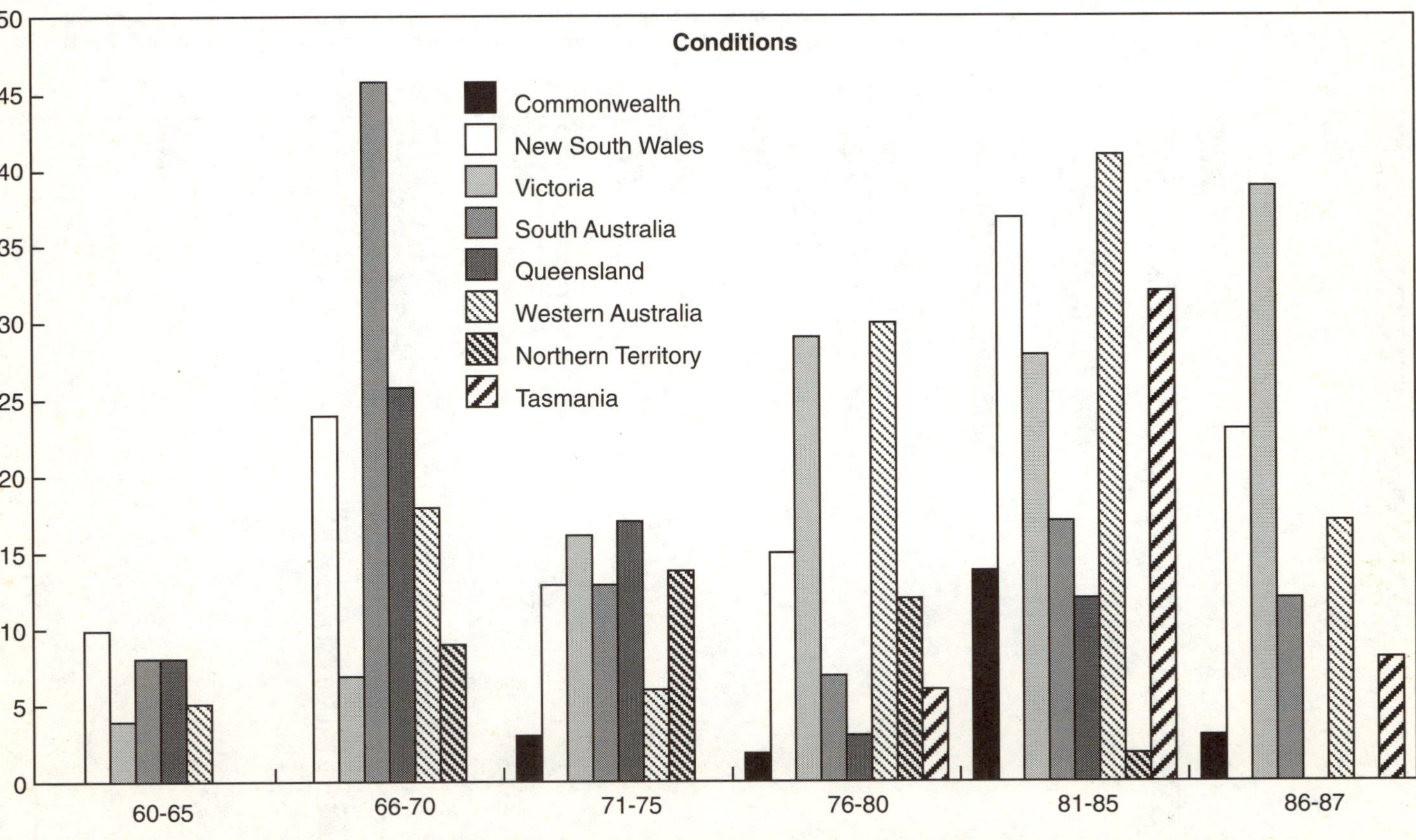

Fig. 6.1(a) Numbers of references in Commonwealth and state parliament between 1960 and 1987 to nursing conditions. Reference indicates each time a nursing issue arose as an item of parliamentary procedure (debates, questions, petitions).

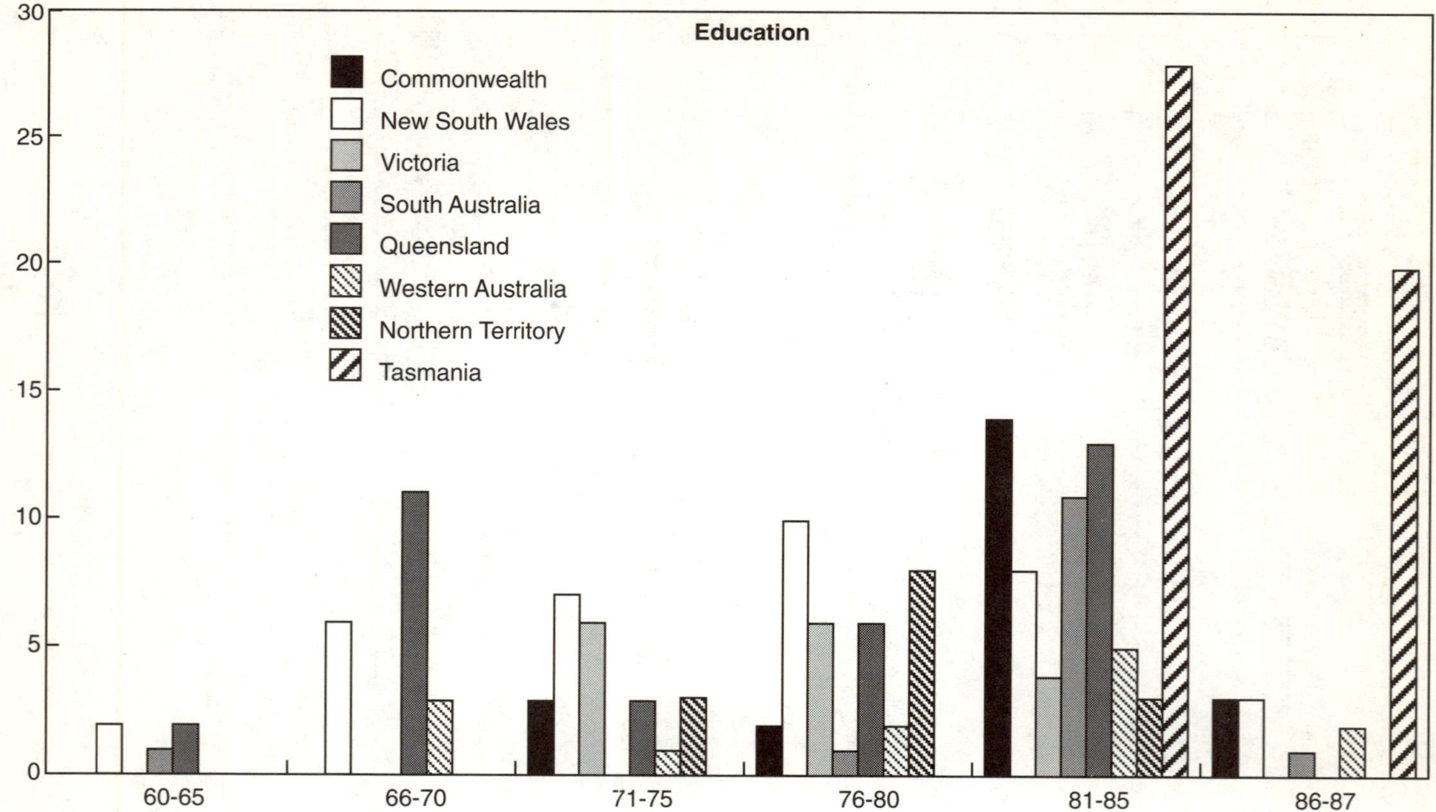

Fig. 6.1(b) Numbers of references in Commonwealth and state parliament between 1960 and 1987 to nursing education. Reference indicates each time a nursing issue arose as an item of parliamentary procedure (debates, questions, petitions).

Nurses are becoming counsellors. Nurses are becoming educators. Nurses are working with doctors and with other health workers, and with patients in the family setting. They are working with a whole human being...The nurses are the safety checks on the inexperienced, overworked, tired and incompetent doctors, but they are not given recognition by doctors in many instances... (Hatton *NSWPD* 1985:8569).

And while traditional values died hard there was acknowledgment of this: 'I am aware that some frown upon the use of the word dedication with regard to nurses, but I have witnessed their absolute dedication...' There was acknowledgment also from the same speaker that nurses were actively constructing a changed definition of nursing: 'They are entitled to be treated by each and every person as equals and as health professionals. They demand and will accept nothing less' (Anderson *NSWPD* 1987:12265).

The social construction of nursing and nurses changed during the decades between 1960 and 1990 and that change came about as a result of nurses themselves collectively changing the rules as to who had the right to make those definitions. While Bonawit (1989) argues that many nurses are reluctant to accept a changed definition of themselves, and that this has implications for the future, the process cannot be reversed. The very real gains made by nurses to the beginning of the 1990s will be consolidated in the next decades. The achievements show remarkable political acuity and persistence in the face of the attitudes outlined, and are even more remarkable given the societal constraints which had created the structured dependency of nursing.

The trend to militant action among nurses has seemed to some observers an especially radical development, since a group of previously submissive workers now appears to be challenging some fundamental tenets of male dominated social structures by trying to gain control over the services they give, rather than being controlled by others, such as doctors and managers (Gavin 1989). The entry of Australian nurses into the industrial arena shows that they have given up their previous stance of hostility towards the union movement (Dickenson 1975:11-12), and union membership has continued to increase (Table 6.1).

In the 1980s the health industry in Australia employed approximately 257 000 health workers who accounted for about 4% of the total workforce.

Table 6.1 ANF membership: State and Territory Branches

	1986	1987	1988	1989	1990	1991	1992
ACT	1380	1486	1513	1466	1421	1513	1476
NSW	2224	2036	2066	31060	31381	32840	35348
NT	867	888	897	891	893	1110	1030
SA	8765	8902	8816	9639	9025	10092	10192
Qld	2067	1976	2002	12050	12058	15534	15747
Tas	3569	3712	3434	3305	3265	3358	3392
Vic	23676	21215	16600	15712	14195	15887	17829
WA	6415	6707	6952	6186	6931	7289	7290
Total	48963	46922	42280	80309	79169	87210	92304

Source: Australian Nursing Federation. Reproduced here by kind permission.

Registered nurses made up the most numerous part of the health sector labour force, making up nearly 54% (Grant & Lapsley 1988). Federal government expenditure on health was approximately 10% of the annual budget, the largest single component after social security, but health costs were maintained at 7.6% of GDP for the decade (Australian Institute of Health 1988).

The Australian health sector had been remarkably cohesive until sporadic outbreaks of nursing discontent in the 1960s and 1970s suggested that nurses were no longer willing to accept low pay, long hours, overwork and inadequate education. Dissatisfaction, however, was expressed in the main by individual nurses simply leaving nursing and going into other employment, contributing to a shortage of nursing staff and increasing the workloads of those who remained. Job satisfaction was reduced as nurses tend to perceive patient care to be the most rewarding aspect of their job and it became impossible to provide even adequate patient care as staff turnover and workloads increased. This is not a phenomenon exclusive to Australia. In England in 1987 nurses 'voting with their feet' had meant that 'even those most emotive of areas—leukemia units, dialysis units, and paediatric intensive care were closing beds and refusing admissions' (Delamothe 1988:25-28).

Nursing is an interdependent activity, the interdependence arising from nurses' co-operation with other health professionals in actions on behalf of the patient or client. Such interdependence can produce conflict when the work of one person affects the work of another. This is exacerbated when there are changing or even opposing beliefs about appropriate technology; when the unequal status, education and expertise of the various occupations lead to conflicting beliefs about the way resources should be used for patient care; and when conditions of scarcity prevail, so that resources are insufficient to meet demands, and allocation to one area deprives another (Pfeffer 1981).

Health care in the latter half of the 20th century has become both more complex and more differentiated, and nursing work has changed as a result. Nursing specialties have developed, often mirroring medical specialities, such as paediatric, geriatric or oncology nursing, or more distinctly nursing specialities, such as stomal therapy and infection control. Changes in technology have led to the development of critical care and intensive care nursing in specialised units. This has affected nurses in the wards, as patients are admitted for shorter periods and require more elaborate care. In short, more patients are more seriously ill, the turnover of admissions and discharges is faster, and pressure on nursing staff is increased. Nurses in Australia had little or no control over the rate of patient admissions and discharges, which is crucial for matching nursing staff to demand. With nursing shortages, high staff turnover, insufficient qualified staff for supervision and the number of 'non-nursing duties' (the clerical and domestic tasks) that nurses were required to perform, even adequate patient care became more difficult.

At the same time, cuts to hospital funding in the 1970s and 1980s by both federal and state governments had affected nursing staff directly by imposing a freeze on staffing levels, and indirectly by hospitals reducing their own budgets for ancillary staff. With resources for health care scarce in general, not every need or even every area can be satisfied. This has tended to mean that medically popular 'high tech' areas have received, nurses believe, disproportionate amounts of funding relative to, for example, community health, casualty or outpatients (Beaumont 1988). Nurses had not been involved at the policy and decision making levels deciding these issues which affected both their work and their beliefs about appropriate patient care.

The frequent changes in health sector policies, funding and programs throughout the decade from 1975-1985, exacerbated by a federal system with both levels recognising the worsening conditions for nurses and the deteriorating conditions of the hospitals but each 'passing the buck' to the other level, created instability in the health sector, thus potentially leading to heightened political activity. There was also the added uncertainty about the transfer of nursing education from hospital schools of nursing to the tertiary sector of education. and whether this would further reduce nursing numbers, at least in the short term.

Whether political action will be taken may depend also on the perceived importance of the issues, and on the relative power of the participants. None of the issues in the disputes discussed below was seen as trivial by nurses. As for relative power, collectively nurses have resources for the exercise of power because of their numbers, which they used effectively by withdrawing their labour, either by placing bans on certain duties or by the use of the strike. They have a further advantage which they only recognised once they had withdrawn their labour—that they are central to the goals of the organisation (Brown & Everill 1987). The essential nature of nursing work had always been recognised but often that recognition led to no more than hollow praise. Status and rewards were not commensurate with the social value of the work performed. It is not only in Australia that nurses' presence has been taken for granted, to the point of their near invisibility (Oakley 1984:24-27). Paradoxically, they had become 'visible' in the workplace by absenting themselves from it.

Neither state and federal governments nor trades and labour councils accepted initially the entry of a previously apolitical occupational group into the political and industrial arena. That nurses and nursing issues had indeed become part of the political system in the 1980s is shown by the marked increase in debates and questions devoted to nursing in state and federal parliaments (Table 6.1 above). The medical profession was similarly concerned that its hegemony was in question. It would have preferred a compliant and unquestioning nursing staff: one which recognised differences of privilege and expertise and the medical profession's self-proclaimed right to make all the important decisions in health care and to take the leadership role in team or committee work in spite of the changes in nursing work and education which had taken place (Australian Medical Association 1985).

Many nurses argued that the disputes were not really about pay but about recognition for their work, though in Western countries worth is usually reflected in rewards. Lansbury (1980) argues that the gap between higher and lower level white collar workers is expanding and that lower level white collar workers have used industrial action to maintain a traditional distance from blue collar workers. Nursing is different. Its work included much which had it been done by men would have been described as blue collar work. Pay and conditions would similarly not have distinguished it from blue collar work; the vocational nature of the work did. Nurses were and are predominantly female (92%) and the segmentation of the workforce by gender means that traditionally women's work is less well paid than men's and has fewer career prospects. Williams (1988) uses the term 'pink collar workers' to describe women who work in occupations which are predominantly female, and where there is a discrepancy between their work and the widely used definitions of blue and white collar work.

The Australian health care system, as suggested above, provided a turbulent environment which increased the likelihood of political action, and the importance of the issues to nurses ensured that their lack of power in relation to the medical profession and their relative lack of experience in industrial relations would not be a bar to the use of direct political action in their attempts to improve wages, conditions and professional status. The protracted disputes were often maintained in the face of punitive government action and of an often hostile media, whose representatives attacked nurses in general as callous and uncaring, and at least two of their leaders were accused of being aggressive and were subjected to gratuitous references to their sexuality. Nurses individually bore heavy personal and financial costs (Gardner & McCoppin 1987:19-34).

Towards militancy: non-nursing duties disputes

The non-nursing duties disputes had their origins in the nursing shortages which reached a crisis in the 1980s. They were, however, much more than a means of shedding a number of tasks so that the total nursing workload could be reduced. In essence, the disputes were about defining the nurse as a professional. Although criticised for defining nursing by what it is *not* rather than by what it *is*, the definition of non-nursing duties was a critical step on the path to professional status achieved by political means. The experience of nursing organisations in Victoria and in the Australian Capital Territory (ACT) are used here as examples of the fight by nurses throughout Australia to shed non-nursing duties. There are three reasons for this decision. First, the non-nursing duties dispute in Victoria in 1984 deserves analysis in that it represented the first sustained industrial action by nurses in Australia. Second, the Australian Capital Territory provides an example of a small number of nurses in the second smallest division in the Australian federal system who were nevertheless willing to take industrial action in pursuit of their aims. Action, which because of the lack of self government in the ACT until May 1989 and its peculiar relationship with the federal level, meant involving not only the ACT health authority but also the federal government.

Third, both disputes were precursors to more direct industrial action: the 28-day strike in the ACT and the 5-day strike in Victoria in 1985, and the 50-day strike in Victoria in 1986.

Victoria sets the industrial pace

Nurses in Victoria had placed bans on selected non-nursing duties in a systematic way in 1982 to support a new wage claim after they had been awarded a 15% increase. State enrolled nurses (SENs) had received a 29% increase bringing their salaries almost to the level of registered nurses. The dispute was resolved with the change of state government from Liberal to Labor and public sector registered nurses received a further 7% increase (Bessant & Bessant 1991:195).

In this instance, and others, the bans on non-nursing work had been a *means* to an end; a strategy to hasten an industrial wage claim. This is consistent with industrial relations strategies in a broad range of occupations where labour is partially withdrawn and work bans are placed on selective duties only, unlike the complete withdrawal of labour when a strike occurs (although skeleton staff may be maintained in some areas). What was different in the 1984 non-nursing duties dispute was that the ban on 22 non-nursing duties was meant to be permanent. The dispute itself was about non-nursing work. Thus it was indeed a strategy to achieve an agreed outcome but it was also, and more important, an aim in itself. It is an example of an industrial action to achieve a professional aim. The professional status of nursing would be enhanced by the removal of duties which were largely clerical or domestic and thus could be performed by other than registered nurses. The precipitating factors in the dispute were the nursing shortages in acute care public hospitals, evident from the 1970s, but which had been exacerbated by federal and state budget cuts. As nursing workloads had increased and conditions worsened, with nurse-patient ratios, which were in any case not reflective of changes in the complexity of nursing practice, rarely adhered to, nurses in increasing numbers left the health system (Gardner & McCoppin 1986). This only increased the pressure on those left behind. The seriousness of the situation was demonstrated by the threat of strike action by the RANF Victorian Branch in December 1983, prior to the deletion of the 'no-strike' clause from the RANF's federal rules in February 1984.

A mass rally of over 2000 Victorian nurses took place on 1 June 1984 and voted that from 11 June all nurses in Victorian hospitals would no longer undertake non-nursing duties. The distress being experienced by nurses was reflected, however, in the number of issues raised and in the tenor of the meeting. Twenty eight resolutions were passed and the issues included: admission and discharge policies, nurse-patient ratios, decision making, nursing education, salaries and career structure, overwork and stress, and supervision of student nurses. Their distress was evident also from two 'phone-ins' conducted by the RANF in May and June.

The state government's attempts to resolve the dispute proved to be inadequate at best and provocative at worst and the dispute lasted for three months from June to August. The government presented a five point proposal on 22 June which included 360 additional support staff to cost $7.2 million, but this was rejected by the RANF because it was too little and the government had failed to recognise that the ban on non-nursing duties was permanent. Negotiations proceeded during July about what constituted non-nursing duties and bans were eased while a working party met to determine these. In August bans were reimposed, and a 24 hour strike was held at the Royal Children's Hospital when it appeared that funds for nursing staff would be diverted to the employment of support staff against the recommendation of the Industrial Commission (RANF *Press Release* 8 August 1984).

Prior to the strike at the Royal Children's Hospital, a three-day strike by RANF members was imposed at the Hamilton Base Hospital in Western Victoria. This was the first strike by nurses after the no-strike clause had been deleted from RANF rules (Fox 1985:28). Fox argues that the dispute was largely concerned with admission and discharge practices by medical personnel which forced nurses to carry out non-nursing duties when patients were admitted as emergencies after hours.

The RANF agreed to settle the non-nursing duties dispute on 16 August when the government offered an additional $7 million for another 340 support staff and agreement was reached on 22 non-nursing duties. The settlement included also an agreement on admission-discharge policies and a commitment to develop a career structure for clinical nurses.

Nursing shortages leading to impossible workloads were the immediate cause of the disputes in both the ACT and Victoria, but the willingness to impose bans, to engage in widespread industrial action, and the number of issues which were raised suggested that nurses were no longer willing to accept conditions imposed on them by others. Issues such as admission and discharge practices over which they had no control but which affected their work, and nurse-patient ratios which failed to reflect the higher dependencies arising from changes in medical practice, were key concerns in demands for a decision making role for nurses. As yet these issues were not clearly articulated, nor perhaps understood by a large majority of the membership, but the results of not being involved in decision making had been *experienced* by all nurses.

From negotiation to confrontation in the ACT

During 1984, a series of lengthy discussions were held between the RANF (ACT Branch) and the Capital Territory Health Commission (CTHC) to transfer non-nursing duties to other health personnel. When implemented, this would achieve two main aims. First, it would alleviate the staff shortages in nursing and, second, it would ensure that the nurse, 'whose primary concern is patient care would not be prevented from providing this care through preoccupation with non-nursing work' (*ANJ* December/January 1985:40). The non-nursing duties submitted to the Health Commission in October 1984 were grouped under eight headings:

- Cleaning and house keeping work
- Courier/messenger duties
- Food services duties
- Clerical duties
- Maintenance of supplies
- Escort duty
- Laundry duties
- Medical duties

The detailed list of duties under these headings which would no longer be performed by registered and enrolled nurses was ratified by a general ACT branch meeting in November and accepted by the CTHC. The discontinued duties, numbering 42, ranged from routine cleaning of sinks and furniture to recording doctors' orders in patients' notes and ensuring resident medical officers kept medication and intravenous fluids orders up to date. Nurses voted to cease non-nursing duties on 4 February 1985. The Commission agreed also not to reduce nursing numbers but to increase support staffing levels.

The RANF branch secretary was understandably pleased with the outcome of the negotiations but her pleasure was shortlived. Nurses in all ACT hospitals and hostels did indeed cease non-nursing duties on 4 February but it was as an industrial action against the Health Commission which had made a last minute decision not to engage the necessary support staff for the effective transfer of non-nursing duties.

The issues of non-nursing duties, nursing shortages and heavy staff workloads remained throughout 1985. A new health department, the Australian Capital Territory Health Authority (ACTHA), replaced the Capital Territory Health Commission but its relationship with nurses deteriorated, culminating in a strike in November 1985. Non-nursing duties, as in Victoria, had proved to be the catalyst for nurses to bring to public attention through industrial means their despair about their continued exploitation.

Strike action in the ACT

Industrial action began on 8 November 1985 with a strike being imposed from 13 November to 6 December. The strike was ostensibly about the need for increased staffing levels to reduce the unbearable workloads imposed on nursing staff by the ACTHA and the federal government, but the dissatisfaction of nurses was much broader than this. It concerned a general lack of job satisfaction arising from poor pay and conditions, and the low staff morale engendered by fewer staff attempting to carry out more complex tasks with the accompanying risks of unsafe patient care. The federal government had acknowledged the staff shortage but had proposed major cuts to health services to balance the ACT budget.

Nurses agreed to return to work when a comprehensive approach to nursing problems in the ACT was offered by the government. These included an independent inquiry consisting of Dr. Sidney Sax from the ANU Research School of Social Sciences and two nurses: a director of nursing from Adelaide and the assistant secretary to the Nursing and Health Services Workforce Branch in the federal Department of Health. The inquiry's terms of reference were to make recommendations to the health minister on matching nursing workloads to the level of nursing staff, and the nursing resources needed to provide health services in 1986/7. In addition to the inquiry, the government undertook to see that rates of pay would be considered by the Conciliation and Arbitration Commission, and a working party of equal management and nursing union representatives would be set up to establish an effective admission and discharge policy. Workload monitoring committees would be established to review staffing levels and workloads, with bans on elective admissions to be put in place if workloads exceeded available staff. Permanent positions would be increased and relief staff employed as required (*ANJ* February 1986:14-15).

But what had happened to non-nursing duties in all of this? ACTHA made an undertaking to finalise the transfer of agreed non-nursing duties. It agreed also to arrange a joint review of nursing to consider among other matters nurse recruitment, a career structure, provision of child care facilities, flexible rosters and continuing education.

It appeared that the RANF (ACT Branch) had had a remarkable victory and that the rational processes put in place would address the ongoing issues, but again, as in Victoria, implementation of recommendations and agreements proved not to match expectations. In relation to the Sax report there was serious concern over implementation of the recommendations for increased nursing numbers in Stage I of the report, and Stage 2 was disappointing in its limitation of staff to current levels (*ANJ* May 1986:22).

1986 and 1987 were taken up with political and industrial activity in pursuit of improved wages and a career structure for ACT, NT and Commonwealth employed nurses beginning with the Comparable Worth Test Case in early 1986. But nurses in the ACT, as in Victoria, had learnt much from the non-nursing duties dispute and the four-week strike over staffing levels:

> RANF ACT Branch has grown into a strong and viable union capable of fighting for, and gaining, the conditions for which we are all striving...We have realized our individual strength as nurses and our mass strength as a united and confident union (*ANJ* February 1986:14-15).

They would need all their strength and commitment in the following two years, but what often fails to come through in descriptions of what are traumatic events is the sheer good humour and fun which nurses found in political activity. In participating in the power structures, and in challenging accepted views of nurses as generally apolitical, they found that not only is 'power O.K.' (Fatin 1983) but it is also fun. This is not in any way to denigrate nurses and how they viewed the seriousness of the issues but it contributed to their inventiveness. For example, when the ACT branch secretary found that the only way she could speak to the ACTU Secretary, Bill Kelty, was to 'kidnap him' at the airport and drive with him to his destination, she did [PP/88]. The delight with which this story was recounted was comparable to a respected director of nursing in Sydney telling how nurses had in December 1985, in order to maintain college education for nurses, chanted 'Neville, Neville' all day outside the NSW Parliament [PN/89]. Neville Wran was ALP Premier at the time and had apparently decided after 12 months to reverse the government's decision on college education which led to 'the four-day war' (Ch. 3). The government did not proceed to reverse its original decision.

Both Victoria and the ACT had had government inquiries into nursing but neither had solved the long term problems. In Victoria, the Committee of Enquiry into Nursing was established in July 1983, that is prior to the dispute. Its terms of reference were, according to Fox (1985), 'encyclopaedic' including 'all aspects of nursing establishments and methods of employment but also: a review of staff levels; work content...organizational structure and decision-making in nursing divisions; causes of nurse shortages...and impact of new technologies and new services'. The enquiry was overtaken by the events of 1984 and in any case did not report until May 1985 (McClelland 1985). In the event, it was not able to prevent further industrial action in Victoria. In the ACT, the Sax inquiry was established as a result of the 4 week strike in 1985 but while its terms of reference were relatively broad (staffing levels, admission and discharge, non-nursing work, rates of pay) its recommendations were limited and implementation of additional nursing staff by the health authority was grudging. But as the secretary of the RANF (ACT branch) said: 'Despite these reactions [of ACTHA], RANF now has a 2 volume independent Report which supports its case' (*ANJ* May 1986:22). In the ACT, local concerns were overtaken by the national ACTU test case to establish the comparable worth of female dominated occupations using Commonwealth employed nurses as the example.

The development of a career structure for clinical nurses with improved pay and a decision-making role became imperative once it was realised that relinquishing non-nursing duties would not solve the problems. While nurses continued to be exploited as vocationally dedicated members of the health workforce without professional or financial recognition, they would continue to leave nursing. Further, the widespread involvement in the industrial sphere in pursuit of their objectives had begun to politicise nurses and had shown them that issues were not individual, nor even located in individual work places, but were common. They had demonstrated that they could be effective in pursuing their aims and that their numbers, as the largest single occupation in the health sector, combined with their indispensability in providing 24 hour care, were a powerful asset.

The increasing militancy of nurses was a gradual process as we have seen, but 1984 had established a precedent in their ability to sustain industrial action: an ability which governments and employers were reluctant to acknowledge. The 1980s as a whole, however, demonstrated that nurses are not the reluctant militants in the white collar labour force but are rather in the vanguard of pink collar workers.

The non-nursing duties disputes in 1984 and 1985 can therefore be seen as mere preludes to what became a decade of unprecedented political action by nurses in all states and territories throughout Australia in pursuit of professional recognition through new pay and career structures.

The discarding of non-nursing duties and the pursuit of new pay and career structures are both issues which are related to professionalisation. In turn they are closely linked to the campaign to transfer nursing education from hospital schools of nursing to the tertiary education sector and to achieve an undergraduate degree, instead of a diploma, as the first qualification for the registered nurse. The prolonged political campaign for tertiary education began in the 1970s and was finally achieved after an in-principle decision on the transfer had been given by the Commonwealth government in September 1984. Degrees for undergraduate nurses took almost another decade and were implemented in 1992. The pursuit of changes in education used political and industrial strategies which often overlapped, as in the non-nursing duties disputes. The campaign for tertiary education itself is discussed in detail in Chapter 3. For this Chapter, it must be seen as complementary political action which contributed to the increasing political awareness and ultimately militancy of Australian nurses. Decades of neglect meant that nursing issues coalesced in the 1980s into a surge of unprecedented action on a number of fronts. In the second half of the decade pay and career structures dominated.

Nurses and the Comparable Worth test case

It is not surprising given the overwhelming predominance of women in nursing work, that nurses' awards were selected by the Australian Council of Trade Unions (ACTU) to pursue a national test case to establish the comparable worth of predominantly female occupations with predominantly male occupations. The national test case opened in November 1985 before the Commonwealth Conciliation and Arbitration Commission to seek a ruling on 'comparable worth'. The ACTU advocate argued that nursing was undervalued because it was a 'traditionally female occupation in which gender had played a part in the valuation of nurses' work' (The *Age* 27 November 1985).

In February 1986, the Commission rejected the notion of comparable worth but reaffirmed the 1972 decision on equal pay for work of equal value, and argued that this principle was still able to be applied in awards where it had not already been implemented. That is, that the existing wage fixing guidelines did not prohibit work value claims. The Commission ruled that nurses were a special case, an anomaly, and could apply separately through the Anomalies Conference of the Commission: 'it appears that all parties acknowledge that a number of special factors may be relevant to a review of nurses' salaries' (quoted *The Lamp* March 1986:9). Under the anomalies principle, the ACTU and the RANF could argue that being a predominantly female industry, nursing 'wage rates had not kept pace with those other employees in predominantly male industries, for work of similar or equal value'. In order to claim that wage rates should be increased under the principle of work value, arguments must be provided showing that there have been changes in the nature of the work, in skills and in responsibilities so that there is a significant addition to work requirements warranting a new classification (Deery & Plowman 1985:313).

Historically, rates of pay for females in Australia had been set at a proportion only of the male rate because they were not considered to be the 'breadwinner'. The proportion had increased incrementally but differences in pay between males and females was still substantial. In 1969 in the Equal Pay Case, the principle of equal pay for equal work had been established but had proved difficult to implement and effectively excluded applications from occupations where the work was largely performed by women but could also be performed by men. Nursing, along with teaching, banking and other predominantly female occupations was therefore unable to secure wage rises on the basis of equal pay for equal work. The subsequent Equal Pay Case in 1972 had gone some way to achieving a reduction in the disparity, or wage differentials, between male and female wages (Ch. 5). The principle of equal pay for work of equal value had been adopted, which meant that award rates were fixed on the basis of comparing the work performed irrespective of sex:

> This requirement made it possible to compare the work value of predominantly female classifications (for example typists) with mixed or predominantly male classifications of related areas of work (for example, clerks and administrative assistants) (Deery & Plowman 1985:311).

The 1986 Comparable Worth test case was rejected because the commission believed it to be confusing in the Australian context and to have been applied differently in different countries. Further, it could be applied to any classification which had been 'improperly valued...with no requirement that the work performed is related or similar' (quoted Deery & Plowman 1991:369).

The ACTU and the RANF successfully argued in March 1986 that the salaries claim for nurses employed by the ACT, NT and Commonwealth should go to the full bench of the Commission in September. The RANF/ACTU detailed the unique role of the nurse and referred to supporting documentation by RANF: *Nursing: a statement* and *Standards for nursing practice* and sought to establish a new national salary rate and a professional career structure for Commonwealth and Territory nurses. In May 1987 the Full Bench handed down its favourable decision, but it was not until the end of 1987 after a concerted political campaign that success could be claimed.

Militancy rewarded: new pay and career structures

While the heading suggests that new pay and career structures were achieved as a result of the increased militancy of nurses, this was not the case, at least not directly, throughout Australia. In New South Wales a decision on a new wages and career structure was handed down in June 1986 by the Industrial Commission of New South Wales without prior industrial action, with the case relying primarily on the principle of changes in work value, that is on the 'nature of the work, level of skill and responsibility involved and conditions under which the work is performed' (Fox 1992:2, 8).

How much are you worth as a nurse in NSW?

In December 1985 a statement from the Premier's Department, suggesting that nurse education should be transferred back to hospital programs to alleviate nurse shortages, had far reaching consequences beyond education. The demonstration and march by nurses immediately following the release of the statement resulted in a meeting of the NSWNA with the Premier, the Minister for Industrial Relations and the Minister for Health and their advisers. The initiatives which resulted contained seven ways of increasing registered and enrolled nursing numbers and the related funding support which would be required. The eighth initiative stated:

> Furthermore in recognition of the need to provide a better deal for nurses, the Government proposes to make a reference to the appropriate Conciliation Committee seeking an early hearing to determine appropriate salaries and working conditions of public hospital nurses in line with the wage fixing principle (quoted *The Lamp* February 1986:8).

The case was referred to the Commission in January 1986. The Assistant General Secretary of the NSWNA, Patricia Staunton, acknowledged 'that the demonstration which occurred on 17 December significantly accelerated plans by the association relating to career structure negotiations and wage increase applications' (*The Lamp* February1986:9). Thus the stage was set by industrial action for a negotiated outcome.

The NSWNA claim used the career structure proposals previously approved by its council, and began preparing evidence to put before the commission from a comprehensive cross-section of registered and enrolled nurses. The aim was to demonstrate that there had been significant changes in the nature and responsibility of work undertaken by nurses since 1981; in other words changes in work value. Inspections of work places were then organized for the senior conciliation commissioner. Over the next six months agreement was reached progressively between the Department of Health and the NSWNA on the career structure classifications and conditions of employment; agreement on salaries, however, was delayed. The day before the case was due to be finalised in June 1986, the Health Department made its offer on salaries.

This proved to be totally unacceptable and was rejected by the assistant general secretary on behalf of the NSWNA. The offer was provided at the same time as the decision in Victoria and was almost identical in rates for registered nurses in the first four years. The offer prompted the assistant general secretary to ask members: 'How much are you worth as a nurse?' (The Lamp July 1986:8).

Negotiations continued on the guidelines for new classifications such as the clinical nurse specialist and nurse unit managers, and the flow on to nurses outside public sector hospitals. These continued for more than a year, but by September 1987 the NSWNA could report that there were only three private sector awards still outside the June 1986 decision (*The Lamp* September 1987:13). Implementation had been achieved through a grading committee, and the association and the Department of Health had established an education program on the new award (and on the 38 hour week).

Rational and comprehensive policy making in South Australia

In South Australia, the development of the career structure was the outcome of five years of research 'based on contemporary management and nursing literature and research, an analysis of the problems identified by nurses and projection of the future needs of the profession' (Silver 1989:228). In what became the prototype for all the other states and territories, except Victoria and New South Wales, the nurses of South Australia had the support of the South Australian government. In December 1985, the Government agreed to a trial and evaluation of the structure after agreeing in principle to the RANF (SA Branch) career structure committees' framework. It also agreed to finance the trial, to take place over seven months and to involve half the state's public sector nursing workforce. The new award was ratified on 16 December 1986, with implementation to occur on 16 July 1987.

This is not to suggest that the RANF (SA Branch) had not had to work hard for the historic decision, nor that it was achieved easily but rather that the South Australian Government participated in what was a rational and comprehensive policy process (Gardner & Barraclough 1992). After the career structure and salary claim had been lodged with the South Australian Health Commission on 3 September 1985, the RANF resolved to make nursing an issue at the forthcoming state election and to launch a public awareness campaign on the problems confronting nurses (*ANJ* November 1985:26-27). It also 'voted unanimously to congratulate and support our Victorian colleagues in the leading role they have adopted in the pursuit of increased remuneration and a career structure for Australian nurses'. Immediately prior to ratification South Australian nurses expressed their disappointment at the government's delays in reaching agreement and showed that industrial action was not out of the question.

Five thousand nurses marched in support of the new career structure and salary claim on 5 November 1986 with placards demanding 'Wage Justice

Now' and 'A New Career Structure Now'. The RANF reported South Australian nurses would 'never be the same again' and that they had:

> now demonstrated to the world at large that they are a large and powerful group, and that although slow to anger they will exercise their power in a responsible and united way for the betterment of nursing and for improved care for their patients (*ANJ* December 1986/January 1987:15).

The flavour of the demonstration however was in stark contrast to the anger being displayed in Victoria, where nurses were engaged in what seemed to be an interminable strike over their new pay and career structure. This is how the RANF described the march in Adelaide:

> There was a feeling of excitement as nurses gathered outside the Royal Adelaide Hospital. Thousands came from both metropolitan and country Government worksites and were joined by their colleagues from the private sector and the psychiatric area...The chanting reached a crescendo as the column, which took over 20 minutes to pass a point, approached the South Australian Health Commission...

The public joined in the enthusiasm and showed support by clapping and cheering:

> Office workers opened their windows and shouted support as the nurses passed by. Reporters and police later indicated that the march and rally was one of the best attended in Adelaide in many years, and they commented on the quality of the organization and the good natured response of nurses who exhibited a wonderful feeling of camaraderie (*ANJ* December 1986/January 1987:15).

The obvious goodwill on all sides must not however detract from the importance of such a march as a political strategy. That the RANF (SA Branch) could demonstrate that nurses were serious about their claim, and more important that the ANF could 'deliver' its own support from a large number of nurses is crucial in influencing governments. A strategy of divide and rule then becomes a no-win option for governments and keeps them on the 'straight and narrow' in future negotiations. As the South Australian RANF branch secretary said:

> I think I could pull nurses out in this state if they try and take those positions [nursing management] away from us...If they [the Government] want to believe that I can blow the whistle out there and get 10 000 people on the street, fine...I fuel it deliberately—regularly. [LS/88]

She was aware also that simply withdrawing labour is only one part of industrial negotiation. It is the public face of industrial relations but for successful solutions more is required from a union leader:

> Withdrawing your labour is the easy bit. The difficult bit is the timing of it, the development of adequate and informed public sympathy, and political sympathy, and then the question of what skills and solutions you will bring to bear on the aftermath. [LS/88]

In December 1986, the South Australian Industrial Commission handed down its decision on the new career structure and associated salaries claims for public sector nurses in South Australia. In relation to general salary increases the decision was justified by the Commission on the grounds that the equal pay principle of 1972 had not been applied to adjust wage rates in the nursing award and that an anomaly had existed. For the rates associated with the new classifications under the career structure, work value salary increases were awarded. Five work levels were identified: registered nurse; clinical nurse; clinical nurse consultant and nurse manager; assistant director of nursing (clinical) and assistant director of nursing (management); and director of nursing. This provided for three career paths for promotion: management, clinical and education. The Industrial Commission argued that:

> The essential nature of the new structure...is to provide an additional career path...and to more clearly identify the roles of nurses at each level of the organisation...so that the 'hands on' clinical nursing duties are clearly separated from such managerial tasks as planning staff allocation and cost control... It is the belief of the parties...that this structure will provide greater job satisfaction, attract qualified nurses back into the profession, overcome staff shortages and provide a higher standard of health care (quoted *ANJ* February 1987:13).

All positions above those of registered nurse were declared vacant and nurses had then to apply for those positions. In the event, this proved to be one of the most traumatic features of the new award. It provided yet another example of the tension between professionalism and unionism and the increased tension inherent in combining both roles in one organisation—the RANF. As the secretary of the RANF (SA Branch) pointed out:

> The profession from a professional perspective said 'If these are all new positions, new job descriptions, and they really are about changing the way that nurses can work, then we should declare all positions open, advertise them and everyone should compete for these positions.'...From a trade union perspective that is culpable—absolutely culpable. A number of trade unions have just looked in disbelief that we ever did it. [LS/88]

In actuality, a very small number of nurses were unsuccessful in obtaining a position comparable to that which they had held in the previous structure, but as the secretary said this does not mean that the adverse effect on those nurses as individuals was not highly traumatic.

As in the other states, negotiations for nurses in the private and other sectors, such as district nursing, to obtain the same award followed immediately, with a successful outcome in February, in spite of Commonwealth government intervention aimed at blocking the award for application in nursing homes.

The conditions in obtaining the new award in South Australia were very different from those being experienced by the RANF in Victoria over largely the same period. Although in South Australia the union and nurses had been willing to expedite their claims through direct industrial action, the process, as in New South Wales, was one of tireless negotiation through the industrial relations system and without the acrimony displayed on all sides in Victoria. The secretary of the RANF (SA Branch) summed it up appropriately:

> Thank you all and in particular Margaret Silver, who was such a competent witness, who appeared to enjoy the challenge, having an answer for everything even after three hours in the witness box. Thank you also to the thousands of nurses involved in the trial whose work in 1986 enabled evidence to be produced to demonstrate that RANF (SA Branch) Career Structure theory works well in practice, and to the thousands of nurses who came out into the streets to attend rallies and meetings which successfully applied the necessary pressure (*ANJ* February 1987:13).

And after the private sector and nursing homes decision the industrial officer concluded that:

> The negotiating and processing of this matter through the South Australian Industrial Commission has been a very complex and difficult task, made even more difficult by the unexpected intervention of the Commonwealth Government... The excellent attendance of members at private sector meetings indicates the increasing depth of professional and industrial awareness and augurs well for the expansion of our membership in the private sector during 1987 (*ANJ* April 1987:15).

The state then began the complex process of implementation. Rather in the way of the cliché that a woman's work is never done, industrial relations issues are only settled to move on to the next. This was particularly so in relation to nursing in the 1980s, when a positive ferment of industrial activity took place across Australia in a concerted campaign to achieve at last wage justice and professional recognition. In a federal system where each state award claim has to be pursued individually through the state industrial commissions, costs are increased, union personnel differs in terms of style and expertise, and the support or opposition from employers and governments varies. The latter does not necessarily depend on party political persuasion as evidenced by the different attitudes to nurses' career structure claims in New South Wales, South Australia and Western Australia on one hand, and in Victoria on the other. The Australian Labor Party governed in all these states.

The leap frog effect in Western Australia

In mid 1986, negotiations on a new salaries and career structure for public hospital nurses began between the RANF (WA Branch), the Health Department and the Industrial Commission and an in principle agreement was reached. The Fremantle Hospital became the first hospital in Western Australia to implement the new award and career structure in July 1987. In October, the annual general meeting of the RANF Industrial Union of Workers, Perth had approved a motion that the deadline for negotiation on the claims to have reached a satisfactory point would be February 1987. A special general meeting was to be called in the second week of February to report on progress and to decide on further action if necessary (*ANJ*

November 1987:21). But for Western Australian nurses obtaining their new award and career structure had not been easy. The campaign might not have involved prolonged strike action as in Victoria but it had required industrial action and lengthy political negotiation and at no time did it appear a fait accompli. The secretary of the ANF (WA Branch), in 1990, explained why she believed that nurses in WA had been successful:

> We have the best career structure in Australia... It's the most advanced. We fought bitterly for that. We won it because the membership wanted it... When it came to the crunch, and we weren't going to get it, we went out to the workplace and explained what it was about...about keeping nurses by the bedside, having a career path by the bedside. They fought tooth and nail. So we got the career structure because of the support from the grass roots of our membership. [PM/90]

The RANF (WA Branch) was also able to gain the support of the media in an effective campaign where the then President, Marea Vidovich, was the sole spokesperson, so that consistent, factual information was provided. During the campaign, a new Minister for Health was appointed which provided the media with the opportunity to demonstrate the strength of the RANF leadership in Western Australia:

> He, poor thing, was swept into office one or two days after the dispute really commenced. There had been a Cabinet reshuffle because we had a new Premier and so he organised his own Cabinet. The 7.30 Report in Perth did a feature on me, because I was the mouthpiece for the federation during the dispute and they had this wonderful picture, a movie taken by the ABC of the Cabinet outside the Governor's residence after they had been sworn in. It began with that music [sings], 'Maria, I've just met a girl named Maria', and the voice over said 'Yesterday he was sworn in as Minister for Health, today, he met a girl called Marea.' So that was all rather facetious but that was how it was. [MV/88]

The secretary was well aware of the need to provide a balance between the industrial and professional aspects of the ANF, and of the inherent reluctance of nurses to approve industrial action. In the case of the career structure (and indeed non-nursing duties):

> That's a professional issue. Sure, we took industrial action for it, and we had probably one of the best-run and most successful campaigns in nursing in this state on that very issue—but was that professional or industrial? [PM/90]

Providing that balance means educating the membership on particular issues and knowing when to draw back from the industrial emphasis to concentrate on the professional side. Had nurses not supported their industrial organisations in pursuit of new salary and career structures it is doubtful if they would have obtained them. The fact that they were able in each of the states and territories to demonstrate that they could 'bring nurses on to the streets', or impose work bans, was effective in encouraging employers, governments and industrial commissions to take their claims seriously. The arguments presented and the obvious deficiencies in nurses' salaries and career paths are of course important, but that these arguments were acted upon lies in the inherent strength of an industrial organisation which can claim that it represents its membership. This is perhaps the greatest achievement of nursing in Australia in the 1980s.

For Western Australian nurses their new salary and career structure meant that they could at last see themselves as leading the other states. They had 'always had to wait and see what happened elsewhere', were 'never up amongst the top states' and then would 'leap frog a bit' but then 'we almost leapt to the top as far as achievements in wages and conditions went' [PM/90]. They were particularly committed to their own career structure which provided for a research stream (see Fig. 4.2). A more subtle difference, because it is not apparent by simply looking at the structure itself but is inherent in its practice, is that at the ward level no one person is in charge:

> In this state we believe that our clinical nurse, or clinical nurses because there are a number of them, are the people who run the ward, because we haven't designated any one as the leader. That is the big difference. [HA/90]

Unfortunately, for Western Australia, this unique structure and corresponding salaries are threatened by the achievement of professional rates and a federal award.

Federalism does not necessarily work against the interests of a particular state or territory, as individual entities; what it does is to encourage differences between them, which then makes a national approach, or uniformity, more difficult to achieve. When uniformity is the goal, state differences have to be sacrificed. Further, although negotiating claims in each state is costly of resources, slow and cumbersome, there is an advantage in that the state governments tend to follow each other more or less quickly in agreeing to similar provisions. In other words, actions in other states are watched carefully by a particular state government or employer, and indeed, more important, by the unions themselves, and this can facilitate negotiation in a particular state. For example, the secretary of Western Australian branch of RANF, was able to present to the Premier and the Minister for Health the spectre of a strike in Western Australia such as that occurring in Victoria over its pay and career structure:

> The first thing [the newly-appointed Minister for Health] said was 'we don't want to go down the same path as Victoria'... 'We don't want a strike'. I said, 'we don't want a strike either, our members don't want to go down the path of Victoria'... That was always a lovely weapon to use... Certainly Western Australian nurses believed that Victorian nurses had done it for everybody...and we had no difficulty at all raising money for the Victorian strike fund... They had stuck their necks out on behalf of members everywhere. [MV/88]

Industrial relations through confrontation in Victoria

1985 began reasonably well for the RANF (Victorian Branch). The non-nursing duties agreement had provided for phased implementation, so that as an allocation of additional support staff was made to a particular health agency nurses would withdraw from non-nursing duties. Apart from resistance by some hospital managers, either to the withdrawal of nurses from non-nursing duties, or to the appropriate reallocation of funds to support staff, implementation had begun relatively smoothly, although there had been some harassment and intimidation of nurses. The Victorian Government had agreed to make a further $1 million available for support staff in 1985, which in addition to the $14 million previously allocated, would allow the employment of a total of approximately 800 support staff (*ANJ* March 1985:15). This allocation later proved to be insufficient.

The Labor Government elected in 1982 faced an election in March 1985, and the RANF (Victorian Branch) organised meetings with the Minister for Health and the Opposition Liberal spokesperson to discuss their health policies. The issues to be raised gave a clear indication that Victorian nurses would continue to pursue improvements in their salaries and conditions:

> Of particular concern to RANF (Victorian Branch) will be the response and election commitments of both parties to the problems currently facing the profession, such as the growing shortage of registered nurses in the hospital system; the dissatisfaction which nurses have expressed in their current roles; *the poor wages and conditions which nurses are required to accept and the lack of a meaningful career structure within the profession* (*ANJ* March 1985:15 (our emphasis)).

The main issue for 1985 became a concern to keep nurses nursing by improving their conditions. The reasons for their continuing exodus were defined by the RANF as 'workloads, lack of salary recognition and career progression, unsatisfactory award conditions, lack of parking and child care facilities, unsatisfactory rosters [and] a lack of involvement in decision making (*ANJ* August 1985:16). Moreover, the government had extended the deadline for the withdrawal from non-nursing duties from June to October 1985, the number and cost of support staff had blown out, and there was a long running demarcation dispute with the Hospital Employees Federation (HEF) about nursing authority over ancillary staff. The non-nursing duties dispute had not succeeded in reducing workloads to acceptable levels, and nurses continued to leave so that by June 1985 the Health Department estimated that there were 900 vacancies for registered nurses in Victoria. The HEF appeared to have gained more from the dispute, with the additional membership of enrolled nurses and other support staff, than the RANF itself.

In September 1985 a mass meeting of nurses at Dallas Brooks Hall led to a campaign of staggered work bans, and the enforcement of admission and discharge policies and award nurse-patient ratios of one RN to 10 patients during the day and one to 15 at night. This was followed almost immediately by a stop work meeting at the Sydney Myer Music Bowl on 11 October. The 5500 nurses at the meeting resolved to go on strike indefinitely from the 17 October in support of their salary and career structure claim which had been placed before the Victorian Industrial Relations Commission. Other issues were admissions and discharges, nurse-patient ratios and agency staff usage. Following the meeting nurses made an impressive sight as they marched to the Health Department in the midst of peak hour traffic.

The first state wide strike in Victoria was in response to the government's offer on 30 September of $21.5m for pay increases. The government's reaction to the campaign was immediate and hostile. Stand-downs were threatened and the nurses were accused of not waiting for their case to be heard by the industrial commission (*The Sun* 10 October 1985). Nevertheless, the government gave an assurance to the RANF that it would issue a directive to hospitals on workloads, and would implement the recommendations of the commission on the salaries and career structure claim. The mass meeting of 4000 nurses on 21 October voted narrowly to return to work the following day and set January 1986 as the deadline for the first instalment of an increase in salaries (Resolutions RANF Mass Meeting 21 October 1985). The commission did not hand down its decision on the new award until 20 June 1986.

The 'Keep Nurses Nursing—Improve Nurses Conditions' campaign was well organised and executed. Although the strike lasted for only five days, it was a clear indication to the government that nurses were prepared to use industrial action in pursuit of their aims. Fox (1991:33) argues that nurses gained nothing from the strike as workloads were secondary to the central issue of wages, and the government could quite correctly argue that it had made an offer and 'it was now appropriate for the tribunal to hear arguments to decide if nurses deserved more than had been offered'. She is critical of the then nursing leadership in Victoria for its handling of the strike and its equivocation at the mass meetings. But more important, Fox (1991:31-33) is critical of the union in its handling of the linkages between increased wages and a new career structure. A more sympathetic treatment is provided by Bessant and Bessant (1991:199-202).

During the non-nursing duties dispute, the government had agreed to establish a career structure working party and a sub-committee of this worked on rewriting the registered nurses award. Fox argues that the January 1985 wages and conditions claim lodged by the RANF had 'displayed a healthy concern with nurses' wages at all levels vis a vis wages of other health sector employees' but that the union had let 'this sound approach slip away some time around May 1985' (Fox 1991:32). One of the reasons may have been that the RANF was too preoccupied negotiating on non-nursing duties and 'lost control of the early direction of the wage/career structure case'. In the event, increased wages became separated from the new career structure, rather than being closely interdependent, so that the career structure was seen as a separate professional issue. The career structure working party reported on 24 October 1985, that is after the five-day strike, and after the government had made its initial wages offer. The government's position had been that the career structure details must be finalised before wages could be considered. This decision was pre-empted by the industrial action. The lack of an agreed award structure, and the ambiguities about classifications in the wages offer remained and contributed significantly to the major confrontation with government which was to occur 12 months later.

In the midst of the 1985 campaign, Barbara Carson was re-elected as secretary of the RANF (Victorian Branch), with a record 45% of members voting. The president of the RANF (Victorian Branch) commented on the increased awareness by members of the work of the RANF, and acknowledged the 'good campaign' run by Irene Bolger, then an industrial organiser with the Branch (*ANJ* January 1986:11). Barbara Carson resigned in January 1986 and Irene Bolger was elected as secretary in May. The style of leadership changed and this contributed also to an emphasis on confrontation, not least because of the leadership style of the Minister for Health, David White, who had replaced Tom Roper after the October strike. That the leader of the RANF and the Minister were totally unable to work together in a negotiated settlement is an understatement of the apparent antipathy between them.

The new award handed down on the 20 June 1986 after extensive proceedings in the Industrial Relations Commission which took 58 sitting days, heard 77 witnesses, looked at 309 exhibits, and produced 3105 pages of transcript, proved to be 'a lemon' (Fox 1991:34, 41). The RANF had argued that there had been changes in work value from increased turnover of patients and their higher dependency, the increased complexity of drugs and their administration, the removal of non-nursing duties and the introduction of specialised nursing in general areas. The anomalies and inequities provision was used to argue that the registered nurse award did not take account of the 1972 Equal Pay Case decision of equal pay for work of equal value so that nurses were underpaid when equated with other professionals on knowledge, skills, educational requirements and responsibility. The Commission agreed that there were anomalies in terms of equal pay principles but that the only major work value change was patient dependency, and this apparently did not affect Grade 1 nurses.

There was failure to gain agreement on definitions of the classifications, particularly relating to the splitting of RN base grades into Grades 1 and 2. What was Grade 1 nursing work? The government saw it as that of an experienced practitioner, but the union as a beginning practitioner requiring supervision (Fox 1991:36). It was inevitable therefore if the government view prevailed that in implementation experienced nurses would be classified as Grade 1. Further, Grade 1 nurses, student nurses and enrolled nurses would not receive wage increases. The deputy (later associate) charge nurse classification, qualification allowances, and the low increases awarded to Grades 3–6 in the six level structure, remained as unresolved issues for the RANF.

With hindsight, it would appear that successful implementation was impossible for three main reasons. First, and most important, nurses themselves had not seen the new award and classifications prior to its release. Second, senior management, which would have to make decisions on classifications at an agency level, were not consulted. Third, the Commission's support for the government's position on no increases for student nurses and Grade 1 registered nurses, and the open ended nature of the award classifications which left them open to interpretation. This, when combined with government costings, which were approximately $14 million below those of the RANF, and budget constraints did not bode well for the long and anxiously awaited new salaries and career structure in Victoria—the first nursing career structure to be awarded in Australia.

Implementation was to be complete by 31 October 1986. Instead 31 October 1986 became the first day of a 50 day strike. Thus the first career structure turned into the reason for the longest running strike in nursing history.

Unlike the professional rates case there had been no resort to a combined approach to a new wages and career structure in New South Wales and Victoria. The experience in New South Wales, which was occurring at the same time as the Victorian claim, stands in sharp contrast to that of Victorian nurses. Considering that the career structures were almost identical, much pain could have been avoided had the two governments, the Industrial Commission, and the nursing organisations worked together to achieve some sort of parity. Federalism, and the fact that nurses in the two states were covered at this time by different industrial organisations, militated against this happening.

'David made me do it'—the 50 day strike

> Ignoring the submissions prepared through the joint processes of individual hospital managements and RANF representatives, the government instead undertook a massive downgrading exercise in its translation of individual classifications from the old to the new structure. Several thousand nurses were underclassified at the lowest level, Registered Nurse Grade 1... At the same time, the number of supervisory positions was reduced to about half the previous number in some instances (Kyle 1987:5).

While the Commission and the RANF can be criticised for a failure to tie existing positions to the new classifications, there can be no doubt that the Health Department Victoria (HDV) undertook a cynical exercise in its translation of positions from the old to the new structure. The downgrading of experienced nurses who had exercised a supervisory role to Grade 1, compounded by relatively small increases and reductions in qualification allowances, which meant that some nurses actually lost pay, resulted in the most profound dissatisfaction, which steadily grew into a grass roots revolt (*ANJ* September 1986:11). By August the dissatisfaction with the implementation of the award, with what nurses saw as a betrayal by the government, led to stop work meetings in all major metropolitan hospitals, the enforcement of admission and discharge policies, the imposition of bans on elective admissions and a refusal to wear uniforms. The government responded by imposing stand-downs. The RANF then instructed nurses who were stood down to continue to perform their duties. At St Vincent's

Hospital 162 nurses resigned over stand-downs at their hospital, and nurses at Sunbury Private Hospital went out on strike when three colleagues were sacked (*ANJ* October 1986). Throughout this period, meetings were held constantly with the Industrial Commission, the Health Department, the Victorian Trades Hall Council (VTHC) and the Australian Council of Trade Unions (ACTU), with the Minister for Health and with private hospital employers.

On 28 August a stop work meeting voted to continue the bans and carried a motion from the floor to call for the resignation of the Minister. In early September, in an attempt to break the impasse, RANF members agreed to lift bans so that a conference could be held before the commission to attempt to resolve differences in interpretation of the award. If this failed nurses would call for stronger action.

Meanwhile, it was becoming increasingly clear that the Health Department's career structure implementation committee had treated hospital submissions on classifications with contempt. For example, the Alfred Hospital classified only 1.45 effective full time positions at Grade 1, the HDV's response was 230.87 at Grade 1 (*ANJ* November 1986:25). In general, many charge nurses were classified as associate charge nurses, clinical specialists and nurse teachers were under-classified and submissions on designated areas of specialist skills were not accepted. The commission referred matters back to the nurses board but by now the number and complexity of the issues under dispute defied negotiated resolution (see Fox 1991:54-56 for details). Even the Commission commented that 'this piecemeal business of shuttling backwards and forwards between the Commission and the Board really is very messy' (quoted Fox 1991:54).

It was now October and nurses too were 'running out of patience' (Brown & Everill 1987). The current secretary of the ANF (Victorian Branch) explained how she and others in an RANF initiative had painstakingly been talking to nurses across the state on how they believed the career structure should be interpreted and implemented:

> We went around the state explaining that structure and I think that sowed the seeds... Every hospital was visited at least once... We said 'if you are at this level you will be a Grade 2, there will be hardly any Grade 1s'... The submissions came in from hospital managements...and they had equated them with where we were saying. So *then* when White came out and said 'Everybody's a Grade 1', that's when they went berserk. [BM/93]

At the stop work meeting on 30 October 1986, 5000 nurses voted to strike indefinitely from 31 October. This time it would not be a 'Claytons strike', although it began as a limited strike as in 1985 with minimal safe staffing for critical care and reduced staffing in other areas. Picket lines were established. The responses by the government, the nurses board, the VTHC, and the commission, which directed nurses to resume normal work, were less than constructive. The ANF had listed 20 'outstanding issues that must be resolved' and members marched after the meeting to the Health Department. A delegation went to the Minister's office but not surprisingly he refused to discuss the issues with them (*ANJ* December 1986/January 1987:13).

Western General walks out

The strike escalated on 5 November when nurses at Western General Hospital walked out leaving staff in critical care areas only. Perhaps only nurses can understand the emotions which they felt as they left the hospital, many of them in tears. Other hospitals followed. The dramatic nature of the walkouts is poignantly and strongly demonstrated in the film *Running out of patience,* which shows in sequence wave after wave of nurses in their different uniforms leaving the main exits of the hospitals. Curlewis (1991) describes how one nurse felt:

> She was so indignant at the way she had been treated by those 'peanuts' in the Commission. She vividly remembers that day on Monday, 10 November when 'she and two other nurses decided to make a stand, leaving their patients to those nurses who stayed behind, and proudly walked from the top floor ward collecting other nurses on the way down. At the entrance 800 nurses were preparing to walk out.

By 12 November, nurses had walked out of 19 metropolitan and country hospitals, public and private, and many more were to follow.

This was an unusual strike, not only because it concerned nurses, who as an essential service caring for the sick are not expected to walk out (McCoppin 1989), but because it was generated from the grass roots. The RANF leadership had not called for the mass walkouts, but the Victorian RANF Secretary, Irene Bolger, supported the rank and file nurses when they did. In most cases, nurses in individual agencies held their own stop work meetings and voted by secret ballot to walk out.

The RANF job representative at Western General Hospital, believed that the mood of nurses had been changing since the 1985 strike: 'I know they are going to walk, because more and more people are talking about it' [IC/88].

The RANF secretary described the walkouts as 'shock moves':

> Feelings among members have run high [but] the unity and solidarity of members has been overwhelming. On Friday November 7...members spontaneously took to the streets to support one another as they walked off the job (ANJ December/January 1986/1987:14).

The nurses marched through the city and then to the Victorian Trades Hall 'in the first protest aimed at the Trades Hall Council since 1971'. In the short term, intervention by the Trades Hall proved fruitless and compulsory meetings before the full bench of the Industrial Commission without the presence of Ministers or employers, making negotiation impossible, merely ended in an order to nurses to return to work. Irene Bolger refused to recommend a return to work and Fox (1991:78) believes that the 'resolute stance of RANF before the full bench' and the legitimation of the leader's position by rank and file members meant that the government should now 'have been revising its estimates of the costs of disagreeing with RANF demands'.

The government only managed to anger nurses more by gratuitous statements and advertisements calling for them to return to work on the basis of 'vocation'. The HEF and the RANF were virtually at war on the picket lines, and the media continued to misreport the strike, fuelling the anger of nurses:

> At Western General we never stopped food to patients, not once, and we never stopped linen, once the linen got low we let it through... And then [management] went on the TV and said we were stopping linen, and they actually emptied the linen out of linen shelves to film the empty shelves...I have never seen nurses so angry. [IC/88]

By 21 November, the statewide strike was in its fourth week with some 46 public and private Victorian hospitals involved. Hospitals were still functioning, but at extremely reduced levels. Acute patients were still being admitted, and some patients were transferred from public to private hospitals. The concern for patient safety placed enormous stress on those nurses who were still working and on the enrolled nurses and volunteers. If the stress became too great, nurses on strike could surreptitiously leave the picket lines and re-enter the hospital. There was a feeling amongst the striking nurses that sections of the media and even management wanted someone to die to demonstrate how unprofessional the nurses were being.

The government, supported by the Industrial Commission, was still refusing to negotiate while the nurses were on strike and hoping that nurses themselves would respond to pressure and return to work. But the RANF was receiving support from other industrial unions, and the dispute could have escalated into power blackouts when key unions in the La Trobe Valley endorsed industrial action if the government continued to refuse to negotiate with the nurses. The Industrial Commission then overturned its earlier decision that the dispute could not be settled by negotiation while the nurses were on strike, and convened a private meeting of all parties:

> It is quite common in arbitral proceedings for parties to discuss at least some agreed matters and we encourage the parties to engage in such discussion (quoted *ANJ* February 1987:20).

This remarkable change came too late, and only served to intensify the strike when the RANF presented its case on the 24 November and was accused by the Health Department and the commission of presenting a 'new claim'. The RANF said that its claim and the principles involved were the same as those endorsed by members in August and at further mass meetings later in August, and in October and November. The RANF was further incensed by the HEF's submission 'to vary the Registered Nurses Award which would effectively restore the structure of the old award over which nurses, initially took strike action in 1985' (*ANJ* February 1987:21).

Intervention at this time by the ACTU was initially unproductive when it presented a career structure and salary proposal with unacceptable salary rates. However, after the RANF secretary had met with the ACTU Secretary,

Bill Kelty, the ACTU presented submissions in early December which were acceptable to the RANF, including the proviso that nurses' wages should be moved to professional rates in 1988 (see below). The Commission and the Minister for Health conceded that problems existed but further talks failed to make any progress and nurses walked out of some previously exempt areas such as casualty, labour wards, and intensive care units. The government then further inhibited resolution when it attempted, with the support of the HEF, to extend the duties of enrolled nurses by invoking powers in the nurses' legislation. This was later withdrawn because of RANF pressure. The RANF and the ACTU continued to negotiate on an acceptable agreement with some concern by the RANF over details put before the commission by the ACTU in mid December.

Victory for nurses

Nurses showed no signs of returning to work and demonstrated their solidarity at a mass meeting of 6000 members on 15 December where they gave the RANF Secretary, Irene Bolger, a standing ovation and resolved that they would return to work when the government accepted the joint ACTU/RANF proposal (*ANJ* February 1987:21). To demonstrate their bona fides, the RANF recommended that nurses who had walked out of critical care areas return to work. Rather than accept the ACTU/RANF proposal the government released outside the Industrial Commission its own offer of a new structure and pay rates, which the RANF described as 'laughable'. This proved to be a 'last ditch stand' by the government and the strike reached a somewhat sudden conclusion when nurses voted on 19 December to return to work to allow the Commission to consider the ACTU/RANF proposal. The Commission had found that there were 'inequities in the new Award and injustices in its implementation' (*ANJ* February 1987:21). Had it really taken 50 days to come to this conclusion?

'Victory' was claimed on 23 January 1987 when the Industrial Relations Commission handed down its decision on a simplified career structure and showed that it had addressed many anomalies and inequities which had been outlined by the RANF: student nurses and Grade 1 registered nurses received increases and after the first year of registration, they would automatically progress to Grade 2. All associate charge nurses would be classified at the Grade 3 level, and charge nurses at Grade 4. Qualification allowances were restored, no nurse would suffer a demotion as a result of the award, and those nurses who had gained more from the 20 June award than the 23 January award would have their salaries maintained. The RANF did not gain everything it had demanded, for example, the Commission maintained the distinction between major public and private hospitals, and other hospitals, in determining rates for associate charge and charge nurses, and as is usual in industrial decisions there remained for future submission and negotiation classifications relating to other areas of nursing, such as maternal and child health nurses. The RANF had to agree in writing that it would not make further claims on those issues already addressed for two years, but the professional rates case would proceed from October 1987. It was also agreed with the government that a six month study into professional issues in nursing, chaired by Fay Marles and with RANF representation would be conducted (see Marles 1988).

Recriminations and adjustment

There is no doubt that nurses in Victoria suffered during those 50 days. Those on strike lost pay and were threatened with loss of homes. The then State Bank of Victoria was inundated with calls from nurses unable to keep up payments on home loans. The strike fund was well organised by the RANF and was well supported, but this could provide only temporary relief. They suffered too from media and government claims of a loss of vocation and unprofessional withdrawal of labour from those most in need—the sick. The public itself did not seem to be particularly hostile and the RANF received hundreds of letters and phone calls expressing support. The tent cities erected on nature strips outside some hospitals often evidenced a cheerful contingent of striking nurses receiving the supporting 'tooting' of passing motorists. This was in stark contrast to the television portrayals of picket line brawls. Nurses themselves, however, according to a survey conducted after the strike, appeared to believe that the strike had reduced public support for nurses but that they had gained in their influence with government (Gardner & McCoppin 1989). Nor did this survey suggest that nurses believed that they had been too militant.

It was perhaps within actual health agencies on a personal level that recriminations were felt most keenly. There were mixed feelings about senior nursing administrators who had continued to work, although some of these had resigned from the RANF, believing that if they were not on strike, they should not be able to claim membership. Nurses who had gone on strike were resentful of those who had not and who in some cases received promotions. There was criticism of the RANF for not providing professional counselling support *after* the strike. Above all there was a tremendous feeling of guilt:

> You can't be conditioned to care for people and then walk out on them...and then go back in and feel the same. [IC/88]

There was too a sense of denial. Nurses themselves it will be remembered made the decision to walk out and yet one of those involved described the change which had taken place once the strike was over:

> They wanted to make the decision. They didn't want to be pushed into it, and yet now the opposite has occurred. They don't want to claim responsibility for any of it. It's almost as if there is a denial that we actually did it. [IC/88]

There was certainly a backlash against the RANF with a loss of membership, since restored, but this could also be linked to a growing dissatisfaction with the 'peacetime' management of the branch by its secretary (see below).

Did David White, the Minister for Health, make nurses go on strike and remain on strike for 50 days? The answer is 'yes', but that it was not only the Minister's intransigence, it was also:

> the failure of White, his advisors and members of the Commission to understand the dynamics of the dispute from the start... The reality is that despite the Commission's stated view that the strike 'was at all times unnecessary and futile', ultimately it was *only* the strength of that action which afforded the RANF the leverage it needed in its dealings with the government, the Commission and the ACTU (Kyle 1987:6).

Nurses could no longer accept that they should as a predominantly female profession be accorded such esteem for their caring role but be denied wage and career justice:

> I think for many nurses they were just so frustrated with the system, and their perception that the system was collapsing and that the work was increasing and that it was unrelenting, that they meant to have it out in an almost—a very angry bloody-minded way. They tolerated it for such a long time but then the energy was released like a hurricane, which is quite different from the dynamics of what males do in unions—for them it's much more controlled and more calculated. There was a huge emotional reaction I think with the nurses. So I think many meant to tough it out and be as bloody-minded as they could be, and still after fifty days there were people on the floor who were prepared to continue striking even though it might have killed them—they were that angry. [GF/92]

> Victorian nurses *were* more politicised. They'd had the marches, they'd had the stop works, I mean they'd got into the flow of things [industrial]. [BM/93]

Gender issues were apparent in media reporting and the fact that female workers had never before challenged male dominated organisations to the same extent led perhaps to the misconception that they could be forced to retreat:

> The Minister's basic problem is that he is sexist. The Minister thought he could con the basically female nursing profession (Shadow Minister for Health quoted Fox 1991:103).

Apart from personal antipathy, political affiliation contributed to the absolute inability of the Minister and the RANF secretary to work together. He was on the right of the Australian Labor Party while she was closely aligned with the left. Perhaps for White it became in the end a determination to win, to dominate, but there were too many nurses to find a liftwell large enough (a reference to White's reputed propensity to cast opponents into liftwells).

Tasmanian private sector nurses on the Australian map

The experience of achieving a new pay and career structure for nurses in Tasmania differed little from the experience of nurses in the other states and territories. Whether the state government was Labor or Liberal (as in Tasmania) negotiation was protracted: 'in Tasmania we are no different from other states in that we have had to fight for a suitable career structure over many months through negotiations and ultimately industrial action' (*ANJ* October 1988:34).

What was different was that while a strike by public sector nurses had been averted, over 300 private sector nurses went on strike to obtain the same pay and career structure agreed by the Tasmanian Government for public sector nurses, in what was described as 'the first strike by private hospital nurses in Australia' (*Mercury* 1 August 1988). The strike lasted 9 days, from 27 July to 4 August 1988, and public and private sector nurses demonstrated their solidarity by marching together through Hobart on the 28 July. Although brief, the strike engendered the same sort of recrimination from the media, employers, the AMA, and other health unions, which was now familiar to nurses:

> The employers' representative, the Tasmanian Confederation of Industries, said that the Premier 'should demand that nurses return to work' and that the ANF's executive should be 'brought to account for its actions' (*Launceston Examiner* 30 July 1988).

The AMA was reported to have 'warned that unnecessary suffering or even a death could result from the lack of adequate services' (*Sunday Tasmanian* 31 July 1988).

The state secretary of the Hospital Employees Federation was reported as accusing the 'RANF of incompetence and industrial inexperience in crippling the private hospital system and jeopardising the jobs of other hospital employees' (*Mercury* 5 August 1988).

Headlines in the media invoked the Florence Nightingale tradition: 'Plea for nurses to light lamp in impasse', and 'Peace in the wards' (*Mercury* 1 August 1988 & 5 August 1988).

In general, however, the media reported the dispute fairly, and public opinion appears to have been supportive:

> In many respects the march by nurses who were already on strike was a particularly brave thing to do. Marching through the streets exposed striking nurses to possible public criticism... With their applause and greetings marching nurses were in no doubt about the general public's support for equality between the private and public sector nurses (*ANJ* October 1988:34).

The career structure in Tasmania was modelled on that of South Australia and was finally implemented in July 1990, with the manager of the nursing advisory unit in the Department of Health Tasmania commending nurses 'for the level of professionalism demonstrated in the appointment process' and reporting that 'nurses were slowly adapting to the new roles created by the structure (*ANJ* February 1991:27).

Queensland reforms: career structure 1991

Achievement of a new pay and career structure for registered nurses in Queensland was delayed by the presence in state government of the reactionary, idiosyncratic and unsympathetic National Party under the leadership of Joh Bjelke-Petersen. Prior to the state election in December 1989, the Queensland Nurses' Union (QNU)[2] conducted a campaign aimed at finding out members' views on professional and industrial issues. It encouraged nurses to use their votes wisely and asked members living in marginal electorates to lobby candidates from the National, Liberal, and Labor parties about their intentions, if elected, on the professional and industrial concerns of nurses.

The National Party Government had, since being elected to govern in its own right in 1983, consistently refused to participate in nursing policy forums, which had been attended by members of the opposition Liberal and Labor parties; nor would it provide its policies on nursing to the union. The union claimed that co-operation, consultation and negotiation with the government had been impossible even though nurses were enduring:

- the worst understaffing in Australia;
- the lowest wages in Australia;
- the doubtful distinction of being the only state without a career structure for nurses;
- poor working conditions;
- poor access to education and in-service training (*The Queensland Nurse* November/December 1989:2).

Members' responses to the ballot seeking their views on award restructuring wage rises, a new career structure and professional rates were not surprisingly overwhelmingly supportive with 97.28% (of the 40.42% who voted) in favour of all three. The union pointed out that a return of 40.42% is higher than average in union ballots (*The Queensland Nurse* November/December 1989).

The QNU published the nursing policies of the Labor and Liberal parties and the views of candidates were provided to members. The Labor Party outlined its commitment to professional rates, award restructuring and a new career structure, accepted the principles of the ANF's policy on career structures and stated that it would 'rely upon the intent and text of the QNU *Strategy Document on Award Restructuring* and the QNU career structure model' (ALP address to QNU Annual Conference March 1989, reproduced in *The Queensland Nurse* November/December 1989:4). Further the Labor Party argued that it would not 'oppose a QNU application to the industrial commission for professional rates and parity', so that nurses in Queensland would not be paid less than in other states and would be paid at the same rate as other equivalent professionals. The Liberal policy was less detailed in relation to wages and a career structure and provided only a brief statement at the end of its nursing policy:

The Liberal Party will work with professional associations to establish career path structures in both clinical and non-nursing practice working towards better remuneration (Liberal Party reproduced in *The Queensland Nurse* November/ December 1989).

The Labor Party was elected and in its annual report for 1990/91 the QNU could report that nurses had secured 'new skill-related career structures and consequent pay rises' without industrial disputation but after an 'intensive political and media campaign' so that preparations were 'well advanced for the implementation of the 5-level Registered Nurse career structure by 4 November 1991' (QNU *Annual Report* 1990/91). The new award for public sector nurses in Queensland had at last aligned them with nurses employed in Tasmania, South Australia, Western Australia, the Australian Capital Territory and the Northern Territory. Award restructuring for private sector nurses followed more slowly with resistance from the Private Hospitals Association of Queensland.

There is no doubt that nurses in Queensland benefited from the experience of nurses in other states in developing and implementing career structures, and from the advent of a Labor Government, but while this was acknowledged the relationship between the QNU and the Queensland Government became tense over the abolition in December 1990 of the position of chief nursing officer in the Health Department and consequently the loss of direct nursing advice to government on policy and planning. The restructuring of the health system into 13 regional health authorities under clinical advisors also caused concern. A clinical advisor in nursing would report to the assistant regional director of community services but would not have direct access to the regional director or to the regional health authority. The QNU would have preferred to have a regional director of nursing. (*The Queensland Nurse* March/April 1991:2, 5; Submission by QNU to Queensland Minister for Health March 1991). Similarly, proposals by some regional directors to introduce management structures on the Johns Hopkins model of clinical teams under medical supervisors, was opposed by the union and advice was sought from the NSWNA from their experience (*The Queensland Nurse* July/August 1991). This again highlights the commonality of continuing issues for nursing in Australia.

Nursing is a professional occupation

We have seen how in the 1980s there was widespread support for industrial and professional concerns and how the two are not separate but overlapping, often resulting in a professional achievement through industrial action. The achievement of professional rates for nurses is yet another example of the close linkage between professional and industrial issues in aims, process, and outcome. The aim of the campaign for professional rates of pay for registered nurses in NSW and Victoria was to adjust their rates to equal the rates paid to other health professionals such as physiotherapists, occupational therapists and medical scientists, who in general earned approximately $100 per week more after six years of employment with smaller differentials at the lower levels. The basis for the professional rates claim was that as nurses had achieved tertiary education for pre-registration nurses, the higher educational standard and utilisation of sophisticated skills entitled them to equivalent rates as professionals in the health industry. Improved rates of pay is of course an industrial issue but to be recognised as having equivalent status to these other groups is a professional outcome.

The existence in nursing organisations of skilled, sophisticated, persistent, and experienced union representatives and organisers is crucial to the successful pursuit of industrial claims. While overt political activity such as strikes and work bans involving the mass of the membership is the more obvious public face of unionism in Australia, this is neither the most time consuming nor the more important part of the industrial process. The mass membership represents the power base for union claims, which can be mobilised (or not), depending on the success or otherwise of ongoing discussion and negotiation in the state and federal industrial relations commissions and the courts, with employers, with governments and government departments, and indeed with trade union peak organisations, such as the ACTU and state trades and labour councils. The 38 hour week for nurses achieved between 1985 and 1987 after protracted industrial negotiation on a state by state basis, is an example of this process.

Nor does negotiation end when there is a decision handed down by an industrial commission or court. Ongoing negotiation then ensues as the new award fixing principles are implemented and extended to other awards covering, for example, private sector nurses or nurses not working in the mainstream of nursing employment. This usually involves further hearings before the commission. Negotiating implementation in the particular employing agency is similarly often a long and complicated task for the industrial organisation representing employees. This was the case, particularly in relation to retrospective payment with the 38 hour week. All these stages require detailed preparation of evidence and submissions and the careful arguing of the case or claim. Negotiation within the nursing organisation precedes any such claim and support from the membership must be gained by the dissemination of information through journals, newsletters, news releases and meetings, right down to the health agency level. Overt support from the membership cannot be guaranteed unless the claim is consistent with the expressed views of a large number of nurses and is something for which they feel a sense of ownership and appropriateness.

The process for the achievement of professional rates, beginning in 1987, was again one of protracted industrial negotiation using arguments based on the professional equivalence of nurses to the other health professionals. The threat of overt industrial action provided the background to what was essentially a negotiated claim. The claim for professional rates in New South Wales exemplifies the process.

In July 1987, the New South Wales Nurses Association formally, that is, in writing, raised the issue of professional rates in that state with the NSW Department of Health as the employer of public sector nurses. A series of discussions followed and documentary evidence supporting the claim was provided. After the department had indicated a willingness to enter into negotiation with the NSWNA, the association filed its claim with the Industrial Commission of NSW as an anomaly within the wage fixing principles. As Patricia Staunton, the General Secretary of the NSWNA, explained to members:

> The wage fixing principles relating to the determination of an anomaly require that both parties i.e. the Department and the Association, agree that an arguable case exists in relation to the determination of an anomaly. If both parties do not agree then the President of the Industrial Commission is required to hear arguments from both parties to determine that issue (*The Lamp* February 1988:10).

The Department of Health, in October, then failed to agree that an 'arguable case' existed, which therefore required a hearing to determine the issue. In December, the president of the industrial commission provided a determination which was not acceptable to the NSWNA and the association immediately filed an appeal with the full bench of the commission. The determination had made a distinction between college graduates for whom the association would have an arguable case for professional rates and hospital educated nurses for whom it would not. The determination was particularly galling as it included a sentence to the effect that 'The Nurses Association can not have cake in 1986 [career structure claim] and eat it again in 1987' (quoted *The Lamp* February 1988).

The association sought and gained support from its membership for planned industrial action, including a one day walk out in all nursing areas except intensive care without provision of skeleton staff, should the Government not agree that an arguable case existed and that there was an anomaly in nurses' rates of pay. On 22 January 1988, after a number of discussions with the Premier and the Minister for Health, the government agreed in writing to support the principle of professional rates of pay, that an anomaly might exist, and that therefore the association had an arguable case, that there should be no disparity between differently educated nurses, and that the appeal should be heard as a matter of urgency by the commission (*The Lamp* February 1988:11). The planned industrial action was then called off.

The appeal by the NSWNA was upheld before the full bench in March 1988 and the claim could now be considered as an arguable case of anomaly or inequity. So far, so good, but even following the progress of the claim from March 1988 onwards is exhausting and it was not until October 1989 that some agreement was reached on phasing in of professional rates for nurses employed under the Department of Veterans Affairs in New South Wales; that is, over two years after the case had begun.

During 1988 and 1989, negotiations with the NSW Department of Health, punctuated by presentation of evidence to various hearings before the Industrial Commission took place, and there was a change of government. The professional rates case in New South Wales was running concurrently with the one being pursued by the RANF (Victorian Branch). This both assisted and slowed the case in New South Wales. In mid 1988, the Victorian Industrial Relations Commission handed down a decision on principles stating that 'nursing is a professional occupation' and 'that there should be no salary differentials whatsoever on account of the different training systems. To award different salaries for the same work would not only be unjust but would be imprudent and would be the cause of needless industrial unrest' (quoted *The Lamp* September 1988:3). In order to avoid 'industrial unrest' either in Victoria or New South Wales, and to achieve a 'coordinated and consistent approach' in setting professional rates for both states, a series of joint compulsory conferences of the two industrial commissions, the two unions, representatives of both health departments, and private sector employers were held. The first historic joint sitting of the industrial commissions took place on the 28 October 1988. Federalism, in addition to division and conflict, provides also for co-operation when it is in the interests of the states.

The 'interim agreement' in December 1988 provided for professional rates in New South Wales to be introduced in three phases, the first phase to be paid to nurses employed in the public and private sectors commencing in December 1988. Thus Victoria and New South Wales had secured professional rates in part. Negotiation on the other two phases then began in both states. Professional rates for nurses employed by the Commonwealth Department of Veterans Affairs in New South Wales and Victoria could now be pursued with increased vigour through the Australian, or federal, Industrial Relations Commission, to ensure that they would receive the interim adjustments paid to their counterparts in each state. Finally agreement was reached in August 1989 on the second and third phases of professional rates of state employed nurses to be paid in two equal instalments in September 1989 and September 1990. Second phase increases were granted also for nurses employed by the Department of Veterans Affairs in New South Wales and Victoria after agreement on the first phase in June, but the third phase remained in limbo for future negotiation.

Given the protracted nature of the claim, it is not surprising that the monthly reports from the general secretary of NSWNA to her members increasingly reflected her frustration.

In March 1989:

> That progress has been slow is due entirely to the reluctance or inability of NSW and Victorian Departments [of Health] to arrive at any coordinated position. In order to put this matter back on to the 'front burner' the Association relisted before the Full Bench... On that occasion the Association registered the strongest objection to the delays... (*The Lamp* March 1989:6).

In June 1989:

> I wish to emphasise that...there are still a number of matters which require to be finalised before this matter can finally be put to bed (*The Lamp* June 1989:6).

In September 1989, the president of the NSWNA joined in:

> The Association has been involved for a considerable period of time in pursuing professional rates of pay for registered nurses (*The Lamp* September 1989:6).

Even when professional rates had been achieved for nurses throughout Australia there was reason for dissatisfaction. For those states which had already entered a federal award (South Australia, Tasmania, Western Australia, ACT and NT) this meant a levelling out of wages and conditions with winners and losers, and perhaps a tendency to move to the lowest common denominator. The federal Industrial Relations Commission set the agenda by terming a 'professional rate' the 'national rate' of pay, with the aim of also standardising conditions. Existing penalties differed between the states so that the ACT and Tasmania, for example, had a 30% penalty rate for permanent night duty, and Western Australia had 12.5%; the Commission standardised the rate at 15.0%. While Western Australia gained here, it lost in relation to professional rates. In the midst of the ANF (WA Branch) negotiations with the state government for a professional rate it entered into the federal award. The professional rate under negotiation in that state was higher than that ultimately achieved under the national rate. The equivalence provision under the Western Australian professional rates claim would have meant higher rates because allied health professionals there were paid at a higher rate than in the other states. Further, the national rate for nurses was not equivalent to professional rates for allied health professionals, even in the other states.

The achievement of the national rate and the standardisation of conditions holds implications for the different career structures across Australia, but particularly for Western Australia, as apart from New South Wales, which is not as yet under a federal award, and Victoria, all the other states and territories, had adopted the South Australian model. The main problem for Western Australia is the Level 3 position where the scope of authority is wider (with responsibility for two or three wards rather than one) than the level 3 positions in the other states. It should therefore be paid at a higher rate than a national rate would allow. It would be unlikely for the Western Australian government to agree to make up the difference. Standardisation could mean making the career structures the same in all the states: something which would be hotly contested by the state branches of the ANF.

The professional rates case in New South Wales, and in Victoria, is important for all nurses, in the achievement of significant increases in rates of pay and recognition at last as having parity with allied health professionals. The case also demonstrates how industrial relations requires persistence, expertise and commitment by the leadership and paid officers of the union, and support and patience from members. It must also be remembered that professional rates was not the only major issue at that time in NSW or Victoria. The implementation of the new pay and career structures, harmonisation of the NSWNA with the RANF, the National Wage Case, and demarcation disputes with other unions, not to mention providing a day to day service to members and annual conferences, all had to be attended to by the unions. The change of government from Labor to a Liberal/National coalition in March 1988 in New South Wales and the need to establish new relationships in the midst of negotiations for professional rates added to the uncertainty of the outcome.

Power tends to be cumulative and there is no doubt that previous successes by both unions contributed to success in the professional rates case. Nurses had received recognition as a political and industrial force.

A radical leadership

'Leadership' is perhaps one of the most frequently used concepts in the organisational literature, so it is hardly surprising that the leadership of nursing organisations has played a critical role in achievements for nurses, and in the internal style and operation of the organisation. In a federal system, much of this is apparent at the state level.

Different styles of leadership are, however, appropriate in different contexts and situations (Robbins 1989). The leadership style of Patricia Staunton, as General Secretary of the NSWNA during the professional rates case, was in sharp contrast to the leadership style of her predecessor, Jenny Haines. Haines had much more in common with her counterpart in Victoria, Irene Bolger.

These two women—Jenny Haines, General Secretary (1982-1987) of the New South Wales Nurses' Association (for over 50 years the largest independent nursing union), and Irene Bolger, Secretary (1986-1989) of the Victorian Branch of the Royal Australian Nursing Federation—each initiated an experiment in radical leadership, which produced the kinds of strong emotion, debate and publicity that had previously been unusual in Australian nursing. They were instrumental in achieving major gains for nurses through industrial action in the two most populous states (NSW with approximately 34% and Victoria 25% of the national population total).

The growth of the political awareness and influence of Australian nurses, which gathered strength with the campaign for tertiary education, a professional goal, was further consolidated by the industrial activity from 1984 by an emphasis on the 'union' side of the so called 'professional-union' dichotomy (Gardner & McCoppin 1987). The appearance of the two leaders during the period contributed to this apparent shift of emphasis to a more radical approach to nursing issues. 'Radical' is used here in the sense of desiring 'root and branch' change.

The most obvious parallels between Jenny Haines and Irene Bolger are that both were elected on reformist platforms, both came from the left of the political spectrum, they experienced stormy and controversial periods in office during which their influence declined, and they were eventually rejected by their members. In both cases there were elements of tragedy, in the classic sense of people occupying high office, achieving prominence and even acclaim, over-reacting, and then falling from grace.

Both Jenny Haines and Irene Bolger took over as secretaries of their respective unions from predecessors who had held office for relatively long periods: six years in Victoria for Barbara Carson, and 14 in New South Wales for Mary Henlen. Irene Bolger's election in 1986, with 37% of members voting, was not particularly controversial although it was realised at the time that the new secretary had radical views. The election of Jenny Haines took place, by contrast, after a 'long and bitter leadership struggle', preceded by a campaign against the incumbent leadership carried out by Haines and her nurses reform group (*The Lamp* July/August 1982:32). This group, founded by Haines and others with the explicit aim of changing the association, operated among the association's members, but outside its formal authority structure. The association, the group claimed, could become 'a modern and effective trade union' under Haines, with a more democratic constitution; and it would also campaign against the Wran government's reduction of funding in public sector health services more effectively than the group considered the Henlen leadership was then doing (Nurses Reform May 1982). The nurses reform group campaign against Henlen and the 'established leadership' was successful with Haines defeating the 'establishment' candidate, Patricia Staunton, with a record 40% of the membership voting.

Irene Bolger's previous political experience had been in her local branch of the Australian Labor Party, and she had also been active at her work place during the 1984 'non-nursing duties' dispute. At the time of her election she was an industrial relations organiser for the RANF (Victorian Branch), and listed 'politics and reading about politics and sociology' as major interests (RANF Victorian Branch *News* March 1985). Her 1985 and 1986 policy statements referred mainly to democratising the branch and to achieving improved pay and conditions for nurses.

Both women thus came to office with previous experience, and a commitment to reform and political action. 'Political' is used here to mean conflict between competing interests, demands and values rather than the narrow reference to competing political parties. This broad usage is often avoided by nurses, amongst others, in the belief that there is something unwholesome about political activity, that one can put around it a *cordon sanitaire*. But political activity is not always overt and it is most certainly not confined to public demonstrations. It includes the sorts of activity which achieved tertiary education for nurses, and before that the gradual raising of educational standards and entry qualifications.

Nurses can avoid pointless agonising over whether they should or should not be 'political' by recognising that they already are, and that it is this political activity which has helped them to achieve their recent advances. The education transfer campaign showed that many nurses saw the need for political action at least by the early 1980s (Cochrane 1989). It was then too that nurses began to question the RANF's 'no-strike' rule, seeing it as a barrier to wage justice though there had been isolated comments even earlier (e.g. Barratt 1975).

At least some nurses have been politically active for much longer than the public, and probably many nurses, are aware. Although both Haines and Bolger were seen as noticeably more radical than their predecessors, this does not mean that Mary Henlen and Barbara Carson were conservative in the usually accepted sense of conservatism: maintaining the status quo. They were however more moderate as union officials, and their political beliefs appear to have been less ideologically radical than were those of the women who succeeded them. Their achievement was to raise nurses' expectations by showing what could be won through collective action, so that when each of the two stood down, their members were prepared to gamble on a different kind of leader who was younger, from outside the established union officiate, and a departure from the traditional authority figures—both Carson and Henlen had been directors of nursing.

'Leadership' can be described as the outcome of the interaction between the personal qualities of the leader, the characteristics of the followers, and the perceived demands of the current circumstances in which they find themselves (Robbins 1989). Haines and Bolger between them introduced a more radical, more ideological leadership style to Australian nursing, which was now acceptable to their followers (nurses) from their perceived grievances about pay and conditions of work.

A political ideology interprets reality in a particular way. It criticises that reality and offers a guide to a preferred state of affairs and is not confined to either the left or right of the political spectrum, although such labels as 'left' and 'right' are imprecise, and subject to contested interpretations. Both Haines and Bolger were widely reported to belong to the 'left wing' of the union movement, although there were differences between them, probably attributable to differences in individual style.

Haines gained national prominence at the prices and incomes conference held by the Australian Council of Trade Unions (ACTU) before the 1983 federal election, as the only delegate who voted against the adoption of the ACTU's wages restraint policy (Cadzow 1983). As a result of her stand she faced censure by the NSWNA Council, with which she confessed to having only 'indifferent' relations (Taylor 1983). Haines explained that, although 'strongly favouring the election of a Labor Government', she 'conscientiously' believed that the prices and incomes agreement might 'in some circumstances, work against the interests of nurses' (*The Lamp* January/February 1983:3). Haines thus showed early in her period of office that she was reluctant to compromise over what she judged to be nurses' interests, in spite of pressure from other unionists.

Irene Bolger received more publicity as Secretary of the Victorian Branch of the RANF than did Jenny Haines as her equivalent in the NSWNA. Bolger achieved national prominence and the sort of constant media coverage usually reserved for celebrities, initially as a result of the Victorian 50 day strike; and her fall was more dramatic, because swifter and more humiliating. Bolger seems in retrospect to have spent much of her three years in office either riding high on a wave of popular acclaim, or being ignominiously 'dumped' by it and trying to cling to the wreckage.

The Victorian 50 day strike had begun on 31 October 1986 following a mass meeting and a march to the Health Department. The decision to strike at first meant that services were maintained by a 'skeleton' staff in each hospital. Then, beginning with Western General Hospital, by the end of November nurses had walked out of 42 hospitals, leaving only critical care areas fully staffed. But the decisions in favour of the 'walk-outs' had been made by nurses themselves and not by Irene Bolger (*Nurses Action* February 1987:6):

> So it wasn't Irene, and I think that's often not remembered. But she gave full support to Western once those kids had made that decision, and from there it snowballed. And I think her tenacity has to be recognised... You've got to give recognition to Barb Carson and to Irene. [BM/93]

The spectacle of a determined woman, backed by a large number of nurses, tackling a phalanx of male politicians and forcing them eventually to make concessions captured public attention. Reactions were often hostile, though this may not necessarily mean that a majority of the public were equally critical of the nurses' actions. Those who did criticise, as Bessant and D'Cruz (1989) demonstrate, often resorted to extreme, even sexist, language in political and personal abuse of Bolger.

Disenchantment

Neither of the leaders escaped criticism from their respective membership and enthusiastic support deteriorated ultimately into condemnation. The issue which perhaps did most damage to Jenny Haines' standing in the NSWNA was the union's 38 hour week campaign, conducted within the new wage indexation system, following a 4.3% wage rise. At the association's 1984 annual conference Haines reported that on the question of the 'offsets' required by the Health Department, she was resolutely opposed to compromise on several proposals. The government, she said, refused to recognise that nurses had already contributed to cost savings as a result of government reductions in hospital funding. By early 1985 it was apparent that there were differences between Haines and two other NSWNA officials, including Patricia Staunton (then legal officer), about the reasonableness or otherwise of the 'offsets', especially increased costs for living in nurses' homes. Staunton argued forcefully in favour of accepting that 'offset', and of negotiating on the question of part time loadings (Staunton 1985). When members wrote to complain about the delay in achieving the 38 hour week, Haines (1985:38) defended her position by blaming the Health Department for not funding the increased staff required, and argued that no group of nurses, such as students in nurses' homes, should be disadvantaged by the introduction of the 38 hour week.

The campaign proceeded with Haines losing ground, having to accede to a Council decision to accept the accommodation charges 'offset' in spite of reported votes against such acceptance at members' meetings. In response she attacked 'a small group within the Nurses' Association', which, she said, was pursuing a campaign for power by supporting the government's 'whittling away' of part-time loading (*The Lamp* August 1985:6-7). At this time Patricia Staunton was elected Assistant General Secretary with a clear majority over the nurses reform candidate, and the reform group also failed to win any seats on the new Council. Haines was under attack from the state ALP for her opposition to the Wran government's health policy (Cruikshank 1987), and for her continued opposition to the federal accord between government and the trade union movement. At the 1985 ACTU congress she and Bronwyn Ridgway, the other Assistant General Secretary, voted against the accord. For this they were criticised by the association's two vice-presidents, and by an irate member, who accused them of 'brainless adventurism' (*The Lamp* February 1986:7).

Haines next clashed with her critics in 1986 over the new career structure and its associated wage claim. The case was conducted by Staunton, and the NSWNA Council restricted public statements about it to her and to the president (*The Lamp* August 1986:10). Haines also demanded that the association should claim a 39% 'across the board' minimum wage increase for nurses, an action which led to her being 'gagged' by Council (*The Lamp* July 1986:7). When some members wrote to criticise the disparity in wage gains for junior and senior nurses in the new award, Staunton defended the lesser gains for juniors, saying that:

> The NSWNA claim was never an across-the-board claim. It could not be, if we were to introduce...the new career positions into the middle of the nursing structure. To do that, as we have, necessitated graduated wage increases in order to ensure that relativities were maintained (*The Lamp* August 1986:4).

The existence of serious differences between opposing factions within the association had now become obvious through the press and at a mass meeting. A branch delegate wrote to complain of 'personal political grandstanding'. Staunton responded by denying any attempt on her part to 'push political barrows', but admitted to belonging to the nurses for unity faction, soon renamed the 'Pat Staunton team'. She dissociated herself from any intransigent and inflexible commitment to '39% across the board or nothing', and deplored the 'personal abuse and vilification' to which, she said, she and others had been subjected. Haines in her turn defended differences of opinion within the association, attributing them to 'a legitimate difference of approach' rather than to personal ambition, though she did refer to a 'marked lack of tolerance by certain individuals and groups for legitimate points of view held by other members' (*The Lamp* August 1986:4-5; November 1986:4). At the close of this turbulent year the retiring president criticised the attempted use of mass meetings for decision making, and even canvassed the idea of appointing, rather than electing, senior union officials (*The Lamp* December 1986:8). Haines, her editorials now confined to uncontroversial subjects, replied by letter in which she rejected both positions, seeing them as 'an attack on a certain faction within the Association and the democratic forms of the expression of membership will' (*The Lamp* March 1987:5).

New elections for the association were announced for May 1987. It was clear by this time that the general secretary was excluded from the major activities of the association. Her position was further weakened by the rift between herself and Ridgway, elected on the same nurses' reform ticket in 1982 but now standing on a separate ticket. The April-May campaign received press coverage as a 'bitter, heated fight for supremacy'. Haines faced attacks from both left and right of the labor movement, publicity about alleged racist bias in the NSWNA, and, she said, misinformation about both nurses' reform and her private life (Cruikshank 1987; Larriera 1987). Even so, she made a personal statement in which she defended her association opponents against charges of racism:

> I unreservedly assert that I have never heard any of these officers, my opponents though they be, make the racist statements of which they are accused (Haines 1987).

Against this unhappy background and a divided opposition, the Pat Staunton team won its predicted victory with 60% of the votes, giving it the three elected officers and all 21 Council places (*The Lamp* July 1987:7).

Six months after the Victorian strike had ended Irene Bolger reflected on the lessons nurses had learned. She assured members that in spite of the inevitable expense of the strike, branch finances were satisfactory, but warned them that some former full-time officers were 'circulating rumours concerning various aspects of RANF's operation during the strike' (*Nurses Action* June 1987:3). This was probably the first intimation to members that the unity achieved during the strike was already threatened. A few months later both her assistant secretary and branch president had resigned after disagreements, and allegations were being made in the press that branch finances were not in order (Donohoe 1987). Bolger accused a 'section' of the Branch of distracting members by spreading rumours, thus creating 'a false state of disorder' (*Nurses Action* August 1987:3). Later in 1987 she became embroiled in a serious argument with the federal RANF (*Nurses Action* November 1987:3). A major difference between Bolger's position and that of Haines was the (then) independent position of the NSWNA, in contrast to that of the RANF (Victorian Branch), which had the added complication of being part of a larger body with which it had to co-exist.

The Victorian secretary's attack on the federal RANF in 1987, appears to have been sparked initially by the federal body's attempts to have its own superannuation scheme accepted in Victoria in preference to the local scheme. She went further however, telling Victorian members that in her view they received too little from the federation in return for the financial support they gave. Early in 1988 she had a further criticism, this time of the negotiations on 'harmonisation' between the RANF and the NSWNA, especially the proposal that the NSWNA would not have to be covered by a federal award, and would not be required to subscribe to the *Australian Nurses' Journal* (*Nurses Action* February 1988). Another objection may have been that the arrival of a New South Wales Branch in the RANF might not appeal to a Victorian official who had hitherto led the largest branch of the federation. Bolger's view contrasts here with that of Jenny Haines, who thought the possibility of an Australia-wide union for nurses was an 'exciting concept' (*The Lamp* September 1985:19). An additional consideration for Bolger was probably that the NSWNA was now led by Patricia Staunton, who was associated with the right of the labour movement (Higgins 1989).

Early in 1988 it emerged that the Victorian Branch owed over $200 000 to the federal office for ANJ subscriptions, so that the journal shrank from 64 to 40 pages. Once again Bolger accused others, this time the federal secretary, of fomenting division.

By mid-1988, it was obvious that Irene Bolger had problems with her branch council and with many of her own members, including people from whom she had formerly received support. At a June mass meeting her financial management came under attack, and in September she used a court order to abort a mass meeting called by the council to discuss the federal award. She was now reported to be 'embattled', and defending the branch against 'attempts by state council...to overturn democratic decisions of the members without notice' (Reddy 1988).

Jenny Haines had opposed the federal RANF when it applied in 1983 for a federal award to cover all nurses, seeing such a move as threatening the NSWNA (*The Lamp* August 1983:5). At the mass meeting to decide Victoria's position Bolger also opposed seeking the award but her case against it was overwhelmingly rejected. This was not, she said, a threat to her leadership, but the result of a 'numbers game' organised by her opponents (Davis 1988). The alleged 'numbers game' intensified however, and in the October council elections Bolger's opponents, described as 'an alliance of pragmatic left elements and some centre and right candidates', won all positions. This time she blamed 'outside interference in the elections, the opposition's seemingly unlimited finances and the media's campaign of personal vilification against me' (Arnold 1988).

By early 1989 Irene Bolger, as Jenny Haines had been, was isolated within her own organisation. She pointed out to members that no charges had been laid against her, but said that financial management was 'a classic way of attacking union officials, particularly troubled ones like me. I have obviously been seen as a threat to the Labor Government, the ACTU, and some within our organisation' (*Nurses Action* January 1989:3). The new branch council did decide however to bring charges against Bolger. In May it sacked her as secretary and expelled her from the branch. Amongst the charges which were upheld, a majority related to financial management (ANF Victorian Branch *Letter to members* 29 May 1989).

Only her reinstatement as a member of the branch now interrupted Bolger's string of defeats. She failed to attract enough support to have council's decision overturned and finally took court action. A settlement reinstated her as a member and restored her salary after it was revealed that the new (appointed) secretary had withheld pertinent information from council (Innes 1989). In the prelude to the October election for the secretary's position , one reporter judged her to be optimistic, and predicted that the election would be close: 'Ms Bolger, with her high personal profile, has a good chance of winning the election...' (Davis 1989). In the end, in spite of the apparent bungling over the court case, the contest was not as close as predicted. In a 48% poll Bolger gained 43.6% of the vote, losing to Belinda Morieson, her former professional officer (ANF Vic. Branch *Newsletter* December/January 1989-90).

Haines and Bolger were ideologues of the left who found it difficult to accept the necessity for compromise and accommodation in the labour movement, given that the ALP is not a revolutionary party but works within the capitalist system. Haines, for example, considered that the unions were duped by the Labor Government's 'social wage' campaign, which she saw as 'just a sell-out to big business' (*The Lamp* March 1983:9), while Bolger regretted that the senior unionists who wrote *Australia Reconstructed* should be 'so unimaginative, dwelling so slavishly on re-creating a more productive capitalist economy...' (Bolger 1988). Both were consequently against the Accord, and Bolger in fact saw clearly that the 1986 strike had threatened to subvert it (ABC Broadcast 11 September 1988).

Both women advocated more democratic procedures within their unions, though Haines was more successful in their achievement. These were later adopted by the Queensland Branch of the ANF (*ANJ* February 1992:33). Both supported gains for nursing's lower ranks. Connected with the democratic principle was the tendency of both to rely on votes at mass meetings, in contrast to decisions made by their councils. Many left wing ideologues prefer 'direct' or participatory democracy to the representative or 'indirect' kind (Christenson et al 1981). In addition, Bolger appeared to believe that a vote against her at such meetings was the result of manipulation. As both leaders became alienated from their councils, which had the power to control them, they seemed to forget that, like themselves, those bodies were elected, and by the same electorate. Under attack, Bolger's criticisms of her opponents appear to have been more virulent, a contrast with Haines's magnanimity in her personal statement.

Both Secretaries, Irene Bolger in particular, experienced the applause of their massed members, and it is perhaps not surprising that Bolger apparently thought she could translate the acclaim of nurses at mass meetings during the unusual conditions of a strike into the support she needed to stay in office. She seemed not to understand that after the strike nurses needed a different style of leadership, moderate and supportive, so that they could recover from their experience. Both women failed to consolidate their positions by establishing a reliable group of supporters within their organisations. Haines because her support came from her own group outside the union office, and Bolger because she alienated her supporters within. They also failed to adjust to the need for compromise and accommodation in routine political life.

The actions of Haines and Bolger during their terms of office suggest that they put greater stress on the industrial side of their responsibilities, but they did not wholly neglect professional issues. Haines wrote positively of the education transfer several times, and in 1983 referred to her plans for professional as well as industrial gains (*The Lamp* December 1983:3). Bolger supported the RANF position that professionalism must be maintained, though she realised that it had been used in the past to keep nurses submissive (*Nurses Action* April/May 1988). The image they presented however tended to be that of the militant union leader rather than the conventional one of the professional nurse. There seems therefore to have been some connection between their radical beliefs and their emphasis on industrial action, so that they must both have contributed substantially to nurses' growing readiness to take collective action.

The election to office of Haines and Bolger marked the desire for a change in the style of nursing union leadership in the major states. It does not however demonstrate a radical swing to the left among the nursing rank and file. Nurses have become more militant, but 'increasing union militancy, including the use of strikes by non-manual workers, need not imply greater support for socialism, let alone revolution' (Rawson 1978:116). The gradually growing disenchantment that marked the terms of office of both Haines and Bolger, and their final rejection by their members (though both retained a significant degree of support), suggest that nurses have mostly *not* become radical, certainly not to the point of accepting the uncompromising political orientations of these two women. It is significant that both were succeeded by leaders reputed to be politically more moderate.

After defeating Jenny Haines, Patricia Staunton asserted that the image of the new, radical nurse was mistaken:

> Because nurses are starting to professionally assert themselves does not mean they are more industrially militant or radical. The manifestations of so-called radicalism are only ordinary people reacting to the community at large taking nurses for granted (Casey 1987).

So when nurses appear to be acting in a purely 'industrial' or 'trade union' fashion, they are not aspiring radicals, but are in fact demonstrating the new found assertiveness of a formerly oppressed and undervalued professional group. Staunton's statement is probably an accurate account of where most nurses are now politically: they see political or industrial action as a way of improving their professional status and conditions of work, so that the two theoretically antagonistic 'wings' of their associations are in practice reconcilable.

Some leading nurses knew this already: '...it is agreed that the industrial aspects and the professional aspects cannot be effectively separated (and indeed it would be a pity if this were to happen)...' (Henlen 1975); and 'it is becoming more and more difficult to allocate matters on the basis of being purely professional or purely industrial' (Patten *ANJ* 1976). The federal secretary has spoken unequivocally against separation: 'Professionalism and unionism are not mutually exclusive, they are interdependent' (Beaumont 1989:247).

Haines and Bolger showed that nurses can be inspired by radical ideals, but that at the same time they want their leaders to work within the established systems. It would be unfortunate however if nurses forget these former leaders. They may have failed to achieve all that they could have wanted, but they did make an ineradicable impact, as a new approach 'precipitates a partial reorientation of the previously dominant outlook, bringing about a new emphasis...' (Shils 1968:73). As Irene Bolger said of the strike and its aftermath: 'It's there. It can't be taken away' (Debelle 1988).

The nursing leadership in the 1990s recognises the contributions made by their predecessors and that they have enabled them to pursue nursing issues with stronger, more professional, more experienced nursing organisations at state and federal levels. Some of the leaders of the state or territory branches are still there and have shown that they can adapt their styles and strategies to the experiences of the time. Some, like Marilyn Beaumont, Patricia Staunton and Marea Vidovich have gained prominence at the federal level. All have a distinctly professional style, in the sense of being expert in their jobs, and while they are quite able to withdraw nursing labour when necessary, they appear to prefer an emphasis on negotiation.

One union or many

Industrial coverage of nurses in the Australian states and territories has historically been divided between a number of unions. In the 1980s, it became apparent that a strong national organisation was required if nursing was going to achieve improved pay and conditions of work. This had two elements—first, a strengthening of the national organisation, the Royal Australian Nursing Federation, and second, and following from this, coverage by the RANF of registered nurses through state branches in all states and territories. Although the RANF was the largest single union covering registered general nurses, the state branches of the RANF had had a great deal of autonomy and the national, or federal, level was relatively weak.

This was exacerbated by state registered nurses in the largest state in terms of population being covered by a different industrial organisation altogether. In New South Wales, the New South Wales Nurses Association had covered all but the very few nurses employed by the Commonwealth Government in that state. In Queensland, the Queensland Nurses' Union (QNU) had formed as a breakaway organisation from the RANF in 1982 and became the state registered union representing nurses in that state. The RANF continued to represent Commonwealth employed nurses. Interestingly, both the NSWNA and QNU believed themselves to be more industrially focussed than the RANF. Division was not confined to different organisations representing registered nurses. In order for the RANF to be able to make claims on behalf of both state employed and Commonwealth employed nurses, 'dual registration' was necessary in the other states—that is registration by the RANF with the Australian Industrial Relations Commission and with the relevant state industrial relations commission. In South Australia, this led to a split into federal and state sections of the RANF state branch between 1984 and 1985 (McCoppin 1989:270).

In 1988 the NSWNA 'harmonised' with the ANF, to be followed, in 1989 by the QNU. Both organisations retained their names and separate journals, *The Lamp* and *The Queensland Nurse* respectively, but the memberships were integrated with the ANF by individual application for reciprocal membership. The Federal Council Meeting of the RANF in April 1985 had resolved to seek formal communication between nursing unions, and meetings followed between the RANF, the NSWNA and the QNU with the intention of forming a national nurses' association. RANF Rule 50 was added in recognition of harmonisation with the NSWNA, and in 1988 the Queensland Council of the ANF resolved unanimously:

> That the Queensland Branch supports harmonisation with the Queensland Nurses' Union of Employees on the same basis as the harmonisation achieved with NSW Nurses' Association and RANF NSW Branch in the form of RANF Rule 50 (*ANJ* August 1988:33).

The newly formed Queensland ANF/QNU Branch adopted the local branch structure of the NSWNA to provide increased opportunities for participation in decision making by members (*ANJ* February 1992).

The benefits for nurses of having one national industrial and professional organisation were perceived to be the driving force behind the (belated) rapprochement (Ch. 5):

> Obviously, NSWNA would not have taken the step that it did to harmonise with the ANF if we didn't see some sense in having one organisation looking after nurses. Certainly, our view was that the ANF could not properly state that it was *the* major union for nurses in this country, when all the nurses in New South Wales were outside it, with the exception of maybe 1000. At the same time, the NSWNA was being fairly shortsighted if it felt it could influence events nationally, it wasn't part of it, so there was a mutual benefit for both. [PS/90]

For an industrial and/or professional association to be effective and able to argue that it is representative of its members and therefore can legitimately act on their behalf, it must have close to 60% of its potential membership. For the RANF to be perceived as a national organisation representing nurses it could not afford to have New South Wales and Queensland largely outside its jurisdiction (see Table 6.1).

Coverage of enrolled nurses and mental health nurses remains a problem but is being addressed. The RANF in most states, while not disallowing membership, had not pursued coverage of enrolled nurses but had perceived itself as the professional and industrial organisation representing registered nurses. With growing recognition of the need to protect nursing as a whole, combined with trends in the industrial arena to fewer and larger industry-based unions, the ANF has attempted to increase its membership of enrolled nurses. In the Australian Capital Territory and the Northern Territory, where ENs are few, they are largely members of the ANF.

Coverage by different unions of registered nurses on the one hand, and of psychiatric (mental health) nurses and enrolled nurses on the other contributed to a lack of cohesion in industrial disputes in the 1980s. This was apparent in the 1986 nurses' strike in Victoria where the HEF (now the Health Services Union of Australia, HSUA), which covered enrolled nurses, did not support the RANF (Victorian Branch) and allowed supplies to bypass picket lines, and generally acted 'in their role as spoiler' (ANF *News Release* July 1992). Demarcation disputes over coverage of nurses is a continuous feature of industrial relations in the states and dissipates resources.

The Australian Council of Trade Unions (ACTU), which is the peak, national union organisation on industrial relations policy and practice, in 1987 proposed a radical reform of the organisation of unions in Australia. The ACTU argued that for a more effective union movement there should be fewer and larger unions, which would be based on industries rather than on craft or occupation (ACTU 1987). This was endorsed at the ACTU biennial congress in 1987 and involved 'specific proposals for union amalgamations and a strategy for the reconstruction of the labour movement into seventeen broad industry groupings' (Deery & Plowman 1991:239). This was supported by the ANF delegation to the congress (Fox 1989), but it would be fair to say that that support was equivocal at best.

On the one hand, the ANF believed strongly that nurses' interests were and are best served by an organisation solely made up of nurses as a nursing industry union, rather than being part of a health industry union. On the other, it could not afford to be left out in the rush for coverage of nurses by other unions and the amalgamations which would ensue. The federal secretary argued that 'ANF...will not allow the nursing profession to be carved up by predators', and that unions such as the Federated Miscellaneous Workers' Unions (FMWU), the Australian Workers' Unions (AWU) and the Public Services Federation (PSF) 'are not organizations which can or will represent workers in the nursing industry in the future' (*ANJ* February 1991:11).

She viewed with concern moves to amalgamate the Hospital Employees Federation (HEFA) with the HREA, the FMWU with the Federated Liquor and Allied Industries Employees Union of Australia, the Victorian Mothercraft Nurses with the Allied Employees Association, and the Australian Workers Union with the Hospital Employees Union in Queensland. Any reorganisation which would confirm coverage of enrolled and psychiatric nurses outside the ANF was anathema:

> We say that psychiatric nursing is an integral and special component of the multiskilled work of nursing. Separating this out from mainstream nursing services diminishes nursing's quality and completeness. It deskills psychiatric nurses as they become more marginalised and fragmented between many unions (*ANJ* February 1991:11).

And in relation to enrolled nurses the federal secretary reaffirmed ANF policy that 'enrolled nurses are important members of nursing teams and nursing organizations'. Quoting an article in the *Financial Review*, she was obviously heartened by the ACTU's position in its overhaul of union coverage in major industry sectors that 'the Australian Nursing Federation is seen as the principal union for nurses, although there remain some issues to be negotiated over which union will cover psychiatric and enrolled nurses in some states' (*ANJ* February 1991:11).

The ANF made tentative approaches to other unions in the health industry with a view to establishing a health industry confederation and individual state branches also pursued 'association' and 'co-operation' rather than 'amalgamation' with other health unions. For example, in Victoria an agreement on matters of mutual concern was reached between the Medical Scientists and Pharmacists Association of Victoria, the Hospital Administrative Officers Association of Victoria and the Victorian Psychologists Association (*ANJ* February 1991:34). As cuts to health budgets in the states intensify, there will continue to be a need for all unions representing health sector workers to cooperate in opposing threats to health services, but it is doubtful if nursing will become subsumed under a health industry union; rather it will continue its efforts to become the nursing industry union.

A federal award for nurses: a long and tortuous path

More female than male workers have historically been covered by state unions and awards because women tend to be employed in service areas such as nursing, teaching and clerical work. The High Court had interpreted the Constitution (s.51 XXXV) to mean that employees in service areas were 'not engaged in an industry or in work of an industrial nature [so that] unions covering such occupations were not able to obtain federal awards' (Deery & Plowman 1991:98), nor to engage in industrial disputes. In 1983 the High Court interpreted 'industrial dispute' to mean 'a dispute between employees and employers about the terms and conditions of employment', which also gave access to federal awards for employees in service areas, like nursing (Deery & Plowman 1991:98).

Attempts by the RANF to gain a federal award for registered nurses brought the issue of union coverage to a head.

The RANF commenced its campaign for a federal award for regulating the wages and working conditions of nurses in August 1982, and served a federal-award log of claims on public and private sector employers throughout the country. The proceedings in the Australian Conciliation and Arbitration Commission (now the Australian Industrial Relations Commission) were then delayed for a number of years when the NSWNA and the Hospital and Research Employees Association of Australia (HREA) argued that the eligibility rule of RANF precluded RANF from creating a dispute on wages and conditions of employees who were enrolled nurses or student nurses (Kyle 1988). In 1985, the NSWNA and the HREA appealed to the full bench of the High Court after their appeal to the commission had been dismissed. In 1986, this application was also dismissed. The Hospital Employees Federation of Australia (HEFA) which covered enrolled nurses had applied for a federal award for nurses in 1984. Thus the stage was set for what Kyle (1988:21) described as the 'long and tortuous path of a Federal Award for nurses'.

The RANF was committed to 'the view that nurses performing the same work, utilizing the same skills, having been subject to similar educational preparation and similar licensing requirements should not be subject to dissimilar rates of pay and conditions of work' (Kyle 1988:21), irrespective of the state or territory in which they happened to work. Pursued by the RANF with support from most of the states and territories, access to a federal award for registered nurses was achieved piecemeal throughout Australia during the 1980s and into the 1990s, so that by 1992 only NSW and Victoria remained under state awards.

In New South Wales, where the cost of living is higher than elsewhere in Australia, the NSWNA/ANF (NSW Branch) has been consistently opposed to a federal award. Its General Secretary, Patricia Staunton, explained why NSW was opposed to a federal award which on the face of it appeared rational:

> The general attitude to industrial relations [of the ANF] was that they could be described as the Girl Guides of the industrial relations arena. They rushed around making all sorts of pious statements with no thought given to industrial outcomes... There was a statement by the ANF that there should be...one rate of pay for nurses in Australia. That the nurse in Western Australia should earn the same amount of money as a nurse in Queensland and a nurse in Tasmania.
>
> That statement has almost alarming simplicity in its attractiveness... The Federation embraced that view with not one iota of consideration about what it meant industrially... If you want one rate of pay for nurses in Australia, you can have it, but you'll have it at a cost [which is] the lowest common denominator outcome. [PS/90]

She argued that this would not be confined to rates of pay but to conditions of employment as well. This view was supported by Fox (1989) who believed that the ANF was making a mistake by pursuing a federal award, which would ultimately reduce its bargaining power by creating a monopoly in a single tribunal (the federal tribunal) which would decide on all award rates. Nurses would 'have lost the important tactical advantage of playing one tribunal off against another to get improved benefits for nurses' (Fox 1989:4). Further, once a federal award was in place it could only be reversed by the federal tribunal itself, as under the Australian federal system, federal laws take precedence over state laws.

In 1988, although opposed by the then state secretary of the Victorian Branch of the RANF, Victorian nurses voted to support a federal award and it appeared that NSW would be the only state to remain outside. Indeed, harmonisation of the NSWNA and the RANF (NSW Branch) had depended in part on NSW being allowed to maintain a state award.

In Western Australia, the ANF in 1990 and 1991 sought a federal award for psychiatric nurses which was opposed by the Western Australian Psychiatric Nurses Association, the HEFA and the FMWU. Similarly in South Australia the FMWU opposed the ANF's federal award application for psychiatric nurses. At the same time, applications by the ANF in both these states for a federal award for enrolled nurses were objected to by the State Public Services Federation, the FMWU and the HEFA (*ANJ* February 1991:11-12). The conflict however has more to do with which union or unions should represent nurses than with the achievement of federal awards per se.

By 1991, with the decision by the Australian Industrial Relations Commission to refuse the Queensland Government's objection to a federal award for public sector nurses in Queensland, most nurses in Western Australia, South Australia, Tasmania, the Australian Capital Territory and the Northern Territory had achieved a federal award, that is that they would be under one federal tribunal.

The achievement of a federal award for Victorian registered nurses became critical in October 1992 when the newly elected Victorian Liberal Government set in train industrial reforms based on individual employee contracts with employers and the eventual overturning of the centralised award system for determining wages and conditions.

The Victorian Branch of the ANF moved quickly to further federal jurisdiction over award rates, and joined with 200 000 other workers on 10 November 1992 in a one day strike and march in city centres across Victoria to protest Liberal Premier Kennett's 'reform' of industrial relations with its emphasis on individual employee/employer contracts and the removal of the central award fixing system from 1 March 1993.

On 16 July 1992 the Australian Industrial Relations Commission had handed down its favourable decision on the ANF's application for a federal award for public and private sector Victorian nurses. This decision entitled the ANF to a federal award for registered nurses and excluded the Health Services Union of Australia (HSUA formerly the HEF) from covering registered nurses in Victoria. State enrolled nurses would be entitled to be covered under a federal award by either ANF or HSUA. The deputy president of the commission in making his decision referred to the role of the ANF as a professional and industrial organisation and said:

> Having considered carefully all of the evidence about the ANF's professionalism, I am satisfied that much of it does reflect a goal of enhancing the benefit which the community derives from nurses' services... The professional activities of the ANF, especially at the national level but to some degree also at the Branch level, are impressive (quoted *ANJ* September 1992:7).

ANF then requested that the HSUA should be excluded from access to the award for all registered nurses, including psychiatric nurses. HSUA appealed in an attempt to stop implementation of the commission's decision, but agreement to withdraw this appeal was reached in October 1992. Implementation was further delayed by opposition from the Victorian Government and from employers. The Victorian Employers' Chamber of Commerce and Industry, the Victorian Hospital Association, the Australian Chamber of Manufactures and the government argued in essence that the case should be delayed because of the new Victorian industrial legislation. The Victorian Government then took the case to the High Court to postpone the implementation of a federal award until the possible election of a Liberal/National coalition government at the federal level in March 1993, when, if this occurred, all federal awards would be replaced by individual or collective enterprise contracts (*ANJ* December/January 1993:10). The commission upheld its previous decision and decided that a federal award should take effect from 23 December 1992, but that employers should be given the opportunity in 1993 to argue again that the award should not be made. In March 1993, the High Court dismissed the Victorian Government's appeal, and the federal Labor Government was re-elected, not least because of a lack of public support for the opposition's industrial relations policies.

The participation of nurses in the one-day general strike in Victoria in November 1992, which included the issue of a federal award for other public sector workers as well as nurses, was reminiscent of industrial activity in 1986. This time not only nurses but the health system as a whole was under threat. The federal ANF, recognising the seriousness of the situation in Victoria, and of proposed changes should a Liberal/National Party coalition be elected federally, issued a special edition of the ANJ covering industrial issues (December/January 1993). It reported that thousands of nurses from metropolitan and country hospitals, community health centres, maternal and child health nurses and students of nursing had joined the Victorian strike to protest legislative changes, including massive budget cuts to the health sector, the loss of the protection of the award system and the erosion of a uniform career, the dismantling of WorkCare, and the loss of minimum staffing levels contained in current Victorian nursing awards. A mass meeting of ANF (Victorian Branch) members on 25 November voted for a campaign of rolling bans in metropolitan and regional centres, including bans on elective admissions, and to hold rallies outside the offices of members of parliament.

The situation in Victoria from October 1992 and the nursing response means that the political and industrial activity of nurses in the 1980s cannot be seen as an aberration, and that the increased sophistication and experience gained will be necessary for the 1990s if nurses are to maintain their overdue recognition in the health and education systems.

A decade of achievement

The 1980s can be seen as a decade of achievement for nurses where issues which had been simmering for the previous two decades came to the boil. The achievements came about through the combined efforts of organised nursing, that is through the organisations which represent nursing professionally and industrially. The campaigns in the 1980s have made gains for nursing throughout Australia, both in terms of improvements in salaries and professional recognition through concerted political and industrial action. It must not however be taken as a complete catalogue of all that was happening in nursing, nor indeed of all the organisations which represent nurses. For example, the Royal College of Nursing, Australia, and the Florence Nightingale Committee of Australia were active in nursing education and research, and in other professional concerns, often working in conjunction with the ANF. Nor must the special interest groups within nursing organisations, which collectively attempt to improve both the conditions in which nursing work takes place and the health status of the community, be forgotten.

There appeared to have been considerable recognition of the coming together of industrial and professional concerns and the linkage of these conceptually. It is difficult to know however whether this is widespread; whether it is confined to the nursing leadership or whether it has been accepted by the membership. The ANF is very much aware of the need to strike a balance between industrial and professional activity, particularly in response to members' reactions to the unprecedented and often traumatic events in the 1980s.

That organised nursing is now stronger and more united is undoubted. The ANF through its state branches and nationally can now legitimately claim to represent registered nursing in Australia. Organised nursing would be helpless without the support of its membership, as we have seen, not least from membership dues which buy in the expertise of its permanent staff. If the leadership becomes separated from its membership, support declines and has to be rebuilt. This distracts the organisation from acting on behalf of its members and dissipates energy for more useful activities.

Nursing organisations have now developed their internal infrastructure and expertise, and have gained substantial political and industrial skills. They will need all these to provide them with the strength to withstand the budgetary, structural, and managerial onslaughts with which they will be faced in the health system. Nursing in the 1990s has lost a key source of the political influence which it was able to use in the 1980s. There is no longer a shortage of nurses but a surplus, in part as a result of funding reductions. It therefore becomes even more imperative that the ANF should gain control of nursing as a whole, or it will be undercut by less qualified staff. In this it is thwarted by other equally determined industrial organisations. Demarcation is often the most hotly contested and vicious aspect of industrial disputation.

The entire wage-fixing system for all Australian employees is itself in the process of fundamental change. In 1988 the Secretary of the ACTU revealed details of award restructuring which would provide a two-tier system for wage increases. The first tier would provide for fixed wage increases but the second tier would be dependent on establishing improvements in productivity. As opposed to workers in manufacturing industry, it is difficult for workers in service industries like nursing to establish measures of structural efficiency and productivity. The changes were intended also to remove rigid job demarcation and to provide for multiskilling and retraining (*The Age*, 2 December 1988). The ACTU has maintained a commitment to centralised wage fixing through 'National Wage Case determinations, but ACTU strategy includes also enterprise agreements ratified by the [federal] Commission as part of its incomes agreement...with government' (Simms & Singleton 1993:291–292).

Organised nursing has demonstrated that it can negotiate the complex industrial and political processes involved in improved wages and conditions. Nurses have shown that they can act collectively and that cohesion is possible. This must be maintained in the future as conflict is unfortunately the reality, but traditions within nursing have not and should not disappear. As the secretary of the ANF (Victorian Branch) said:

> I don't think you can take away the effect of the women's movement on the advancement of nurses... Nurses today are more articulate and more assertive, just as professional, just as caring for their patients. The fact that they don't have the corners of the bed folded as exactly as we were taught [has been] replaced with more appropriate care.
>
> The way I describe what nursing is...is when you walk into a hospital, and you see this young girl...hurtling...down the corridor and she sees old Mr. Smith sort of struggling along in his hospital pyjamas and they are falling down and his bum's bare, and as she races past with the injection tray in her hand, she manages to pull his pants up, do them up, say 'How're you going Mr. Smith?' He's not even aware of what she's done and she's off, and that to me is what it's about. And they still do that. [BM/93]

Note: The sections in this chapter, 'A more radical leadership' and 'Disenchantment', is a revised version of the paper by Brigid McCoppin, 'Two experiments in radicalism', in Proceedings of the 12th National Conference, Royal College of Nursing, Australia, Sydney, May 1990.

They are reproduced here by kind permission of the RCNA.

1. The Royal Australian Nursing Federation became the Australian Nursing Federation (ANF) in 1989. The abbreviations RANF and ANF are used as appropriate to the time.
2. The Queensland Nurses' Union becomes the main union representing nurses in Queensland when it had broken away from the RANF in 1982.

REFERENCES

Amos J J 1984 Tasmania: parliamentary debates. 28 March:189

Anderson P T 1987 New South Wales: parliamentary debates. 14 May:12265

Arch M, Graetz B 1989 Work satisfaction, unionism and militancy among nurses. Community Health Studies XIII(2):172-175

Arnold S 1988 Bolger vows to fight on after nursing election rebuff. The Age 21 November

Australian Institute of Health 1988 Australia's health. AGPS, Canberra

Australian Medical Association 1985 Policies of the Australian Medical Association and Directory for 1985-86. Australian Medical Association, Glebe

Barratt P D 1975 Letter to the editor. The Age 7 April

Beaumont M 1988 Learning about 'Qualys'. Australian Nurses Journal 17(11):16

Beaumont M 1989 The professional role of a national nursing association. In: Gray G, Pratt R (eds) Issues in Australian nursing 2. Churchill Livingstone, Melbourne

Bessant J, Bessant B 1991 The growth of a profession: nursing in Victoria 1940s-1980s. La Trobe University Press, Bundoora

Bessant J, D'Cruz J V 1989 When nurses and teachers strike: public perceptions of 'the betrayal'. Australian Journal of Advanced Nursing 6(3):26-33

Bolger I 1988 Australia reconstructed: a personal view. Arena 83:160

Bonawit V 1989 The image of the nurse: the community's perception and its implications for the profession. In: Gray G, Pratt R (eds) Issues in Australian nursing 2. Churchill Livingstone, Melbourne

Bonner R 1987 Private sector breakthrough. Australian Nurses Journal Vol 16(9) April:14-15

Borthwick W A 1966 Victoria: parliamentary debates. 22 March: 2949

Boyd J C 1983 New South Wales: parliamentary debates. 19 October:1897

Brereton L 1983 New South Wales: parliamentary debates. 8 November:2643

Brown C, Everill S 1987 Running out of patience. AFI, Australia Video

Cadzow J 1983 The rebellion of the handmaidens. The Weekend Australian 28-29 May

Casey A 1987 Divided left the casualty as conservatives sweep nurses' election. Sydney Morning Herald 19 June

Christenson R M, Engel A S, Jacobs D N, Rejai M, Waltzer H 1981 Ideologies and modern politics, 3rd edn. Harper & Row, New York

Cochrane J 1989 Influencing the politics of health reform. In Gray G, Pratt R (eds) Issues in Autralian Nursing 2. Churchill Livingstone, Melbourne

Considine M 1992 Policy: managed or expert? In: Gardner H (ed) Health policy: development, implementation and evaluation in Australia. Churchill Livingstone, Melbourne

Collins P 1987 New South Wales: parliamentary debates. 14 May: 12263-64

Crabtree W F 1962 New South Wales: parliamentary debates. 6 September 1962:204

Cruikshank M 1987 Some issue that should be considered by those attending tonight's fund-raiser (leaflet from Nurses' Reform Group). 15 March, Sydney

Curlewis R 1991 Oral history conference. Brisbane

Davis M 1987 Nurses, unions and the arbitration system. Australian Society 7(2):14-16

Davis M 1988 Bolger loses key vote on federal industrial award. The Age 16 September

Davis M 1989 Nurses' ballot gives Bolger hope. The Age 14 October

Debelle P 1988 Sick, and tired of gossip, Irene talks. The Herald 17 October

Deery S, Plowman D 1985 Australian industrial relations, 2nd edn. McGraw-Hill, Sydney

Deery S, Plowman D 1991 Australian industrial relations, 3rd edn. McGraw-Hill, Sydney

Delamothe T 1988 Nursing grievances I: voting with their feet. British Medical Journal 296:6614, 25

Dickenson M 1975 Nurses and their unions. The Lamp 32(4):11-12

Donohoe B 1987 Nurses' strike fund in order, says Bolger. The Age 19 August

Fatin W 1983 Australian nurses and politics (or power's OK). College of Nursing, Australia and the NSW College of Nursing Joint Conference, Sydney 21-22 November

Fox C 1985 The non-nursing duties dispute. Carol Fox, Melbourne

Fox C 1989 A federal award for nurses: salvation or folly? Carol Fox, Melbourne

Fox C 1991 Enough is enough: the 1986 Victorian nurses strike. Australian Studies in Health Service Administration No 43. The University of New South Wales, School of Health Services Management, Kensington

Fox C 1992 Tribunal policy and dispute settlement: the nurse's case 1986/87. Management Paper No 41, August. Graduate School of Management, Monash University, Melbourne

Freidson E 1970 Profession of medicine. Harper & Row, New York
Freidson E 1974 Dominant professions, bureaucracy and client services. In: Hasenfeld Y, English R A (eds) Human service organizations. University of Michigan Press, Ann Arbor
Gamarnikow K E 1978 Sexual division of labour: the case of nursing. In: Kuhn A, Wolpe A M (eds) Feminism and materialism: women and modes of production. Routledge & Kegan Paul, London
Game A, Pringle R 1983 Gender at work. George Allen & Unwin, Sydney
Gardner H, Barraclough S 1992 The policy process. In: Gardner H (ed) Health policy: development, implementation and evaluation in Australia. Churchill Livingstone, Melbourne
Gardner H, McCoppin B 1986 Vocation, career or both? Politicization of Australian nurses, Victoria 1984-1986. The Australian Journal of Advanced Nursing Vol 4(1) September-November: 25-35
Gardner H, McCoppin B 1987 The politicisation of Australian nurses: Victoria 1984-1986. Politics 22(1):19-34
Gardner H, McCoppin B 1989 Emerging militancy? The politicisation of Australian allied health professionals. In: Gardner H (ed) The politics of health: the Australian experience. Churchill Livingstone, Melbourne
Gavin N 1989 The missing link. Nursing Times 85(1):62-63
Grant C, Lapsley H 1988 The Australian health care system 1987. University of New South Wales, Sydney
Grant C, Lapsley H 1991 The Australian health care system. Australian Studies in Health Service Administration No 74. The University of New South Wales, School of Health Services Management, Kensington
Haines J 1987 A personal statement by Jenny Haines, General Secretary of the NSW Nurses' Association about the recent allegations in the NSW Parliament, daily newspapers and the weekly Tribune alleging that National Action and racists have infiltrated the offices of the NSW Nurses Association. 8 April, Sydney
Hatton J E 1985 New South Wales: parliamentary debates. 23 October: 8569
Henlen M V 1975 Editorial. The Lamp 32 July: 3
Henn G G 1968 Western Australia: parliamentary debates. 10 October: 1645
Higgins E 1989 Staunton tests unions' equality policies. The Australian 10 March
Holding C 1975 Victoria: Parliamentary Debates. 26 March: 4628, 7 May: 6140
Innes P 1989 Bolger victorious as union reinstates her as member. The Age 5 August
Jenkins D H 1964 Victoria: parliamentary debates. 9 December: 2461-2462
Keneally G F 1984 South Australia: parliamentary debates. 5 December: 2190
Kyle F 1987 Victorian nurses strike. Scarlet woman. Issue 23:3-6
Kyle F 1988 The tortuous path of the federal award. Australian Nurses Journal Vol 17 (8) March: 21
Larriera A 1987 High passions in nurses' poll. Sydney Morning Herald. 26 May
Landa D P 1980 New South Wales: parliamentary debates. 24 September: 1403
Lansbury R D 1980 White-collar and professional employees in Australia: reluctant militants in retreat? In: Ford G W, Hearn J M, Lansbury R D (eds) Australian labour relations: readings, 3rd edn. Macmillan, Melbourne
Law G 1980 I have never liked trade unionism. In: Windschuttle E (ed) Women, class and history. Fontana, Melbourne
Manning W A 1968 Western Australia: parliamentary debates. 10 October: 1643
Marles F 1988 Report of the study of professional issues in nursing. Government Printer, Melbourne
McCoppin 1989 The use and abuse of industrial power. In: Gray G, Pratt R (eds) Issues in Australian nursing 2. Churchill Livingstone, Melbourne
McClelland J E 1985 Report of the Committee of Enquiry into Nursing in Victoria, Vol 1. Department of Health, Victoria
Muetzelfeldt M 1992 Economic rationalism in its social context. In: Muetzelfeldt M (ed) Society, state and politics in Australia. Pluto Press/Deakin University, Leichhardt
Muff J (ed) 1982 Socialization, sexism and stereotyping; women's issues in nursing. Mosby, St. Louis
Oakley A 1984 What price professionalism? The importance of being a nurse. Nursing Times 12:24-27

Patten M E 1976 The role of the RANF. Australian Nurses Journal 5(12): 37
Pfeffer J 1981 Power in organizations. Pitman, Boston
Rawson D W 1978 Unions and unionists in Australia. George, Allen & Unwin, Sydney
Reddy M 1988 Embattled Bolger to fight for her position, seek electoral change. The Age 22 August
Rimmer S M 1991 Occupational segregation, earnings differential and status among Australian workers. The Economic Record 67(198)September:205-2165
Robbins S 1989 Organizational behaviour: concepts, controversies, and applications, 4th edn. Prentice-Hall, Englewood Cliffs
Salvage J 1985 The politics of nursing. Heinemann Nursing, London
Shils E 1968 Ideology: the concept and function of ideology. In: Sills D (ed) 1968 International Encyclopedia of the social sciences, Vol 7. Macmillan-Free Press, New York
Silver M 1989 Career structure for nurses: the South Australian experience. In: Gray G, Pratt R (eds) Issues in Australian nursing 2. Churchill Livingstone, Melbourne
Simms M, Singleton G 1993 Trade unions. In: Smith R (ed) Politics in Australia, 2nd edn. Allen & Unwin, Sydney
Speedy S 1987 Feminism and the professionalization of nursing. The Australian Journal of Advanced Nursing Vol 4(2) December 1986-February 1987: 20-28
Taylor J 1983 Nurse asked to explain. Sydney Morning Herald 24 February
Townsend P 1981 The structured dependency of the elderly: a creation of social policy in the twentieth century. Ageing and Society, Vol 1:5-28
Williams C 1988 Blue, white and pink collar workers. Allen & Unwin, Sydney
Willis E 1990 Medical dominance, revised edn. Allen & Unwin, Sydney

7. Living with reality

Australian nurses have achieved much in the last 30 years, often as a result of their own effort and determination, but also because they were carried along by social and political change. The advent of the binary education system in the 1960s opened the way to tertiary education for a few, then for all nurses, while its demise in the late 1980s put nurses in the universities. But their work in promoting education had prepared them for this opportunity, and their developing political skills enabled them to seize it. Nursing students now receive an education comparable with (though still not equal to) that of other health occupations. Nurses have also made themselves part (though again, not yet an equal part) of the decision making structure in their workplaces. The rise of the women's movement in the 1970s forced government and management to accept advances towards equal opportunity for women workers, and the presence of Labor governments in most states and federally in the 1980s brought a relatively sympathetic hearing for women's issues. Nurses have built on these changes, and through sustained political and industrial action they have achieved improvements in rates of pay and working conditions which have implications not only for wage justice and comparability with other health workers, but also for their recognition as equal colleagues in the health sector. They have unified their associations into a national body, and public policy makers are beginning to listen to them.

These achievements are interdependent: the education transfer campaign forged a political alliance and taught many nurses how to act effectively in the policy arena; the added status attaching to tertiary graduates should support and reinforce the gains of hospital trained nurses who have made themselves heard in the workplace; and the unity of their major association, the Australian Nursing Federation (ANF), builds on the demonstrated industrial strength of its various state branches, giving nurses a channel of power for making their policy preferences known. An older nurse who has witnessed these changes comments:

> Nursing has achieved a great deal. It's come a long way in the last 10 years, the progress has been quite incredible. Sometimes you get depressed and think it's still a long way to go, but when you look back and see how far we've come...five or ten years ago we were struggling for a degree, and here we are

setting up units for Ph.D. studies and Master's studies—it's just marvellous! So it's not going to go back, but...nurses really will have to stick together...[MP/88]

A former secretary of the British Royal College of Nursing (RCN) believes that 'the prerequisite for effective political participation by a profession is the ability to speak with one voice in public' (Clay 1989). Behind the public voice however there must be nurses who understand the issues and support the position their representatives take, otherwise nursing's impact on health policy will be reduced (Meppem 1991).

There is some agreement that nurses should figure prominently in the health policy arena. According to a senior WA nurse:

> Our greatest strength and a source of exploitation is the fact that we are the largest, most diverse and eclectic group in the health care system...and [are] arguably very cost-effective, multi-skilled flexible providers of health care services. But, [she warns] it is not sufficient just "being there"; there is increasing pressure to demonstrate what difference our activities make (*ANJ* 1991 April:22).

The paradox of nursing today, a British nurse believes, is that although nurses form the largest part of the workforce of a major public sector service industry and, owing to the growing political skill of their associations, have a higher profile than ever, neither doctors nor lay managers, let alone the public, have much insight into or knowledge of current nursing issues. These remain invisible to 'everyone except nurses' (Robinson 1989). In addition, many nurses fail to see their work within a broad policy framework, so nursing looks inwards, preoccupied with its own affairs, while doctors and others stay on the outside 'unable or unwilling' to understand (Robinson 1992). And many nurses still 'fail to question who holds or acquires power, and underestimate their own potential power as a group' (Jolley 1989). These comments suggest that they are not making an essential connection between 'nursing policy' (policy about nursing) and 'health policy'—the broader framework within which nursing should play an influential part. The two cannot be separated: the content of nursing policy will shape the kinds of health policy that nurses decide they want, and health policy (and beyond it, social conditions and policy in general) at any particular time will affect the developments that may be possible in nursing.

An American nurse regrets that US nursing, less united than Australian, has failed to mobilise its collective strength to pursue the ideal of better health care for all (Moloney 1986:268). A New South Wales nurse who took part in the education transfer campaign thinks that failure to maintain such a policy goal would be to abandon the campaign's ultimate aim:

> I believe that the whole move in nursing education from the 1970s...was predicated on the need for a better health care system. I think we've lost sight of that somewhere along the line...[KM/89]

A former federal Minister for Health has observed that nurses 'have a very clear idea of the health policy they want' (Howe 1993). In contrast to its earlier tendency to lobby and send submissions on policies which had already been promulgated by government or the parties, the ANF in 1993 published its own health policy, sending it for comment to the major political parties before the impending federal election. The ANF (1993) believes that nurses are 'uniquely placed' to understand the health system and health policy, and that their considerable contribution to health services entitles them to exercise an influence on health policy making. But the 'invisible' nature of nursing work, and nurses' continuing perception of themselves as relatively powerless will make it difficult for them to move towards not just valuing this contribution themselves, but persuading others to do so—especially those who control funding, whether government or private. This problem has worried older nurses: 'The origins and maintenance of the feelings of powerlessness among nurses of all ages...I do not think it's all gender and professional status related. We sure need a new self-image' (Slater 1988); and beyond that, a determination to make that new image (of a powerful and expert occupation) widely known.

Still in the profession trap

Nurses as a group are more influential than they were in 1960, but in Australia there are regular criticisms of their lack of assertiveness: for example, of their 'unquestioned, accepted understandings of what constitutes nursing' and 'uncritical adoption of the language of professionalisation' (Bruni 1991). This uncritical acceptance of received 'truths' accompanies a failure to analyse what power nurses have as a group and how they might mobilise it. They need to look beyond the immediate workplace to examine existing power relations, such as those between doctors and themselves, relations which shape their understanding of society and of health care (Bruni 1991). The power disparity between doctors and nurses is still considerable, a further reason for nurses to examine it realistically. A Victorian nurse describes one of its effects:

> I can go to [the doctors] with a case about a particular patient. I might particularly want some treatment started or stopped...I might have an extensive discussion with the family and with the patient, and I might have a good case that is well thought out...[Now] I don't expect that they will roll over and play dead just because I've asked them to do something...But they can look at my evidence, throw it out of the window and say no, and walk off without a discussion or a debate—and the system will support them still. [AH/92]

The system supports them because medicine holds a legally sanctioned monopoly over central tasks like diagnosis and prescription, a monopoly which has given doctors an institutionalised position of occupational ascendancy that has remained unchallenged even though, as many nurses know, it produces obvious 'fictions' in the doctor-nurse relationship. What is theoretically professional power resting on superior (but fallible) expertise has become in practice quasi-bureaucratic power based on domination of an occupational hierarchy (Freidson 1974). At the same time, there is said to be little supporting evidence in Australia for the 'implicit assumption' that colleague relations and a team approach will improve the quality of patient care (Kenny & Adamson 1992).

Nursing theory has also come under critical appraisal in Australia. Nursing theorists have ignored Marxism, one critic points out—a surprising oversight given the past history of oppression and the new interest in the politics of nursing (Holmes 1991). A consequence of this is that contemporary theory has a major weakness: 'The complete failure to acknowledge nursing's socio-historical embeddedness, and to articulate any political position, never mind construct any specific political program'; and this failure is the result of the pervasive influence of the US nurse theorists, says Holmes, since 'the phenomenological and humanistic philosophies of Paterson and Zderad, Watson and Benner, are products of the fierce individualism ("you are what you make yourself") which underpins the political conservatism of the United States' (Holmes 1991). But if Australian nurses have taken up these theorists, a local nurse academic sees cultural and political differences in Australia which may rule out a general adoption of their conservative ideology:

> I think in this country—and I really do believe this independently of whether we've got a Labor government or a Liberal government—this culture demands a strong social base. We believe in social equity. We believe it's right that everybody should have access to the health care system. We only argue at the margins. [JP/90]

The past stand of nurses against the 'user pays' principle in health services and their publicly stated preference for universal access to health care support this belief. These political preferences can inform the debate on theory, expanding it beyond the 'patient as person' framework often favoured by the theorists. And they may encourage nurses to use research 'to serve those that are exploited and dominated', rather than to dominate others or to legitimate existing élites (Lumby 1991).

Australian nurses may develop a relatively egalitarian approach in their theory and research, but a British nurse advises them to avoid some of the features of what is now called 'New Nursing', the product of the US and British movements in the 1970s and 1980s which developed round an interest in nursing theory. The centrepiece of the ideology of New Nursing is the nurse-patient relationship, especially the idea of a partnership between nurse and patient, most often seen in the method of practice known as 'primary nursing' (Salvage 1992). Yet the reality of past practice has been that, despite the professional rhetoric about putting patients first, many nurses saw their major function as assisting and supporting the doctor (Buckenham & McGrath 1983:64). New Nursing, Salvage thinks, is in fact an occupational strategy for seeking higher status, rewards and power for nurses. Its leaders, she thinks, should 'guard against the seductive assumption that empowering nurses is the route to empowering patients', or that raising the status of nursing will in itself benefit patients, while they avoid awkward issues such as the impact of the division of labour and gender relations (Salvage 1992).

To avoid the implications of gender relations and of the division of labour for nursing practice is to deny the reality of class and sexual oppression. The ANF federal secretary regrets the reluctance of some nurses to see the political dimensions of their work:

> I think that there are not enough nurses who join in the public debate *as nurses*...[For example] they might be an administrator of a centre...there are so many of those who say 'I was a nurse once' to me...They don't say 'I am a nurse and as a nurse my view is'—there isn't enough of that...I think we have to generate a very strong sense that there's a career in being a political advocate for nursing. [MB/92]

While continual political activism is neither usual nor necessarily desirable its opposite is not the apathy that stems from ignorance and feelings of powerlessness. A South Australian nurse worries about that sort of apathy:

> The Miscellaneous Workers' Union had an organiser...I think she was pretty bloody wonderful. She always said that apathy is institutionalised powerlessness. And that's the big enemy for women, for nurses...and it's a whole range of things that cause that, but what's the most effective way of dealing with it? Very difficult. [LS/88]

And a Victorian nurse thinks that in the past some rank and file union members naively overestimated the power of their branch secretary:

> A lot of people don't see that she's an instrument of the union...the average union member doesn't see that. They see Irene [Bolger, ANF state secretary 1986–1989] telling us what to do, and that's not the job of a union secretary. Until they have a perception that Irene can be actually extremely well controlled by a strong Council and a much stronger membership, things won't change. [HV/88]

The changed style of union leadership since the turbulent period of the 1980s should enable union members to see this more clearly. The leadership now tends to be neither 'matriarchal' as in the days of the matrons, nor politically extremist.

Power to the managers

From 1974 to 1984 British nurses occupied senior administrative positions on a par with those of doctors and general administrators, but although some showed themselves to be excellent managers, on the whole they had not been adequately prepared for their new responsibilities. Serious doubts emerged: 'Some nurses were promoted to management simply because they were good nurses—"Manage a unit? She couldn't run a bath!"'. The National

Health Service (NHS) was reorganised as a consequence of the 1983 Griffiths report. Griffiths, the senior executive of a supermarket chain, recommended 'the assertion of central, managerial control, using the full panoply of modern business methods' to replace the previous occupational, especially medical, control of the health service. This 'managerialist' advice usually accompanies an ideological belief in free market forces as the major determinant of social relations. Central to the new system were devolution of decision making authority to the clinical unit with an accompanying accountability for resource management. The evidence a few years later seemed to show however that the new system had not solved the problem of controlling doctors and had left the lay general manager needing advice and guidance from the clinicians, nursing and medical (Strong & Robinson 1988:48 et seq).

Management, being full of uncertainties, is affected by imported (especially US) fads and fashions, and some Australian health care institutions have recently adopted a US and British organisation design which does away with the old tripartite functional structure (medical, nursing, administrative) in hospitals. Tripartite management left the three staff agglomerations relatively independent but failed to integrate them into a co-ordinated service. With the change to a structure of clinical teams under medical supervision, a senior management position may no longer be designated 'director of nursing' and may have no line (direct) authority over clinical nurses, only staff (advisory) authority. One leading nurse thinks that for nurses to give up positions labelled 'nursing' reveals an occupational inferiority complex:

> There's almost an embarrassment among some nurses at [senior] level that they don't want to be seen as nurses any more. They want to be seen as part of this top high-flying participative management team, and 'If you don't call me a nurse, then that's terrific, because I can take my place along with the rest as the Director of Corporate Services', or whatever. That's a shame...[PS/90]

But another sees a two-fold potential in such positions:

> I think the development of nursing, and...the broadening of nursing education will see a lot more nurses in positions that have nothing to do with nursing, but rely on [a nursing] core educational base...and that can only be to nursing's benefit. To have us in the system of management of *health* has to help health. [JH/89]

These two apparently irreconcilable views will need further debate. On the one hand nurses could lose the advantage of having senior positions which cannot be filled by another occupation. On the other, they may gain wider influence over health services as a whole.

A senior New South Wales nurse recognises that there are 'many people who believe that nurses are not required in the top management positions', but she maintains that nurses must remain accountable to nurses (Meppem 1991). The ANF agrees with the principle of devolution of decision making to the clinical unit, but opposes any attempt to remove the director of nursing's job from line responsibility to a merely advisory position (Parkes 1991). This would remove her accountability for the standard of nursing care and her ability to provide 'a single voice for the total nursing service at executive level'; and keeping line authority for the director of nursing does not equate with centralised decision making (ANF 1991)—though it has at least the potential for reviving the old authoritarian hierarchy. Those promoting these structural changes often cite the advent of casemix funding as their reason, though this by itself does not necessarily entail a particular kind of hospital structure and certainly not medical control of the clinical unit (ANF 1991). A psychiatric nurse describes a hospital dispute over this question, where the ANF position on the line authority of the director of nursing was upheld:

> The doctors were saying 'All the nurses will report to us', and senior nurses were saying 'No, no, no! I'm a nurse and I'll report to the Director of Nursing'. Not clinically; it's administratively, it's executive responsibilities. [EC/91]

This comment makes a useful distinction: the nurse is seen to have full responsibility for her clinical decision making (with reference of course to medical orders) and cedes to the director of nursing only the final administrative authority, though this will still leave some 'grey areas' where decisions are a mixture of both. The ANF (1991) believes that nurses must insist on being consulted before any organisational changes are implemented, but the Victorian Branch secretary is phlegmatic about this latest fashion in hospital management:

> We tend to be doing a bit of rearguard action...It really depends whether we manage to hold the breach long enough until there's a change. It's really management flavour of the month. Let's wait and see what the next one is, and if we can stop that being implemented long enough for them to have found some other new thing. [BM/93]

Nurses in the free marketplace

A circumstance affecting nurses in the future is likely to be continuing reductions in government funding for health services. Australian nurses as usual face this in common with their colleagues elsewhere. The British (Conservative) Government's 'market style' changes to the previously sacrosanct NHS, designed to restrain costs, have been attacked by the RCN with 'a ferocity which famously brought one minister close to tears', and RCN president June Clark has declared: 'We have to work with every democratically elected government but we do not have to support political ideologies which conflict with our values' (Limb 1992). For the RCN this was a partisan statement in that it was critical of the government's free market ideology. Such an ideology accompanies 'managerialist' theories such as those of Griffiths (above) which advocate introducing private sector business practices into the public sector, not all of which may be appropriate. British nurses are reported to have borne an increased workload with diminishing resources as part of 'plans to increase productivity and to reduce "inefficiency"' but the plans have been implemented with little thought of the effect on nurses, and their views have been ignored (Delamothe 1988a). An example of this is cited in an Audit Commission report which found that NHS staff have been forced to produce statistics for managers, but that the 'expensive computer systems' installed to support this allowed little consideration for the way nurses work; nurses were therefore 'unenthusiastic' about using the computers since they found that this 'produced more work for them but showed no obvious benefit for patients' (Watts 1992).

Australian nurses may also have to adapt, if not to a market oriented health service such as New Zealand is developing, at least to one which will continue to suffer restricted funding. This will be particularly difficult for a workforce which has traditionally looked to government for jobs and pay. Nursing unions when they have contemplated exercising political influence have usually thought almost exclusively about influencing governments, especially given Australia's centralised wage fixing system. But even Labor governments adopt free market ideas such as privatisation, and at least one (Liberal) state government is considering the British 'internal market' system for health care, which is designed to control costs. The ANF (Victorian Branch) secretary has reservations about this scheme:

> That really worries me...it seems to me that it is just about the ultimate step in putting health care on an economic rather than a care basis. But if somebody can do your hip transplants cheaper than the hospital up the road, I want to know why and I would say that nine times out of ten it's because of a reduction of some sort of care and it's probably nursing care. [BM/93]

The federal (Labor) government is also encouraging decentralised, workplace (or enterprise) bargaining for workers, though unlike the Coalition parties it retains a prominent place for unions in the process. This trend has been evident since the introduction in 1987 of the 'two tier' system of wage fixing. Further, the ANF still sees itself as a craft union, which may make it difficult to adjust to the future emphasis on large industry unions. The federal secretary believes her members like to have elected officials who have had the same work experience as themselves, and that this helps to maintain ANF strength at a time of waning influence for unions in general:

> We read about this research which has been done on the declining number of people belonging to unions, but our membership growth is constant and consistent across the country, and our services are geared to meeting our craft orientation members' needs—and quite deliberately so...they recognise that [their union representatives] have had experience doing the work they're doing...so it's really a sense of connection there...[MB/92]

Who will nurse the sick in 2000?

In Australia the education of the SEN varies between the states. Western Australia and New South Wales educate their SENs in TAFE, though New South Wales reports declining numbers working in the public hospitals (Hyland 1991), while Victoria seems to have retreated from the idea of improving SEN education and the (Coalition) state government has closed the Melbourne school which was running a new 'pilot' program with extended theory hours. In Tasmania, the SENs (or TANs, Tasmanian auxiliary nurses, as they prefer to be called) do an 18 month two stage program which in 1989 replaced a two-year course. The possibility of transferring the course to the further education sector is 'being explored' (*ANJ* 1991 February:26-27). British nursing authorities have decided to eliminate the SEN and augment the registered nurse (RN) workforce by introducing a briefly trained 'support worker' in what will then be a different kind of 'two tier' nursing structure.

A major problem for the RN is that her functions overlap with those of the SEN. Although in theory she supervises the SEN's work, in practice the 'process orientation of nursing work, as well as the team structure within which it occurs, militates against appropriate supervision'. A new and separate identity for the SEN, even a new name, is one suggested solution (Fox-Young 1992). The Royal College of Nursing, Australia (RCNA) believes that nursing care is primarily the responsibility of the RN and opposes any increase in SEN numbers or expansion of their education (RCNA 1990). A senior New South Wales nurse condemns this sort of policy as pie-in-the-sky: 'The ideological stance by some professionals for a single level nurse cannot realistically be sustained. A recognition of other levels, and the integral part they play in the delivery of nursing services must be faced' (Meppem 1991). This statement implies an integration of the SEN into the nursing team, and the possibility of other levels. A Western Australian nurse sees benefits:

> The registered nurse should be able to rely on *every* member of the team...I believe the registered nurses out there *want* accountable, educated, literate [SENs]...If there's more and more pressure going on the registered nurse, that person has to have more and more reliable people under her—or him. [BB/90]

A New South Wales nurse, however, sees a possible threat:

> It's a fairly scary future. That's why we have to keep our eye on the Minister [for Health]. We don't want him saying, 'Here's a way we can flood the market with enrolled nurses. We can get rid of these expensive RNs. And after all there aren't many 18-year-olds coming through, and they don't want to do nursing...' That's the philosophy. [MS/90]

A related question is that of the supply of nurses in the health workforce, especially as health care faces continued financial stringency. In contrast to the position during the nurse shortages of the 1980s (which helped to promote the quest for better pay and working conditions) the job prospects for nurses, especially new graduates, are now more difficult. The demand for nurses in the 1990s, an expert committee concludes, 'is likely to reflect tension between demographic factors [such as greater numbers of aged in the population] making for an increase, and financial factors limiting demand'; but the outlook for the nurse labour market as a whole in the 1990s is one of 'a reasonable balance of supply and demand' (DEET 1991:21,26).

Amongst many other balancing acts, nurses will need to consider how they can maintain their own optimum numbers for giving high quality care, without on the one hand giving politicians (and doctors) a chance to argue for substituting lower paid categories for the RN, or adopting an unrealistically élitist position on the other. One possibility is a rearrangement of nursing work, and two nurses suggest ways of doing this. First in South Australia:

> We could even—this goes over like a lead balloon—start looking at our workloads, and think 'Let's do an absolute minimum between 7.30 and 9.00 am until we can get those married women in here—just hold the fort'. [EP/88]

And in the West, a public service nurse says to her clinical colleagues:

> 'Let's look at your workload: why are you doing everything in the morning?'... there's so much routine attached to nursing...So I ask, 'Why do you roster everyone...on this ward, five in the morning, four in the afternoon, when on Saturday and Sunday your occupancy drops by 12?'...And they keep saying 'We need more staff'. I say to them 'You need to *redistribute* your staff'. [DMcC/90]

The growing field of home care, where untrained relatives carry out much nursing presents further problems. A senior Australian nurse thinks a flexible approach to the boundaries of the nursing 'role' will be required:

> Indeed for a nurse to say that a *nurse* has got to provide [airway] suction [to a child at home] and *only* a nurse can do it, when the mother's doing it during the day anyway—I don't understand the rationale...But in a way because I'm prepared to concede a less complex situation...I believe I'm strengthening my argument when you really *do* need nurses who can make complex judgements in complex situations. [MP/91]

And a British nurse sees possibilities there for the RN as a resource or consultant:

> Nurses say 'We're not going to be needed'. And I say, 'My God!...think of the worst kinds of patients in terms of dependency, there'll be at least five to ten outside being cared for by relatives...' [Who] keep saying in surveys, 'What we want most of all is not a service, but someone to come in and say "Marvellous, you're doing that right", or "Do you think if you try it this way it might be better?"' [JS/90]

The power of nursing to keep control over its domain has somehow to be reconciled with the idea of the patient having some genuine power. Health care is a service industry in which power is monopolised by the providers, especially doctors. A South Australian nurse sees one possibility for reducing nurses' power over patients:

> I don't think we allow patients to be involved enough in their care…we have to turn that power structure around, all that power being exerted on the poor patient to conform…I did a study of the decision making that was allowed to the client by the nurse…Patients weren't asked for preferences: 'I'll be back in 10 minutes to bath you, love'. It's still very much to 'get through the tasks', but if nurses were really committed to…being more flexible, they could do it. I've seen it done. [EP/88]

And a nurse academic thinks:

> …the true mark of the professional of the future is not going to be in that one-up position of 'I've got all this information and knowledge to give to you', but rather 'How can I facilitate things for you, how can we both draw on the different bodies of knowledge that we've got, and how can we put this together?' [JP/90]

In the past nurses' perceived powerlessness in their relations with doctors may have encouraged some unnecessary control over patients.

Holding on or letting go

The dangers of losing parts of nursing work, or 'role erosion', come not just from relatives who can be taught to do dressings or clear airways, or from senior nurse managers joining the corporate élite, or from physiotherapists and occupational therapists who compete for what nurses see as 'their' tasks, but also from specialisation within nursing which creates distinct identities and interests. Further, the new career structure in some states in which the charge nurse position has been divided into separate clinical and managerial positions may bring the danger of 'lay' managers. A South Australian nurse thinks there will be risks especially if there is a shortage of nurses in the future:

> So it would be rational to have all the nurses doing clinical nursing, not 'lose' them to management—especially when you've got non-nurses coming up from administration courses…[SS/88]

Both New South Wales and Victoria, in what would have seemed 10 years ago an unlikely alliance, have retained the charge nurse position. The New South Wales ANF Branch secretary explains her state's opposition to dividing the position:

> ...because I don't believe you can separate out clinical and administrative at that level. That is the linchpin, that nursing unit manager position, the charge nurse, it all flows from there. The degree of autonomy and control you give at that level is critical for the future of the profession...Somebody's in charge is what I know, and that somebody's going to be a nurse, because I think that's very important. [PS '90]

Nurses have a case for keeping hold of different kinds of work where introducing additional occupations might further fragment patient care. They are also entitled to think of group self-interest where, for example, a nurse can carry out the job of stomal therapist as well as a member of a separate occupation is likely to. A South Australian nurse is worried:

> I've worked as a respiratory specialist, and I understand that in America it would be a respiratory therapist who would do that sort of work...[And] stomal therapists—that's another area I could see non-nursing people moving into. I wouldn't want to see nursing give more away—just terrible! [SS/88]

The question of creating one new occupation was answered 20 years ago in the debate over the 'physician's assistant': nurses accepted the extra tasks. When it comes to management, there is a strong case for keeping nurses managing nurses, especially in the matter of professional accountability for standards of practice (ANF 1989). Nurses also have the advantage that they are accustomed to co-ordinating different kinds of specialised care to the patient, a central management function. Defending occupational interest is again a legitimate aim: a Singapore nurse manager reacted forcefully when her hospital proposed introducing 'lay' management to the clinical unit:

> Executives with MBAs and diplomas in business management—they would administer the wards and do the budget. I said 'No!' I fought it, because if they take over the management part, what would happen to our nurse administrators? And then [the executives] would want to dictate to us, tell us where to put the trolleys, or they would order equipment that is not right for us...we would be told to do the bedpans and feed the patients, so we would lose our other skills...And once we let them in, we'll never get them out! [ST-M/93]

Like the New South Wales ANF branch secretary, this nurse saw beyond the issue of who can do a particular job, who has the skills, to the question, can nursing afford to lose such important positions? Her answer was also unequivocal: nurses must fight to keep them.

For nursing as a whole, there are clear dangers of fragmentation, of 'divide and rule' when the specialty groups become separate, the ANF federal secretary believes:

> The government would exploit the divisions. I think the potential is there for that exploitation of different points of view at the advanced [specialist] practice level, and it's that level of work for nurses that will be absolutely the focus for the future. [MB/92]

Specialisation has other implications for nursing unity. The specialties want separate identities so that they are not lumped together under a general nursing 'umbrella'. Midwifery has advantages in seeking this separation, a senior Victorian nurse thinks:

> They've got a very clearly defined field...they can identify midwifery practice in a way that's very difficult to identify for general nursing practice. So in a way what they're doing is capitalising on that. [MP/91]

Midwifery is only one example. Psychiatric nursing also wants to maintain a separate identity to ensure proper recognition of the skills of its practitioners. But if the trend for psychiatric services to be integrated (or 'mainstreamed') into general health services continues, psychiatric nurses may be encouraged to come in from the cold. Psychiatric nursing has been a 'Cinderella' for too long, a New South Wales psychiatric nurse jokes ruefully:

> And being Cinderella, probably the most beautiful part of the health services as well—but that takes a lot of convincing for the ugly sisters!...There are some [general nurses] who want to see [pre-registration] psychiatric nursing in particular shoved into the postgraduate domain, and others who want to see developmental disability nursing shoved right out of nursing altogether, to give them more time in their three-year curriculum for what they believe is medical-surgical nursing. And I think that would be a *disaster.* [GC/90]

The US example, at least in education, shows a preferable method of integration, a Victorian community psychiatric nurse believes:

> I've had the experience of the American system and their graduates have had a good training in psych as well as general. They're equipped to work effectively as psych nurses. The worry here seems to be that the psych they get during their general training just isn't good enough. [AC/90]

And a WA psychiatric nurse believes integration is essential:

> If you look anywhere else in the world, like America...they don't have a single discipline of mental health independent of general nursing. It may well be that there won't be any such thing as a mental hospital in the future. There might be some very small specialised units...[BB/90]

Workplace changes, especially the 'mainstreaming' of mental health, seem likely to force integration, and general nurses may be ready to welcome their psychiatric colleagues.

A related issue is the official regulation of nursing. There are still 'vast discrepancies' in legislation between the different states and territories but the development of the Australian Nursing Council (ANC) should encourage national policy on regulation. Nurses' Acts and other regulatory mechanisms will have to become broader and more flexible, since they will need to allow for adequate delineation of the nurse's responsibilities in order to protect both the nurse and the public, without at the same time closing off future developments (Percival 1992). An Australian nurse believes that the ANC will assist 'the need to be united both within the different branches or domains of nursing, and at a national level as a whole setting aside States' differences' (*ANJ* 1991 February:28). The ANF secretary asserts that nurses themselves must become aware of the disadvantages of the fragmented system:

> ...I see [the union's function as being] to make nurses aware of what the actual organisation is that they are supporting, how it works, what the differences are between the states and territories, and so on, so that they don't think that because they've got an Australian Nursing Council—that's wonderful, and they've achieved it, and that's the end of it. It's only the beginning...[MB/92]

Another problem that nurses face in the future derives from uncertainty about health service needs. If these are to change in the direction of more care in the community, with an emphasis on health promotion, self-care and fewer patients in hospital, nurses will need to contribute to the planning, development and assessment of future services. Yet they face the perception that community work and health promotion are not nursing work. A New South Wales psychiatric nurse thinks that this applies also to his own specialty:

> Developmental disability services have been moved from Health to Family and Community Services [Department]. People say 'You don't need nurses in Family and Community Services, because it's not health', whereas you could argue very strongly that Family and Community Services belongs to nurses because we're the people, whether in midwifery or in paediatrics or infant welfare, and in mental health, developmental disability, we deal with family and community. [GC/90]

Again, the lack of knowledge among policy makers as well as among members of the public hides the real nature of nursing work and thus its potential for extending into new kinds of practice.

Beyond 'role erosion' there is always the possibility of expanding the work that nurses do. An ACT nurse and her public service colleague think so, though they are aware of likely conflict:

> I think the question of allocation of tasks will come up: what the nurses are allowed to do, impinging on the doctor's role...I think there are a lot more things they could take on too. Inserting intravenous drips is one thing, putting in sutures...[Or] that 'gatekeeper' role in community health centres: what proportion of people who come in to a GP's surgery with...a minor complaint, don't really need medical attention? But there'll be a fight. [PS&KK/88]

A nurse and a GP from Queensland have already recommended nurse practitioners as part of 'an integrated team' co-ordinated by the GP (Del Mar & Blue 1992), and the NSW Health Department is setting up nine pilot projects to examine 'the feasibility, safety, effectiveness, quality and cost' of the nurse practitioner, especially working in collaboration with GPs

(Staunton 1993). The Australian Medical Association president has responded by stressing that the major criterion for accepting this innovation must be that it provides a higher standard of 'medical' care rather than merely cheaper services (Nelson 1992). The nurse practitioner movement in the US has expanded since its inception in 1970 to about 18 000 practitioners, and 38 states have amended their medical practice legislation so that practitioners can carry out functions such as performing physical examinations and prescribing medication (Moloney 1986:96-97).

The ANF president has firm views about fighting to defend, even expand, nursing's domain:

> Nursing…first of all has to start off on the premise that it really does have something to defend: is there this identifiable body of work called nursing, that has professional integrity, and has credibility, that has to be defended and can be defended? [So, at one end of the career ladder]…is it a nurse? is it a residential care assistant? is it a child care worker?…I take the broader view that it's all nursing work and I'm not going to enter into semantic debates… because if you don't argue at that end you just keep giving it away. [And at senior levels]…is it a director of nursing? or is it just a manager of corporate services? or what is it?…If you take the word 'nurse' out of the title…does that still take nursing out of the function, out of what it is they're doing? I don't think that it does…I take the view that nursing has got to protect its positions…and it must argue on the 'line' relationship…my view is you must firmly fight for those positions. That's not an issue you should have to think twice about, if you genuinely believe that you've got this body of skill called nursing work… [And in the] long-term view: Is this really going to benefit nurses, or nursing? Is it going to benefit the *patient?*—don't forget the poor bloody patient still sitting in there somewhere trying to get a guernsey! [PS/90]

And a WA nurse who believes there will be three levels of nurse in the future makes a critical point:

> [Personal care attendants] *are* all being trained. We've got to get some control over that. It's *nursing.* OK, so there are these different levels of nursing, different types of nursing, but let us have control over it, let us determine what the parameters of those levels are, and the training that they'll have. And let's make sure there's a career path, so that someone can come in as a personal care attendant…and have a certain amount of training, and by adding to that they can become an SEN, and by adding to that they can become an RN. *We've* got to get control of that. [PM/90]

Not surprisingly, broadening the definition of what constitutes nursing is more likely to appeal to union minded nurses than to a more exclusive (and exclusionary) body like the RCNA, though the ANF has so far resisted having a category other than RN and SEN eligible for membership. A New South Wales nurse sees the difficulty of deciding where to draw the line:

> It would be very hard for [the ANF] to pick up personal care assistants, who are performing duties that were once the domain of the nurse. So we've lost them. And home carers—they are definitely 'non-nurses'. But now this demarcation is: what's nursing, and what's not nursing? [MS/90]

But the ANF secretary speculates on greater flexibility in the future:

> It may be that we have to get beyond the fixation on representing registered nurses and enrolled nurses, so that we could stop fixing on classification titles and begin to think about it as representing the nursing industry and people who are involved in nursing work. That's the big shift…[MB/92]

Such a shift could bring membership growth, but it would make nursing still more heterogeneous. The risk then would be, as in British nursing, that it would be impossible to satisfy both the lesser trained personal care attendants *and* the directors of nursing when, for example, policies for raising standards were under discussion (White 1985).

A related question is that of 'non-nursing duties'. Even if there is not always clarity about which tasks are nursing, at least there is some agreement about those that are 'non-nursing', though a Victorian nurse sees a continuing problem of responsibility:

> Whilst I do not believe that any nurse should have to pick up a dish of water and go and mop all the lockers down every night, I think that we've forgotten how to throw out the food that [patients] have not eaten at the end of the shift, and how to collect medicine cups, and how to throw out the flowers when they're dead. But that's part of the transition. We've changed so fast that we need to spend a few years organising where we are…[AH/92]

Nurses must decide what constitutes nursing work and who should do it while consulting other interested parties, so that they avoid accusations of trying to create a monopolistic position. Their problem will be to decide from time to time what can reasonably be claimed, what is worth defending and what can be defended. A New South Wales nurse asserts:

> I've got a very firm belief that nobody can take anything away from you that you don't want to give away. If nurses are not comfortable in their chosen role, and are not prepared to act,…obviously someone will come along and do for the patient that which you aren't doing. [JC/89]

Like any large and heterogeneous occupation, nursing is cut across by multiple divisions, including state borders, different gradings and educational standards, the many specialties, and the gap between junior and senior ranks. British nursing is similarly fragmented, even without the federal boundaries (Salvage 1988a). Unity will always be precarious and under challenge, and it will take considerable political skill to keep the various state and other divisions even loosely joined. A New South Wales nurse links these divisions, and rank and file apathy, to the difficulty of mobilising nursing power:

> They've never really exercised their quite enormous—numerically—political power. Very often it's because they fight amongst themselves so that there is no unity. New South Wales always stood alone: the battle of the [NSWNA] versus the ANF, it's been going on for the 30 years that I've observed it. From time to time they look as if they're getting really close, and then something happens and they're off again! Then there are the various [ANF] branches. They don't see eye to eye on what they should achieve. What they keep forgetting is that there can only be that number of really dedicated people, but then there's a large number of people who are just content to work,...go back to their family, and collect their money...They can't all be dedicated. [YJ/90]

The harmonisation successes of the 1980s have made the ANF a large and apparently cohesive organisation. The ability to exercise political power depends not only on numbers, however, but also on having a strategic position in the workplace such that other workers cannot be used as substitute labour. This is an asset which nurses have to some degree, though not to the extent that doctors have. Power depends also on group characteristics which are not easy to acquire: structural position in the division of labour, predominantly male composition, and membership of upper social strata. In the absence of these qualities, nursing's numbers and the ability of its leaders to mobilise them become crucial, especially when the centralised wage fixing system is devolved to 'enterprise bargaining', a change which could threaten the national industrial standards that the ANF has achieved (*ANJ* June 1993:17-18.

From a tightrope to a see-saw

The tension between the professional and the union perceptions of what should be nursing's domain, how nurses should consolidate and defend it, has not lessened and is not likely to. Whereas in the 1970s and early 1980s organised nursing was united behind the education 'goals' a South Australian nurse thinks that a distinction has emerged:

> Some people would look to the College [RCNA] to be the professional organisation...The ANF is seen as an industrial body because it's become so much more industrially active—a relative said to me, 'You nurses, you're like the waterside workers!' [EP/88]

The unity of the nursing organisations contributed to their success in achieving the 'goals' in 1984, at the same time that nurses were becoming more industrially militant. The 'goals' campaign began the transformation of nursing into a political force, but the industrial activity of the 1980s was essential to gain the improvements in pay and conditions, including the career structure, without which the educational advance would have risked becoming a hollow victory. Where some nurses saw the 'goals' period as predominantly 'professional', the succeeding years came to be seen as very much 'industrial'. A nurse prominent in the 'goals' campaign regrets this:

> ...personally I think that we put a little bit too much emphasis on these industrial areas and haven't kept the professional aspects to the fore as much as we should have...I must say I have been rather depressed about some of these developments...[such as] more militancy and focus on salaries rather than looking at how the profession can improve its practice, how the profession can perhaps make a better contribution through education...[MP/88]

A Victorian nurse considers that the militancy of the 1980s was necessary to assert nurses' claims for industrial justice, but that events in her own state pushed the union orientation too far:

> Irene [Bolger, former ANF Branch Secretary] did us a favour in making us very well aware that we were a pair of skilled hands rather than people who were 'chosen' to do a particular thing. We chose to do [nursing] ourselves, and we have a particular set of skills which need to be rewarded accordingly. Bringing us down to the level of a trade union was not *such* a bad thing, because...we *are* workers, the same as doctors are, and anybody else who has particular skills. But then to go on perpetuating that sort of image without looking at the professional issues as well...A lot of nurses who saw themselves as special people—and that again isn't such a bad thing—they found that very difficult. [HV/88]

A Western Australian nurse agrees that there is a case for trying to establish a balance between union power and professional assertiveness:

> I've always been a champion for industrial justice...I'm pleased we're starting to get appropriate remuneration in salaries etc. But I hope we...put the professional emphasis as well...[that we're] not just seen as getting the right money for nurses, but [also] being more vocal about health care issues, and starting to stand up. [DMcC/90]

The ANF has always asserted a dual claim to represent both the professional and industrial interests of its members, and many belong to it for either or both reasons. It is therefore constrained to aim at what members will accept as a balance between the two, though the nature of that balance will change over time. A British nurse considers that the more professionally inclined members of the RCN became dissatisfied as it became more 'unionistic' in the 1970s, and remarks that 'the power of the College is based presently on the size of its membership, not on its professional authority' (White 1985). The 'professionalist' nurses, White thinks, could be 'squeezed out' or form new associations, as in the US and Canada. An Australian analogy would be the 'professionalist' nurses supporting the RCNA and the more union minded staying with the ANF. If Australian nurses want to exercise political influence in health policy and to defend their own interests, they may decide however that they have a better chance of doing so if they maintain their major association as it is now, a body committed to the twin aims of professional standards (giving it White's 'professional authority') and industrial strength, the latter depending in large part on membership numbers. These aims are in some ways antagonistic, but many nurses obviously feel that they are two aspects of the one unified aim and are equally essential, even though one aspect will demand more attention and effort than the other as circumstances alter.

A major reason for maintaining these two aims as inseparable is the importance of the ANF as the voice of nursing in health policy making. ANF professionalism is seen in its policy and standards documents, but if these are not backed up by industrial power, politicians may not listen so willingly to nurses' representatives. A South Australian public service nurse saw a first hand example of this:

> Over time, through constant wearing away it is almost, *almost,* automatic now for the [Health] Commission to ensure that any committee that is established has nursing representation on it. It *is* rare now that it doesn't happen. An example was recently where they set up a committee to implement the recommendations of a report...In the preliminary document it didn't have a nurse on it, and the Executive Director...said 'But we've got to have a nurse on it'. I thought, well at last we're educating them. He *then* said, 'Because RANF will go berserk if we don't!' In fact the debate ended up not about whether a nurse should be on it...but how many. [CG/88]

However diligently nurses search for the professional status which has so far eluded them, their political influence, and thus the extent to which they can enforce professional standards in their work and education, ultimately depends on the ability of the ANF to 'go berserk'.

'Professionalist' nurses may be disturbed by the ANF withdrawal from the International Council of Nurses (ICN) after six years of debate, but with only 9% of members taking part in the deciding vote. The question arose originally as a result of the Victorian Branch financial deficit of 1987-88, and the consequent failure of the Branch to pay capitation fees to the federal council. The ANF has faced serious costs (over $300 000) as a result of its federal award proceedings, and of its efforts to protect its coverage of nurses against attack from other unions. Further, the union harmonisations of the late 1980s doubled its membership, thus raising the required ICN affiliation dues (*ANJ* October 1992:10-11; March 1993; June 1993:5; August 1993:9). Failure to remain with the ICN, especially if this was the result of expenditure on industrial activities, might unbalance the even tilt of the 'see-saw' between professional and industrial aims and damage the ANF claim to represent both.

Educating neater

'Australia leads the world in the rational, planned transfer of professional nurse education to the tertiary sector. We have not followed the American path, or the Canadian path, or the British path' (Moorhouse 1988). Australian nursing has achieved a wholesale transfer rather than the piecemeal US variety, and one that puts nursing education squarely within the tertiary sector, rather than alongside it as in Britain.

A major aim of the transfer was to remove education from control by hospital service demands, but this may risk exchanging hospital for academic control. Two issues are central. One is nursing's ability to maintain control over its curriculum, which could be threatened by academics from other disciplines. The leaders of the education campaign always stressed nursing control, given that the purpose of nurse education was to prepare nurses who would give direct care to patients. New nursing departments also face competition from established departments which guard their resources and in some cases do not perceive nursing as a genuine discipline, a view possibly reinforced by the largely female composition of the staff (Speedy 1987). The US Institute of Medicine recommended in 1983 that Congress should establish 'on a federal level, an organizational entity to place nursing research in the mainstream of scientific investigation' (Moloney 1986: 137). Australian nursing and nursing research are similarly not yet part of the academic mainstream. A New South Wales nurse academic saw the effect of entrenched attitudes towards academic credentials:

> Initially people were very jealous because...they thought that [nurses] were getting [senior] positions without adequate academic qualifications. I think what they've learned to realise is that someone may not have the academic qualifications, but they have nursing qualifications and experience...And when they've been on committees with our people...Our staff have really been able to hold their own. [MR/89]

Even so, there is pressure on nurse academics to measure up to the established standards. A New South Wales educationist sees the difficulty for nursing staff whose college of advanced education has merged with a university:

> We've got an old, arrogant university that prides itself on its research component, having amalgamated with it people who never saw research as their prime function—indeed why should they? They were doing something perfectly adequate and socially necessary. And now they're feeling constrained to conform to the ethos of the big institution. I think that's a great pity. [JL/90]

Nurse academics are caught between academic and clinical pressures. Arranging and conducting the clinical teaching program, for which the academic nurse is professionally accountable, are time consuming activities, but the tertiary milieu imposes competing demands: studying for higher degrees, building a publication record, and learning to understand the conditions and power relations in an unfamiliar (and, like the hospital, male dominated) organisation. The nurse academic (like the medical) is required to retain her practice expertise for clinical teaching, but at the same time she is expected to perform the equally demanding tasks of a conventional lecturer and researcher (Botti et al 1991). A Northern Territory nurse academic supports the retention of clinical expertise:

> ...the medical profession got it right: the fact is that if you're a professor of medicine you are actually practising medicine. I believe we need to look at that more in nursing. I think the models that were set up in the United States, where you have the faculty engaged in practice as well as teaching and research, work quite well. We should be looking towards doing that. [KR/90]

Not surprisingly, one study has found that senior nurse academics in particular suffer a significant degree of 'role ambiguity' and conflict, though this can be alleviated by support from peers and superiors (Grundy & Pennebaker 1988). Academic staff in other disciplines are familiar with the low value put on teaching skill as against the more visible and easily quantified research and publication record. Nurse academics have the further handicap that their practice expertise is on show away from the university, hidden from academics in other departments. This also applies to medicine, but in one case separation leads to an overestimation of what doctors do, because their public image leaves out the more routine parts of their work, and in the other it leads to an underestimation of what nurses do, since few university staff are aware of the complexity of their work. Yet a British nurse academic insists that the university departments of nursing must develop the best research standards, not in order to impress non-nurse colleagues but:

> ...so that you can produce highly able researchers with post-doctoral experience who then set the standards for academic work in nursing...And I feel that unless we're careful, we're going to expect too much of academic departments...it's the high-level research work which is eased out, or is not supported sufficiently. [JW-B/90]

And a psychiatric nurse academic sees her colleagues becoming aware of other activities such as going to conferences:

> They keep saying to me 'Oh, you're so professionally involved—how do you do it?'...[And] they are suddenly starting to understand that if you don't do professional things in your discipline, then you may be beaten in the rush for the next position, say senior lecturer...[LS/90]

Perhaps nurses are still trying too hard to prove that they can do everything.

A second issue of control lies in the actual teaching of clinical skills, which mostly takes place away from the nursing department in a hospital or other agency, and is therefore dependent on successful co-operation between direct care agencies and the nursing staff in the universities (McManamny 1987). Already some nurses perceive a service-academic gap, as a WA nurse says:

> [Tertiary education] was the way to go...But I think some nurses have gone a little bit overboard with academia. So we've got an 'academic' group. I think that's necessary, but what we have to recognise is there's another group out

> there who are just as good, as nurses, just as articulate, just as capable, but [who] don't use the jargon. [PM/90]

Nursing departments do not have the resources to supply enough staff for all the labour intensive student supervision in clinical agencies, so they have to use sessional staff and 'preceptors' from the agencies. Both hospital staff and nursing academics need to understand each other's difficulties and collaborate to make sure graduates are prepared for the demands of clinical practice (Meppem 1991), but the different nature of the tertiary programs compared to the old hospital courses can lead to problems, as a New South Wales nurse found:

> One difficulty was being able to orientate the people who were coming from the clinical area...you really need an orientation time to introduce them to the program, what our purposes are...It's not satisfactory having a lot of sessionals, because they're not part of the program. [RP/89]

Even though nurse education no longer takes place wholly in the hospital, it is still influenced by the hospital's goal of maximum patient turnover, especially with today's 'managerialist' ethos in health care, and government embarrassment about waiting lists. This can translate into tension between the nurse who has to fulfil her obligations to her patients and to the hospital, and the student who wishes to maximise her learning. When the students are no longer a useful part of the workforce then agencies may feel less inclined to admit them. In some cases tertiary institutions find themselves in competition for clinical placements, either where these are scarce, or where a particular agency offers superior experience (McManamny 1987).

The clinical-academic pull and push on staff applies also to students. While wishing to expand the student's intellectual horizons to encourage a wider social and cultural perspective, nurse academics also want to maintain the conditions necessary for developing the psychomotor skills essential for daily practice (D'Cruz & Bottorf 1986:31). A New South Wales nurse is worried about this, but optimistic:

> We run some risk of following the North American example, where they acknowledge now that often they throw the baby out with the bathwater in concentrating on intellectual skills and on the knowledge of principles etc. to the detriment of looking at the development of some basic skills for people going into the clinical areas. I don't think we've done that in Australia so far. I think we've sought a balance between the intellectual 'stretching' and the practical know-how that we need to retain. [RP/89]

Important questions now for nursing are how do the tertiary graduates perform as nurses, and will they remain in nursing, particularly as bedside nurses? After examining earlier evaluations of both hospital and tertiary graduates, Lublin (1985) challenged their finding that there was no significant difference between the two kinds of graduate. Further evidence suggests, she says, that tertiary education 'can produce a different sort of practitioner'. In Sydney, Pratt (1989) found that 80% of her sample of college graduates thought their clinical education had prepared them adequately to perform the majority of the psychomotor skills they needed in their practice, most of which were for basic patient care. A study of New South Wales graduates found that in their first year in the workforce they were able to develop and strengthen their clinical performance. Further, their beginning clinical skills did not necessarily correlate with the number of clinical hours in their undergraduate program—the quality of clinical learning experience may be more important than the quantity (Battersby & Hemmings 1991). As for fears that college graduates will not stay in nursing, an early South Australian study found that graduates prefer to remain in direct care positions, are reluctant to seek promotion away from the bedside, and have stayed in nursing despite difficulties that arose because of prejudice against their tertiary program (Pickhaver et al 1985:30-33, 63).

Such findings provide a useful riposte to continuing rearguard attacks on tertiary education for nurses, including those which perpetuate the irrational belief that academic qualifications will somehow disqualify nurses from giving compassionate patient care (e.g. 'A Melbourne nurse', *The Age* 21 November 1990). A South Australian nurse does not believe that the 'expressive' part of nursing work, with its concern for the patient's comfort, has disappeared, though there may be less time for it:

> I still hear people say 'Oh, nursing's not what it used to be, the kids don't care', and so on. But in recent times I've seen the young ones curling up the older [patients'] hair and doing all those nice little things, and I think—where can you criticise?...so I don't know that bedside care has changed a great deal. [EC/88]

A less positive finding from the point of view of nurse academics is that graduates' attitudes towards nursing do not always correspond to those of their lecturers. The hospital trained nurse often failed to act as patient advocate in the way that the school of nursing taught because she was 'socialised into the attitudes of the health team, and her team loyalty takes priority over all other considerations' (Buckenham & McGrath 1983:61). The tertiary education strategists wanted this to change, but a Sydney study showed that '...a prevailing feature of nursing students, even at the end of their educational programs, is a commitment to medical-procedural educational priorities and an associated allegiance to a relatively restricted concept of the scope and nature of nursing' (Higgins 1988). The challenge now for nurse academics, says Higgins, is to devise a curriculum which will help students accept the professional idea of nursing, and will thus enable them to resist the prevailing view as it exists still among the public, in many health care agencies, and in the media (Aber & Hawkins 1992). Olesen and Whittaker (1968) have shown however that the process of moving the student from her 'lay' definition of nursing to the more 'professional' definition upheld by the academic staff is complex, and that students only slowly and reluctantly give up their attachment to their former beliefs. As a veteran nurse academic found in Tasmania:

> They've got an expectation of going in with 'hands on' and looking after people, and they just love that clinical contact. All my experience...since 1974 has been that the students still hold the stereotype of the hospital nurse: you went to a hospital and you nursed sick people...[MP/88]

If today's graduates perpetuate the old image of the doctor's handmaiden then the newly won gains in the workplace may not be consolidated. Some nurses are however hopeful that there will be a new assertiveness, like this ACT nurse and her public service colleague:

> I don't think people who go through a tertiary education will be like us, who were trained from an early age in the hospital system to be subservient. And [they'll have] more experience of the power of collective action—not necessarily through the union, there are other ways: if you work collectively towards a goal, you can have quite a lot of power. I hope that nurses will build on their gains...[KK & PP/88]

A longer period in the university might afford more time to change students' perceptions, but nurse academics have failed to get a pre-registration degree of more than three years. Nursing education is therefore still shorter than that of other occupations such as physiotherapy. In spite of considerable lobbying, the more straitened circumstances of the economy compared to the situation in 1984 discouraged the federal government from embarking on additional expense for such a large number of students, and there was some suspicion among educational authorities about pressures for occupational credentialling. Further, nursing was not united on the question of the three-year degree any more than it had been in 1982 over the degree-diploma question. In 1982 the argument was resolved by the dominance of the 'goals' coalition, but in 1990 the existence of many heads of academic nursing departments in different institutions probably militated against a consolidated view. A New South Wales nursing department head describes the position:

> You see, the profession doesn't agree...The one thing that people agree on is that we *should* have a pre-registration degree. The majority have said that the degree should be *at least* three-and-a-half years long. But there are quite a lot of people who've said 'If I'm offered a three-year degree, I'll take it'. So if the profession is not united, you can't do anything. I think you then just have to work within the constraints. [MR/89]

Leading nurse academics have learned from this setback and have set up the Australian Council of Deans of Nursing, a formal body developed from the nurse academics network established by the RCNA. For the nursing student, an alternative possibility under examination by a national review team is an 'intern year' immediately following registration (AHMAC 1993).

There remain many hospital trained nurses who want university education, many probably because it is now expected for promotion to senior positions, but some perhaps because they see it as an enriching experience in itself, denied them in the past. It is unfortunate that places are limited so many will expect to wait, and some may experience the poignant regrets of a Western Australian nurse when she did a tertiary course after years of clinical and management practice:

> I wish I'd had it 20 years ago, I just wish I'd had that knowledge. I look at that anatomy and physiology...and I keep thinking...it will help me in my position [now]...but it just makes me weep to think I've missed out on 20 years of knowledge. *I could have used it.* [DMcC/90]

Leading women

> Today, the need for leadership in nursing is greater than ever to gain more influence in policy and high-level decision making, to push through reforms in education, to contribute to the effective management of the NHS, and to develop better nursing practice. This requires a new cohort of nurses to create and fill leadership positions not only in traditional fields, but also in general management. Yet there is precious little evidence to suggest that this widely recognised need has been translated into action (Salvage 1988b).

This statement about British nursing was prompted by the RCN not just having to advertise but *readvertise* for a new general secretary after the retirement of Trevor Clay, the man who had 'finally buried the twin set and pearls image and placed the college squarely in the world of politics' (Turner 1989). The ANF has not had to suffer a similar embarrassment, and in any case its most senior job is open to nationwide election by the members, unlike the appointed RCN position. Even so, some Australian nurses are worried about future leadership. A New South Wales nurse concludes sadly:

> ...there's just no leadership emerging in nursing...It seems to me that what's happening is that many of our nursing leaders...those visionaries, and the people who had so much influence, have all retired, or are in the process of retiring, and we're left almost with a gap...I think there are a lot of people who are getting there, but...the Paulina Pilkingtons, the Ruth Whites, the Merle Parkeses, those people who *really had* an enormous amount of influence—where are they? [JC/89]

A former ANF federal secretary thinks however that today's leaders are more likely to emerge from the ranks, a change reflecting the effect of democratic forces:

> It's been a real levelling out process, I think, in the last few years...there's been a sense that the more senior people in the profession have dominated too much. I think up to a point that's true...[And] that has changed. The leadership for the moment has to come somewhere from the middle, probably to get over and get rid of some of that past...[MP/91]

The nursing leaders of today are less often directors of nursing, though they may be professors. In the ANF most seem to have reached their positions as a result of an interest in union affairs and in what union action can accomplish for nurses, rather than from an accustomed position of command—though that does not mean that the Ansteys and Henlens of the 1970s were any less anxious to further the welfare of rank and file members than are today's leaders, or that the present union secretaries are any less authoritative than were their matronly predecessors. Given the events of the recent past, today's leaders are more likely to be overtly political than their precursors, though probably no more wily and astute behind the scenes. The most obviously political leaders of the 1980s, those from the far left, quickly lost office, but a New South Wales nurse argues that the term of office of the radical Jenny Haines as secretary of the NSWNA (1982-1987) was politically beneficial:

> It brought out into the open the political dimension of nursing, which 'wasn't nice'—it was 'never there'. And it was *always* there. It's been there forever, but it's been submerged. And I think that was probably the greatest benefit. We had to face up to the fact that there were political ideologies and political factions, and we were amongst it as much as anyone. [KM/89]

Today's leaders owe a debt to those nurses who, like Jenny Haines and Irene Bolger, were prepared to be openly political at a time when this was less acceptable. Even in 1990 an obviously political statement was not popular: a WA Branch secretary found members shying away from one when the ANJ March issue sported a cover criticising the Coalition health policy just before a federal election:

> [The ANF] had written to all the political parties asking for their response to an agenda that we set. We didn't really get a response [from the Coalition] and that cover was highlighting that. But a lot of members said 'How dare you insinuate that we should vote Labor!' People were saying 'It's so political, we shouldn't be political'. [This shows] our inability to get through to the majority that being political is part of professional growth...you're talking about nursing having an effective voice in decision making and policy, which is being political...[PM/90]

In the future nurses will need to accept the necessity for 'being political', and their representatives will have to demonstrate an even greater degree of political sophistication if they are to consolidate and build on the achievements of all nurses.

The ANF was openly partisan recently for the first time in the 1993 federal election. The content of the federation's new health policy (above) showed members that in its broadly social and environmental ideas about health the ANF was much closer to the Labor Party than to the more market oriented policy of the Coalition (*ANJ* 1993 February, March). As the secretary commented, 'Australian nurses have long supported efforts...to create a health system that assures access, quality and affordability' (*ANJ* 1993 February: 6). The American Nurses' Association was similarly influenced when it officially endorsed presidential candidate Bill Clinton, who was promising to make US health care more accessible and put greater emphasis on primary health and long term care. The ANA was reported as 'actively working to ensure his election' (Seymour 1992).

The dangers of partisanship are illustrated by the Australian Medical Association (AMA) which endured a 'painful metamorphosis' after the 1993 election, brought on by internal recriminations. The AMA, some doctors thought, 'crossed the line' from medical politics into party politics by openly supporting the (failed) Coalition health policy. Like nurses, doctors are affected by health policy so they are entitled to comment publicly, but the AMA problem seems to be that it was perceived as 'too partisan' and was identified with a right wing ideology which voters rejected—perhaps the AMA 'would have got away with it, had it not backed a loser' (Chandler 1993). Nurses will judge whether the ANF's more discreet (and less publicised) partisanship also 'crossed the line' or made a justifiable political choice, given the similarity of its own health policy to that of the (victorious) Labor Party.

Nurses *are* political and they will *go on being political* as long as they continue to exercise their growing political skills in pursuit of their aims, whether in improving their education, in seeking more decision making power in the workplace, in acting through their unions for improved pay and conditions, or in defining and defending nursing work. They may also decide to expand their lobbying activities in the wider sphere of public policy: in environmental issues, including those related to health such as the growing volume of waste generated by the use of disposables, or in support of disarmament and an anti-war position. These activities have been sporadic so far, and have not reflected the potential for influence of such a large number of health sector workers.

The idea that nurses 'shouldn't be political' (above) stems from misconceptions about the nature of political activity, which is not always obvious and is certainly not confined to public demonstrations (or to journal covers). Political activity occurs in any struggle over power, whether in the workplace, in industrial relations, or in the public arena—in any situation in which groups with different interests seek to increase their influence, relative to that of opposing groups, over decisions or over policy. Groups will use various strategies, ranging from demonstrations to much less public negotiation. Their members will inevitably differ on the tactics to be used and even on the goals to be pursued, just as members of the ANF and the AMA have done. Those who argue that nurses should not be political, and who define 'political' as confined to the more obvious forms of such activity, like the strike, are either defending their own interests against those of nurses, or, if they are nurses themselves, are failing to identify and defend their legitimate interests.

Nursing leaders in Australia have always been predominantly female, unlike the position in Britain where nurses have allowed 'a minority of men to fast track into positions of power over them' (Delamothe 1988b). Nursing seems to belie the popular image of Australia as a 'man's country', though it may be an omen for the future that there are for the first time two male ANF state secretaries (Queensland and WA). A former South Australian state secretary has strong views about keeping the union centred on women and on women's issues:

> The men...there's this sense that they're natural leaders...[And a male federal secretary?] Over my dead body. Over my dead body! But part of that is the gender issue. Part of it's the basic bloody stuff like child care...You have a career structure...and then you bloody can't get into anything because it's all part time and there's no child care. And I won't have this union sitting around crowing about the benefits or the great leaps forward we've got whilst ever there's no work based child care. Well, the difficulty is nurses aren't politicised about child care. [LS/88]

Leading nurses (e.g. Wiesel 1984) have been exhorting their colleagues for years to think, organise and act collectively, rather than simply enduring their individual hardships. It seems that feminism as an ideology has not yet contributed to mobilising this potential army. Nursing 'has failed to embrace feminism for a variety of reasons. These include fear, ignorance...and the belief that accepting feminism implies loss of favour with dominant groups. In the case of nursing, it is clear that many nurses derive power from their subordinate relationship with doctors...' (Speedy 1991)—and perhaps there really is 'some strange connection between carrying out chores for doctors and sexual excitement' (Savage 1987:90). A South African nurse criticises her colleagues who continue to accept subservience, but acknowledges the added burden of racial division in her own country:

> I think nurses are responsible for some of their own problems in that they have signed away their authority as unit managers, and instead of being in charge of that unit, they are the carrier out of orders. So the consultant may see himself as being the person in charge, not the sister—simply because the sister hasn't seen her function and said 'I'm sorry doctor, but I will do the nursing care. If you're not satisfied, please come and tell me'. But they can't see that...[And] for a black nurse to say that to a white doctor—that's been very difficult...[BR/89]

There is also a generation gap: a group of young nurses in Melbourne is quoted as saying that 'they value their right to vote, their right to choose between practising their profession or staying at home with children, and their right to equal pay' but they still shun the feminist label, not realising apparently that political action informed by feminism has achieved much that they take for granted (Teh & Gowdie 1988).

Nevertheless, the ANF federal secretary believes that part of her responsibility is to encourage women with feminist beliefs to take leadership positions:

> I think that you invest a big and important section of your life in the organisation, and that it's so important that you have to make sure that you generate interest in others following you, that you don't stamp on that because it threatens you. I believe that I have a responsibility to make sure that nurses with a very strong sense of feminism, and who have integrated that ideology into the way they operate, become involved in this organisation, so that as it becomes more and more effective and therefore powerful, it's not hijacked. [MB/92]

Australian nurses are fortunate to have a less conservative and more feminist leadership than there is in Britain. After hearing the new (female) RCN secretary speak, a British nurse-feminist lamented the conservative thinking among her colleagues:

> People thought her speech was very radical. I didn't, because it contained statements like, 'What women in nursing need to do is to persuade their husbands to help them with the housework'. Well, that is not the feminist position to me! But [other nurses were saying] 'Oh gosh, she's really got it now. That's the way forward'. [CW/90]

This 'Playboy bunny' brand of feminism cannot transfer to the political arena because it leaves women's issues unpoliticised. Nurses will therefore be in danger of continuing to see issues such as workplace child care as purely domestic problems unless they accept at least some feminist ideas.

Part of the work of the leadership in the future will be to persuade nurses that 'there is a clear need for women within nursing to reject the conditioning they have received over the years about gender and to acknowledge their own worth and ability' (Savage 1987:69). This will help counteract the tendency towards destructive power relations within nursing, exemplified in the perception that, as many nurses say, they have been 'their own worst enemy', blaming each other for the effects of their subordinate status (Street 1990). But for nurses themselves to recognise their own worth and ability will not be enough. There has also been an enemy outside: a harsh mixture 'of patriarchy and class oppression has in the past been nursing's worst enemy' (Short & Sharman 1987). Perhaps such enemies offer too convenient a source of blame—some statements and commentary by nurses convey the sense of a continually set (and sat) upon group, the impression of an embattled occupation. Australian nurses have experienced enough successful exercises in the use of collective power to obviate the need to fall back on such images. Recent evidence suggests that they are aware of their continuing subordination to doctors, but are conscious also of their improved education, pay and working conditions (Kenny & Adamson 1992).

A former leader, Pat Slater, looked forward to nurses 'using the experience of the past, holding firmly to the essential values and beliefs of our humanist tradition...our commitment to our own vision of good nursing practice';

but she was not merely nostalgic about tradition. She was committed also to 'overthrowing the useless trappings of the past: our servility, poor self image, powerlessness, desire for conformity and fear of taking risks...' (Slater 1982). Confirming this vision of nurses as a group for whom dedication means not self-sacrifice but the power to act for themselves and for others, a Victorian nurse thinks her colleagues have gained too much to go back to those elements of the past which Slater rejected:

> I can't see them letting go of what they've gained...[Nurses] enjoy being competent and responsible and making decisions and seeing the effects of it and answering for their errors themselves—not having some charge nurse or some registrar roar at them because of the way a fluid balance chart wasn't filled in...But [instead] seeing that the decision they made on admission...or an intervention, has made a positive difference to the patient's life. They really enjoy that, and they see that what they do is good, and what they do is important. But it's not valued enough in the system yet. That's the next step that I think we need to take. [AH/92]

Achieving full recognition of their contribution within the health system and a commensurate influence in health policy will require Australian nurses to maintain and sharpen their political awareness and determination, because recognition will depend on fundamental changes. Some of these can occur inside nursing, such as further consolidating the unity of the nursing organisations. This refers both to the new unity between the states, and the possibility that the ANF may eventually count among its members increasing numbers of psychiatric and enrolled nurses; and it refers to the more elusive unity of professional and industrial aims.

A realistic appreciation of their industrial strength and its sources will help nurses recognise some of the false prophets and promises of traditional professionalism. They can then use that strength to work for a higher degree of autonomy and more job satisfaction in the workplace (Daniel 1990:81). The changes outside nursing which will enable them to be valued 'in the system' are general changes in attitudes to work, especially to 'women's work', such that nurses' practical and expressive skills are not overlooked in the reverence for technical or academic expertise; and changes in attitudes to women so that their qualities as persons are no longer hidden behind objectified physical attributes. Such changes will be resisted by other vested interests in health care, especially medical interests (Mackay 1989:181).

We have tried in this book to describe nurses' achievements and their failures, especially some of the reasons for them. These reasons exist inside nursing, and outside in prevailing social, political and economic conditions. Events outside nurses' control have played a major part in enabling them to achieve some successes, while also helping to ensure that other efforts met with failure. Australian nurses are justified in feeling a sense of pride in their achievements, remembering at the same time how much more there is to do. As the ANF Victorian Branch secretary says:

> I think now for the first time nurses will have to be recognised at a national and state level as a political force; still not with quite the same power that the doctors have, but I think we've certainly demonstrated to both political parties that we can play quite a major part in outcomes. And I think that's a major achievement. [BM/93]

Many nurses are aware that favourable social and economic changes promoted some of their gains, but as the ANF federal secretary points out, they have triumphed also in less favourable conditions—for example in the 1980s when the federal Labor government-ACTU accord held wages down:

> We had extraordinary rises in wages during that period of time. If we had paid attention to [the argument that] 'This is what the Accord is. Wages are essentially frozen', we would not have tried. But we *did,* because we absolutely believed that we did not get equal pay...I don't know whether it was more diligently researched, or whether we were able to use the issues of the day to attach our arguments to, and make them so compelling that you couldn't dismiss them...but many people began to take up the cause.
>
> I'm convinced that we would not have achieved the wage increases if we hadn't had the way opened by the ACTU...if Bill Kelty [ACTU secretary], for example, hadn't sat at the ACTU Executive table and said 'Now, we should all support the nurses as a special case'; and if the ACTU hadn't stood up in the Industrial Commission and said 'The ACTU supports nurses as a special case, and any increases awarded to them will not lead to a "flow on" to other categories of employee in the health industry or beyond'. We achieved what we did through a broad coalition of support, and I think it was the right time to be quite 'up front' about achieving a national agenda for nursing. I think that was important. [MB/92]

This statement illustrates some of the ingredients of success: careful preparation, building support among influential groups (whose members appreciate both the merits of the case and the strength of the organisation presenting it), and recognising the time when a particular change may be acceptable. Nurses are realists when they accept that their own political attitudes and actions are the public expression of their legitimate interests, and that successful pursuit of those interests will depend in part on prevailing social, political and economic circumstances. Their success in the 1990s and beyond will come from judiciously uniting their chosen interests with those circumstances.

REFERENCES

Aber C S, Hawkins J W 1992 Portrayal of nurses in advertisements in medical and nursing journals. Image: Journal of Nursing Scholarship 24(4) Winter:289-93

AHMAC (Australian Health Ministers' Advisory Council) 1993 National review of nurse education in the higher education sector—1994 and beyond. Issues Papers. Department of Health, Housing and Local Government in co-operation with the Department of Employment, Education and Training, Canberra

ANF (Australian Nursing Federation) 1989 Nursing in Australia. A national statement. ANF, College of Nursing, Australia, New South Wales College of Nursing, Florence Nightingale Committee, Melbourne

ANF 1991 Health service organisational structures. Policy statement and discussion paper. ANF, Melbourne

ANF 1993 Australian Nursing Federation health policy. Australian Nurses' Journal February:7-11

Battersby D, Hemmings L 1991 Clinical performance of university nursing graduates. Australian Journal of Advanced Nursing 9 (1) September-November:30-34

Botti M, Duke M, Forbes H, Ho T 1991 Nurse academics in universities: a dilemma. Conference proceedings, Royal College of Nursing, Australia, Brisbane

Bruni N 1991 Nursing knowledge: processes of production. In: Gray G, Pratt R (eds) Towards a discipline of nursing. Churchill Livingstone, Melbourne

Buckenham J E, McGrath G 1983 The social reality of nursing. Health Science Press, Sydney

Chandler J 1993 AMA searches for a way to lose partisan image. The Age 18 March

Clay T 1989 Nursing and politics: the unquiet relationship. In: Jolley M, Allan P (eds) Current issues in nursing. Chapman & Hall, London

Daniel A 1990 Medicine and the state. Allen & Unwin, Sydney

D'Cruz J V, Bottorf J L 1986 The renewal of nursing education. Health Education Occasional Papers No.2, La Trobe University, Melbourne

DEET (Department of Employment, Education and Training) 1991 National nurse labour market study. Volume One: summary report. Australian Government Publishing Service, Canberra

Delamothe T 1988a Nursing grievances III: Conditions. British Medical Journal 296 16 January:182-185

Delamothe T 1988b Nursing grievances V: Women's work. British Medical Journal 296 30 January:345-347

Del Mar C, Blue C 1992 Nurse practitioners in general practice (letter to the editor). Medical Journal of Australia 157 (7):502-504

Fox-Young S 1992 The future of the second-level nurse: extension, elimination or evolution? In: Gray G, Pratt R (eds) Issues in Australian nursing 3. Churchill Livingstone, Melbourne

Freidson E 1974 Dominant professions, bureaucracy and client services. In: Hasenfeld Y, English RA (eds) Human service organizations. University of Michigan Press, Ann Arbor

Grundy O, Pennebaker D 1988 Role socialisation and adjustment of nurse educators to tertiary institutions. In: National Nursing Education Conference, Expanding Horizons in Nursing Education, Conference Proceedings, Perth

Higgins L C 1988 Educational priorities of nursing students: curriculum implications. Institute of Nursing Studies, Sydney CAE, Sydney

Holmes C 1991 Theory: where are we going and what have we missed along the way? In: Gray G, Pratt R (eds) Towards a discipline of nursing. Churchill Livingstone, Melbourne

Howe B 1993 Interview with the federal Minister for Health. ABC station 3LO, 8 January

Hyland D 1991 The enrolled nurse review. Report of the task force to review the education, role and function of the enrolled nurse in New South Wales (chairperson D. Hyland) to the Minister for Health and Community Services, NSW and the Minister for Health Services Management, NSW. New South Wales Health Department, Sydney

Jolley M 1989 The professionalisation of nursing: the uncertain path. In: Jolley M, Allan P (eds) Current issues in nursing. Chapman & Hall, London

Kenny D, Adamson B 1992 Medicine and the health professions: issues of dominance, autonomy and authority. Australian Health Review 15(3):319-334

Limb M 1992 Fasten your seatbelts. Health Service Journal 7 May:10

Lublin J R 1985 Basic nurse education in CAEs—the educational evidence for transfer. Australian Journal of Advanced Nursing 2(2) December-February:18-28

Lumby J 1991 Threads of an emerging discipline: praxis, reflection, rhetoric and research. In: Gray G, Pratt R (eds) Towards a discipline of nursing. Churchill Livingstone, Melbourne

Mackay L 1989 Nursing a problem. Open University Press, Milton Keynes

McManamny S 1987 Issues—clinical education/clinical agencies. Joint Interdepartmental Steering Committee for the Transfer of Nurse Education (discussion paper for the committee). Melbourne

Meppem J 1991 Critical issues in nursing. Australian Nurses' Journal February:16,24

Moloney M M 1986 Professionalization of nursing. Lippincott, Philadelphia

Moorhouse C 1988 Diversity in nurse education: a perspective towards Australia's third century. In: Pathfinders: three centuries of nursing. Conference proceedings, College of Nursing, Australia, Canberra

Nelson B 1992 In reply (letter to the editor). Medical Journal of Australia 157 (7):504

Olesen V L, Whittaker EW 1968 The silent dialogue. Jossey-Bass, San Francisco

Parkes R 1991 Nurses to be invaded? (editorial). Australian Nurses' Journal April:7-9

Percival E C 1992 Contemporary issues in the regulation of nursing. In: Gray G, Pratt R (eds) Issues in Australian nursing 3. Churchill Livingstone, Melbourne

Pickhaver A, Young B, Goldsworthy T 1985 'They seem different somehow': study of the first five graduating cohorts of the diploma of applied science (nursing) from the Sturt College of Advanced Education, South Australia. Commonwealth Tertiary Education Commission, Canberra

Pratt R 1989 Sine qua non: the psychomotor skills profile of beginning practitioners in nursing. University of New South Wales, Sydney

Robinson J 1989 Nursing in the future: a cause for concern. In: Jolley M, Allan P (eds) Current issues in nursing. Chapman & Hall, London

Robinson J 1992 Introduction: beginning the study of nursing policy. In: Robinson J, Gray A, Elkan R (eds) Policy issues in nursing. Open University Press, Milton Keynes

Robinson M 1986 Nurses beware. Australian Nurses' Journal November:30

Royal College of Nursing, Australia 1990 Position statement: provision of quality nursing care. RCNA, Melbourne, 8 June

Salvage J 1988a Professionalization—or struggle for survival? A consideration of current proposals for the reform of nursing in the United Kingdom. Journal of Advanced Nursing 13 (4):515-519

Salvage J 1988b Take me to your leader. Nursing Times 5 October:24

Salvage J 1992 The new nursing: empowering patients or empowering nurses? In: Robinson J, Gray A, Elkan R (eds) Policy issues in nursing. Open University Press, Milton Keynes

Savage J 1987 Nurses, gender and sexuality. Heinemann, London

Seymour J 1992 Healthy states? Nursing Times. 21 October:20

Short S, Sharman E 1987 The nursing struggle in Australia. Image: Journal of Nursing Scholarship 19(4) Winter:197-200

Slater P V 1982 The role of nursing organisations in professional education—challenges for the future. 16th Patricia Chomley Oration. College of Nursing, Australia, Melbourne

Slater P V 1988 Personal communication

Speedy S 1987 Feminism and the professionalisation of nursing. Australian Journal of Advanced Nursing 4 (2):20-26

Speedy S 1991 The contribution of feminist research. In: Gray G, Pratt R (eds) Towards a discipline of nursing. Churchill Livingstone, Melbourne

Staunton P 1993 Editorial. The Lamp November:3

Street A 1990 Cultural practices in nursing. Deakin University, Geelong

Strong P, Robinson J 1988 New model management: Griffiths and the NHS. Nursing Policy Studies Centre, University of Warwick, Coventry

Teh K, Gowdie C 1988 What young women think of feminism. The Age 9 November

Turner T 1989 Winds of change? Nursing Times 29 March:69-70

Watts S 1992 NHS computers 'failing to assist in patient care'. The Independent 15 December

Wiesel E 1984 The whole picture (letter to the editor). Australian Nurses' Journal August:6-7

White R 1985 Political regulators in British nursing. In: White R (ed.) Political issues in nursing: past, present and future. Wiley, Chichester

Appendix: Health Employment Statistics

Table 1 Persons employed in health and health-related occupations, states and territories 30 June 1986

Occupation	NSW	Vic	Qld	SA	WA	Tas	NT	ACT	Aust
Health occupations									
Health diagnosis and treatment practitioners									
General medical practitioners	8 910	5 930	3 590	2 190	1 930	620	230	400	23 790
Specialist medical practitioners	3 350	2 330	1 210	960	750	190	60	140	9 000
Total medical practitioners	12 260	8 260	4 800	3 140	2 680	810	290	540	32 790
Dental practitioners	2 270	1 540	1 030	600	570	110	50	140	6 310
Pharmacists	3 850	2 880	1 770	790	820	280	60	180	10 640
Occupational therapists	880	840	360	210	350	80	20	50	2 770
Optometrists	580	340	260	110	130	40	10	20	1 470
Physiotherapists	2 080	1 410	890	630	590	160	50	130	5 930
Speech pathologists	370	390	240	120	120	50	10	20	1 320
Chiropractors and osteopaths	530	340	220	160	70	20	10	20	1 370
Podiatrists	280	360	100	110	80	40	-	-	980
Radiographers	1 600	880	730	430	380	140	30	80	4 270
Other health diagnosis and treatment practitioners	1 700	900	550	300	240	80	20	90	3 880
Total health diagnosis and treatment practitioners	26 410	18 150	10 960	6 600	6 040	1 790	540	1 260	71 740
Registered nurses	44 480	37 990	21 810	14 070	11 900	4 700	1 220	2 060	138 220
Enrolled nurses	8 640	11 710	4 810	4 480	3 490	1 430	270	390	35 220
Dental nurses	2 800	2 330	1 470	900	870	180	80	170	8 800
Total nurses	55 910	52 030	28 090	19 450	16 260	6 310	1 570	2 620	182 240
Total health occupations	82 320	70 180	39 050	26 040	22 300	8 090	2 110	3 880	253 970

Occupation	NSW	Vic	Qld	SA	WA	Tas	NT	ACT	Aust
Health-related occupations									
Medical testing professionals	2 440	2 620	910	650	730	170	50	200	7 780
Social workers	1 750	1 860	790	940	650	180	60	140	6 370
Counsellors	1 870	880	550	440	380	120	80	170	4 490
Psychologists	1 200	1 010	600	320	480	100	30	110	3 850
Ambulance officers	2 010	1 219	1 110	242	281	145	47	43	5 097
Medical technical officers and technicians	2 670	1 510	1 110	1 100	720	180	80	200	7 570
Total health-related occupations	11 940	9 100	5 070	3 690	3 250	900	340	870	35 150
Total health and health-related occupations	94 260	79 280	44 120	29 740	25 550	8 990	2 440	4 750	289 120

Source: ABS *Characteristics of Persons Employed in Health Occupations, Australia* (4346.0) ABS 1989 Table 1

Table 2 Persons employed in health and health-related occupations, states and territories 6 August 1991

Occupation	NSW	Vic	Qld	SA	WA	Tas	NT	ACT	Aust
Health occupations									
Health diagnosis and treatment practitioners									
General medical practitioners	9 030	6 300	4 160	2 370	2 220	640	260	460	25 450
Specialist medical practitioners	4 650	3 680	2 150	1 220	1 050	280	110	200	13 350
Total medical practitioners	13 680	9 980	6 310	3 590	3 270	930	370	670	38 800
Dental practitioners	2 440	1 580	1 150	600	630	110	60	150	6 720
Pharmacists	3 790	2 990	1 880	770	930	270	70	180	10 880
Occupational therapists	1 070	1 040	520	320	500	100	30	80	3 660
Optometrists	690	440	330	130	140	50	10	30	1 820
Physiotherapists	2 390	1 730	1 140	730	760	170	60	150	7 130
Speech pathologists	530	460	320	160	170	60	20	30	1 750
Chiropractors and osteopaths	560	400	240	170	110	20	10	20	1 540
Podiatrists	320	370	140	120	130	40	-	10	1 140
Radiographers	1 760	1 030	810	450	450	130	40	70	4 760
Other health diagnosis and treatment practitioners	2 500	1 300	940	410	310	130	40	120	5 750
Total health diagnosis and treatment practitioners	29 730	21 330	13 800	7 450	7 420	2 000	710	1 500	83 930
Registered nurses	45 060	37 160	22 460	13 460	12 990	4 640	1 430	2 180	139 370
Enrolled nurses	9 460	12 830	6 650	4 800	3 520	1 550	490	370	39 670
Dental nurses	3 100	2 410	1 660	980	1 000	180	80	190	9 590
Total nurses	57 630	52 400	30 770	19 230	17 500	6 360	1 990	2 750	188 630
Total health occupations	87 360	73 720	44 560	26 690	24 920	8 360	2 700	4 240	272 560

Occupation	NSW	Vic	Qld	SA	WA	Tas	NT	ACT	Aust
Health-related occupations									
Medical testing professionals	2 220	2 300	870	720	880	200	50	200	7 430
Social workers	1 920	2 030	920	1 120	760	170	70	180	7 170
Counsellors	2 870	1 740	1 130	950	660	180	100	270	7 890
Psychologists	1 550	1 230	770	350	590	100	40	120	4 750
Ambulance officers	2 020	1 260	1 350	440	280	120	60	50	5 580
Medical technical officers and technicians	5 080	3 930	2 770	1 700	2 180	400	120	320	16 500
Total health-related occupations	15 650	12 490	7 810	5 290	5 340	1 170	440	1 130	49 320
Total health and health-related occupations	103 010	86 220	52 370	31 970	30 260	9 540	3 140	5 370	321 880

Source: ABS *Characteristics of Persons Employed in Health Occupations, Australia* (4346.0) ABS 1993 Table 1

Table 3 Persons employed in health occupations by industry, Australia 30 June 1986

	Hospitals (excluding psychiatric)	Psychiatric hospitals	Nursing homes	Medicine & optometry	Dentistry, dental laboratories	Community health centres	Other	Total health industry Number	%	Other industries	Total all industries
Health occupation											
Health diagnosis and treatment practitioners											
General medical practitioners	6 760	280	80	14 040	70	390	270	21 890	92.0	1 890	23 790
Specialist medical practitioners	2 440	240	30	5 230	70	110	240	8 360	9.9	640	9 000
Total medical practitioners	9 200	520	110	19 270	140	500	510	30 250	92.3	2 540	32 790
Dental practitioners	220	20	-	180	5 420	40	20	5 890	93.3	420	6 310
Pharmacists	1 300	80	30	30	20	30	30	1 510	14.2	9 130	10 640
Occupational therapists	1 060	190	390	40	10	250	210	2 140	77.3	630	2 770
Optometrists	10	-	-	20	1 340	-	10	1 380	93.7	90	1 470
Physiotherapists	2 160	60	440	280	20	240	2 140	5 340	90.1	5 930	-
Speech pathologists	430	10	60	40	10	150	170	860	64.8	470	1 320
Chiropractors and osteopaths	-	-	-	70	-	10	1 250	1 320	96.1	50	1 370
Podiatrists	110	-	40	230	-	50	440	880	89.6	100	980
Radiographers	2 460	10	10	1 210	50	30	260	4 030	94.4	240	4 270
Other health diagnosis and treatment practitioners	950	30	510	290	110	100	1 020	3 010	77.5	870	3 880
Total health diagnosis and treatment practitioners	17 890	920	580	21 650	7 130	1 390	6 040	56 610	78.9	15 130	71 740
Registered nurses	84 600	6 750	20 030	6 140	440	4 310	3 910	126 170	91.3	12 050	138 220
Enrolled nurses	19 220	1 100	9 760	320	110	480	600	31 600	89.7	3 620	35 220
Dental nurses	250	30	20	260	7 390	60	50	8 060	91.6	740	8 800
Total nurses	104 070	7 880	29 810	6 710	7 940	4 850	4 560	165 830	91.0	16 410	182 240
Total health occupations	121 970	8 810	31 390	28 360	15 070	6 250	10 600	222 440	87.6	31 540	253 970

Source: ABS *Characteristics of Persons Employed in Health Occupations, Australia* (4346 .0) ABS 1989 Table 2

Table 4 Persons employed in health occupations, Australia 6 August 1991

	Hospitals (excluding psychiatric)	Psychiatric hospitals	Nursing homes	Medicine & optometry	Dentistry, dental laboratories	Community health centres	Other	Total health industry Number	%	Other industries	Total all industries
Health occupation											
Health diagnosis and treatment practitioners											
General medical practitioners	6 710	240	80	14 560	100	4 600	850	22 990	90.3	2 460	25 450
Specialist medical practitioners	3 880	230	50	7 240	70	140	570	12 170	91.2	1 180	13 350
Total medical practitioners	10 580	470	120	21 790	170	600	1 420	35 160	90.6	3 640	38 800
Dental practitioners	210	-	-	150	5 790	40	50	6 260	93.2	460	6 720
Pharmacists	1 350	60	30	50	10	30	60	1 590	14.6	9 290	10 880
Occupational therapists	1 180	160	390	60	10	420	500	2 730	74.6	930	3 660
Optometrists	10	-	-	20	1 690	-	10	1 720	94.5	100	1 820
Physiotherapists	2 290	30	520	200	20	330	2 840	6 220	87.2	900	7 130
Speech pathologists	490	20	50	30	10	170	290	1 060	60.6	690	1 750
Chiropractors and osteopaths	-	-	-	30	-	10	1 440	1 480	96.1	60	1 540
Podiatrists	110	-	30	150	-	60	670	1 010	88.6	130	1 140
Radiographers	2 410	-	10	1 430	30	20	510	4 410	92.6	350	4 760
Other health diagnosis and treatment practitioners	1 150	30	990	340	160	180	1 680	4 530	78.8	1 230	5 750
Total health diagnosis and treatment practitioners	19 780	780	2 130	24 240	7 900	1 850	9 470	66 160	78.8	17 780	83 930
Registered nurses	79 900	5 210	19 980	5 710	580	4 420	8 740	124 540	89.4	14 840	139 370
Enrolled nurses	19 750	800	10 010	780	150	890	1 900	34 280	86.4	5 390	39 670
Dental nurses	280	-	10	190	8 030	70	100	8 680	90.5	910	9 590
Total nurses	99 940	6 010	29 990	6 680	8 760	5 380	10 740	167 500	88.8	21 130	188 630
Total health occupations	119 720	6 790	32 120	30 920	16 670	7 230	20 210	233 660	85.7	38 910	272 560

Source: ABS *Characteristics of Persons Employed in Health Occupations*, Australia (4346 .0) ABS 1993 Table 2

Table 5 Persons employed in health occupations by industry and sex, Australia 1986 & 1991

Year	Health occupations	Hospitals (excluding psychiatric)	Psychiatric hospitals	Nursing homes	Medicine	Dentistry, dental laboratories & optometry	Community health centres	Other	Total health industries
Males									
1986	Nurses	6 420	3 150	1 090	120	50	340	260	11 430
1991	Nurses	6 640	2 390	1 320	170	120	480	820	11 940
1986	Medical practitioners	6 670	330	70	15 720	120	280	340	23 520
1991	Medical practitioners	6 870	280	70	16 630	130	300	970	25 240
1986	Dental practitioners	170	20	-	150	4 750	30	10	5 130
1991	Dental practitioners	150	-	-	130	4 860	30	40	5 210
1986	Other health practitioners	2 030	80	80	660	1 120	120	2 350	6 450
1991	Other health practitioners	2 010	70	90	630	1 280	150	3 100	7 330
Females									
1986	Nurses	97 660	4 730	28 720	6 590	7 890	4 510	4 300	154 400
1991	Nurses	93 300	3 620	28 670	6 510	8 640	4 900	9 930	155 560
1986	Medical practitioners	2 530	200	40	3 560	30	220	170	6 730
1991	Medical practitioners	3 720	190	50	5 170	40	300	460	9 920
1986	Dental practitioners	40	-	-	20	680	10	-	760
1991	Dental practitioners	60	-	-	20	930	20	10	1 040
1986	Other health practitioners	6 450	300	1 390	1 550	440	730	3 170	14 020
1991	Other health practitioners	6 920	240	1 910	1 600	660	1 050	4 840	17 230
Persons									
1986	Nurses	104 070	7 880	29 810	6 710	7 940	4 850	4 560	165 830
1991	Nurses	99 940	6 010	29 990	6 680	8 760	5 380	10 740	167 500
1986	Medical practitioners	9 200	520	110	19 270	140	500	510	30 250
1991	Medical practitioners	10 580	470	120	21 790	170	600	1 420	35 160
1986	Dental practitioners	220	20	-	180	5 420	40	20	5 890
1991	Dental practitioners	210	-	-	150	5 790	40	50	6 260
1986	Other Health Practitioners	8 480	380	1 470	2 200	1 560	860	5 520	20 470
1991	Other Health Practitioners	8 930	310	2 000	2 230	1 940	1 210	7 940	24 560

Source: ABS *Characteristics of Persons Employed in Health Occupations*, Australia (4346.0) ABS 1989 Table 9; ABS 1993 Table 10

Interviews

Airey, Rebecca	Psychiatric nurse, South Australia. November 1988
Alexander, Margaret	Professor, Department of Nursing, Glasgow College, Scotland. January 1990
Anderson, Beth	Director of Nursing, Western Australia. September 1990
Andreazza, Marisa	Charge nurse, Victoria. July 1990
Attrill, Helen	President ANF (WA Branch). September 1990
Barrois, Genevieve	Nurse journalist, L'Infermiere Magazine, Paris. December 1989
Bassett-Smith, Diana	Clinical nurse consultant, Victoria. October 1990
Beaumont, Marilyn	Federal Secretary ANF. October 1992
Berger, Gertie	Former nurse educator, Victoria. 1988, and December 1990 [GBa/90]
Booker, Bill	Head, Enrolled Nurse Program, West Australian Department of TAFE. September 1990
Boulden, Heather	Deputy Director, Aboriginal Development and Consultancy Branch, Department of Health and Community Services, Northern Territory. October 1990
Bryant, Rosemary	Head, Nursing Policy and Planning Unit, Health Department, Victoria (former director of nursing, South Australia and President ANF (SA Branch)). January 1991
Burbidge, Gwen	Former matron, Victoria. October 1990
Cameron, Suzanne	Chair, Board of Nursing Studies, Queensland. July 1991
Carter, Evonne	Charge nurse, South Australia. November 1988
Chegwidden, Audrey	Community psychiatric nurse, Victoria. July 1990
Collins, Isabell	Nurse administrator, Victoria (former president, ANF Vic. Branch). October 1988
Connor, Marjorie	Former Secretary, Royal Victorian College of Nursing, 1988, 1990
Cornell, Judith	Executive Director, New South Wales College of Nursing. September 1989
Couglin-West, Val	Director of Nursing, Queensland. August 1991
Crowther, Elizabeth	Director of Nursing (psychiatric), Victoria. December 1991
Curry, Graeme	Lecturer, Faculty of Nursing, University of Technology, Sydney. May 1990
Davis, Anne	Professor of Nursing, University of California, San Francisco. August 1990
Duberley, Janet	Department of Health & Social Security, England. January 1990
Durdin, Joan	Former nurse educator, South Australia. November 1988
Emden, Carolyn	Senior lecturer, School of Nursing, Sturt/South Australian College of Advanced Education-Sturt. November 1988
Fehring, Garry	Charge nurse, Victoria. October 1992
Fox, Stephanie	Lecturer, Canberra College of Advanced Education, ACT. October 1988 (Interviewed with Sandra Trick.)
Frame, Jean	ANF, New South Wales Branch. September 1989

Gaston, Carol	Acting Executive Director Corporate Services, South Australian Health Commission. November 1988
Gibb, Annette	Intensive care nurse, Berkshire, England, February 1990
Glover, Ro	Registered nurse, Victoria. July 1990
Godfrey, Joan	Former Head, School of Nursing, Queensland Institute of Technology. August 1991
Gray, Helen	Secretary ANF (Tasmanian Branch). November 1988
Haines, Jenny	Intensive care nurse (former secretary, New South Wales Nurses Association). September 1989 [JHa/89]
Hamilton, Jill	Director of Physical Resources, Southern Area Health Service, New South Wales. September 1989
Hardstaff, Elaine	Clinical nurse consultant, Victoria. July 1990
Harte, Cecily	Former Secretary ANF (NSW Branch). September 1989
Hawkesworth, Gay	Vice-President Queensland Nurses Union and member ANF (Queensland Branch) Council. August 1991. (Interviewed with Denis Jones.)
Hemingway, Adrienne	Associate Charge Nurse, Victoria. June 1992
Henderson, Tony	Senior Policy Officer, Psychiatric Services Policy Unit, Western Australian Health Department. September 1990
Henlen, Mary	Former Secretary New South Wales Nurses Association. September 1989
Hitchins, Rhea	Executive Officer, WA Nurses' Board, Western Australia. September 1990
Irwin, Lynne	Convenor in Public Health Training, Department of Nursing, Armidale College of Advanced Education, NSW. August 1988
Jayawardena, Yvonne	Former Director, National Nursing Education Division RANF. December 1990
Jennings, Suzanne	Registered nurse, Victoria. July 1990
Jones, Denis	Secretary ANF (Queensland Branch). August 1991. (Interviewed with Gay Hawkesworth.)
Kearney, Ita	Former Head, Melbourne School for Enrolled Nurses. January 1991
Kelly, Kathryn	Policy Officer, Nursing Advisory Section, Department of Community Services and Health, Canberra. October 1988
Knott, Judith	Assistant Director of Nursing, Victoria. June 1990
Law, Roger	Industrial Officer, ANF (Launceston Office), Tasmania. November 1988
Lawler, Jocalyn	Senior Lecturer, Department of Nursing, Armidale College of Advanced Education, NSW. August 1988
Lennox, George	Principal Nursing Officer, Department of Health Services, Tasmania. November 1988
Lublin, Jacqueline	Senior Lecturer, University of Sydney. December 1990
Mason, Janie	Senior Lecturer, Northern Territory University. October 1990
Mathews, Kathleen	Former Director, New South Wales College of Nursing. September 1989
McCarthy, Doreen	Project Coordinator, Health Department, Western Australia. September 1990
McCulloch, Sybil	Head, School of Nursing, South Australian Institute of Technology. November 1988
McGrath, Maureen	Nurses Registration Board, New South Wales (former secretary, Nurses Education Board). September 1989
McKenzie, Regis,	Director, Sydney Home Nursing Service. December 1990
McManamny, Sally	Senior Lecturer, La Trobe University, Victoria. October 1991
Morieson, Belinda	Secretary ANF (Vic. Branch). March 1993
Murphy, Penney	Secretary ANF (Western Australian Branch). September 1990
Nagle, Gabrielle	Chief Executive Officer, community health centre, Victoria. February 1992
Newnham, Phillis	Principal Director of Nursing, Prince Henry and Prince of Wales Hospitals, New South Wales. September 1989

Osborne, Patricia	Former nurse educator, Victoria. December 1990
Parker, Judith	Professor of Nursing, La Trobe University, Victoria. November 1990
Parkes, Merle	Head, School of Nursing, Tasmanian State Institute of Technology, Tasmania, November 1988
Patten, Mary	Deputy Chief Executive, Royal Children's Hospital, Victoria, (former federal secretary RANF). June 1991
Penridge, Joan	Senior Lecturer, Department of Nursing, Queensland University of Technology. August 1991
Percival, Elizabeth	South Australian Nurses Board. November 1988
Pickhaver, Anne	Principal lecturer, School of Nursing, South Australian Institute of Technology. November 1988
Pilkington, Paulina	Former Secretary, Nursing Branch, Commonwealth Department of Health. September 1989
Power, Prue	Secretary, ANF (ACT Branch). October 1988
Pratt, Rosalie	Principal Lecturer and Head, Department of Clinical Studies, Institute of Nursing Studies, Sydney College of Advanced Education. September 1989
Roberts, Kay	Professor of Nursing, Northern Territory University. October 1990
Robertson, Barbara	Professor, University of the Witwatersrand, South Africa. December 1989
Rosenberg, Hilary	Registered nurse, Victoria. August 1990
Rosenthal, Margaret	Head, Institute of Nursing Studies, Sydney College of Advanced Education. September 1989
Rouse-Northey, Suzanne	WorkCare Rehabilitation advisor, Victoria. May 1992
Salamons, Linda	Head, Department of Mental Health Nursing, University of Western Sydney. May 1990
Salvage, Jane	Director, Nursing Developments, King's Fund Centre, London. January 1990 [JSa/90]
Schultz, Sylvia	Assistant Director of Nursing, South Australia. November 1988
Shepherd, Jean	Sister in charge, Oxford. December 1988
Shield, Barbara	Former Education Officer, RVCN, Victoria. December 1990
Sim, Teik-Meh	Nurse administrator, Singapore. March 1993
Smith, James P.	Editor, Journal of Advanced Nursing, London. January 1990
Smith, James	Lecturer, Department of Health Administration & Education, La Trobe University. February 1992
Sneddon, Marilyn	Deputy Director of Nursing, Victoria. July 1991
Spratt, Peggy	Policy Officer, Nursing Advisory Section, Department of Community Services and Health, Canberra. October 1988
Staunton, Patricia	Secretary ANF (NSW Branch) and General Secretary NSWNA. November 1990
Stolz, Karen	Senior Lecturer, Department of Nursing, Queensland University of Technology, Queensland. August 1991
Sudano, Leena	Secretary ANF (SA Branch). November 1988
Sullivan, Margaret	Head, TAFE Division of Nursing, Sydney. December 1990
Taylor, Geri	Director of Nursing and Human Services, Commonwealth Department of Community Services and Health, Canberra. April 1990
Trick, Sandra	Lecturer, Canberra College of Advanced Education, ACT. October 1988. (Interviewed with Stephanie Fox.)
Tunks, Lian	Associate charge nurse, Victoria. July 1990
Veldman, Hetty	Health education nurse, Victoria. November 1988
Vidovich, Marea	Former President RANF (WA Branch). October 1988
Watson, Jenny	Senior Lecturer, School of Nursing, South Australian College of Advanced Education-Sturt. November 1988
Webb, Christine	Professor, Department of Nursing, University of Manchester. January 1990

Wheatley, Dorothy	Former President RANF, and Head, School of Nursing, Sir Charles Gairdner Hospital, WA. September 1989
Wilkinson, Joan	Secretary, ANF (Northern Territory Branch). October 1990
Wilson-Barnett, Jenifer	Professor, Department of Nursing Studies, University of London. January 1990
Wood, Patricia	Assistant Secretary, Health Research and Services Division, Commonwealth Department of Community Services and Health, Canberra. May 1990
Woodruff, Ann	Head, Department of Nursing, Footscray Institute of Technology, Victoria. May 1990

When quoted in the text, interviewees are identified by initials and date.

The authors would like to thank Richard Curlewis for permission to use material from his interviews with Gertie Berger and Marjorie Connor.

Index